HIKES LIST

S0-CFW-313

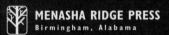
MENASHA RIDGE PRESS
Birmingham, Alabama

"The best book about hitting New Mexico's trails."
—*New Mexico Magazine*

60 HIKES WITHIN 60 MILES

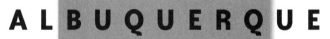

ALBUQUERQUE

INCLUDING
SANTA FE,
MOUNT TAYLOR, AND
SAN LORENZO CANYON

SECOND EDITION

STEPHEN AUSHERMAN

60 HIKES WITHIN 60 MILES: ALBUQUERQUE

Copyright © 2012 by Stephen Ausherman

All rights reserved

Printed in the United States of America
Published by Menasha Ridge Press
Distributed by Publishers Group West
Second edition, second printing 2014

Library of Congress Cataloging-in-Publication Data

    Ausherman, Stephen.
      60 hikes within 60 miles Albuquerque : including Santa Fe, Mount Taylor, and
    San Lorenzo canyon / Stephen Ausherman. — 2nd ed.
       p. cm.
    Includes index.
    ISBN 978-0-89732-600-1 — ISBN 0-89732-600-8
    1. Hiking—New Mexico—Albuquerque Region—Guidebooks. 2. Albuquerque
    Region (N.M.)—Guidebooks. I. Title. II. Title: Sixty hikes within sixty miles.
    GV199.42.N62A434 2013
    796.5109789—dc23

                                     2011046441

Cover and text design by Steve Sullivan
Cover photos by Stephen Ausherman
Interior photos by Stephen Ausherman, except the following: pages 90, 132, 208, 218,
    230, and 249 by Celia Ameline; pages 140 and 320 by Michael Scialdone; and page 238
    by Betsy Dranttel
Cartography and elevation profiles by Stephen Ausherman, Chris Erichson, and
    Scott McGrew
Editor: Ritchey Halphen
Proofreader: Donna Poehner
Indexer: Ann Cassar/Cassar Technical Services

Menasha Ridge Press
P.O. Box 43673
Birmingham, AL 35243
menasharidge.com

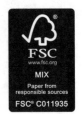
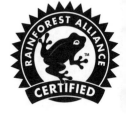

DISCLAIMER

TABLE OF CONTENTS

DEDICATION

To Chuck and Nancy, Judy and Amy, the Boerigters, Dave Shapiro,

Scout Lisagor, Señor Hawley, Mr. Smith, Mr. Death,

Aaron, Celia, Fennel, Tia, Reverend Huston,

Jim Bo, Elzbieta, Scial, Shay, and Betsy (especially Betsy)

for enduring hikes with me when I was less familiar with these trails

and for Gurdin Chapin

(Pasó por aquí)

Special thanks to John Coleman for his

diligent correspondence from the trails.

—STEPHEN AUSHERMAN

FOREWORD

Welcome to Menasha Ridge Press's *60 Hikes within 60 Miles.* Our strategy was simple: First, find a hiker who knows the area and loves to hike. Second, ask that person to spend a year researching the most popular and very best trails around. And third, have that person describe each trail in terms of difficulty, scenery, condition, elevation change, and all other categories of information that are important to hikers. "Pretend you've just completed a hike and met up with other hikers at the trailhead," we told each author. "Imagine their questions, and be clear in your answers." An experienced hiker and writer, author Stephen Ausherman has selected 60 of the best hikes in and around the Albuquerque metropolitan area. From the greenways and urban hikes that make use of parklands to flora- and fauna-rich treks along the cliffs and hills in the hinterlands, Ausherman provides hikers (and walkers) with a great variety of hikes—and all within roughly 60 miles of Albuquerque.

You'll get more out of this book if you take a moment to read the Introduction explaining how to read the trail listings. The "Topographic Maps" section will help you understand how useful topos will be on a hike, and will also tell you where to get them. And though this is a where-to rather than a how-to guide, those of you who have hiked extensively will find the Introduction of particular value. As much for the opportunity to free the spirit as well as to free the body, let these hikes elevate you above the urban hurry.

All the best,
The Editors at Menasha Ridge Press

ABOUT THE AUTHOR

STEPHEN AUSHERMAN has worked as a public-health assistant in Iraq, Nigeria, Kenya, and Tanzania; a teacher in Korea and China; and a journalist in India and the United States. He was a Writer-in-Residence at Buffalo National River in Arkan-

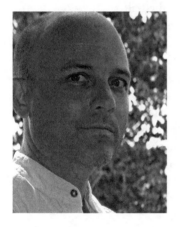

sas, Devils Tower National Monument in Wyoming, and Bernheim Forest in Kentucky, and an Artist-in-Residence for Cornucopia Art Center in Minnesota, Blue Sky Project in Illinois, and Cape Cod National Seashore in Massachusetts. Born in China and raised in North Carolina, Ausherman took an unscheduled detour to Albuquerque in 1996. He has lived there ever since. Visit his website for useful links, maps, and trail notes: **restlesstribes.com/60updates**.

PREFACE

> *May your trails be crooked, winding, lonesome, dangerous,*
> *leading to the most amazing view.*
> **—EDWARD ABBEY**

Sometime in the mid-1920s, New Mexico Governor Arthur T. Hannett placed a ruler on a map and conceived an idea for a shorter Route 66. He drew a straight line connecting Santa Rosa to Gallup, with Albuquerque lying near the half-way point. The planned shortcut was met with less enthusiasm than protest, particularly among those living in the towns it would have bypassed. When Hannett lost the 1926 gubernatorial election, he spent his final month in office executing a retaliatory farewell to the capital city. Without regard for land ownership or what stood in the way, he ordered a new road cut between Santa Rosa and Moriarty. And despite boundary fences, dense piñon forests, blizzard conditions, and sabotaged equipment, road crews completed the unwavering 69-mile roadway in just 31 days. This new segment of Route 66 soon brought travelers to Albuquerque in record time by eliminating the old winding route through Santa Fe.

When I first set out to write this book, I put a ruler on the map and drew straight lines, each a 60-mile spoke radiating from the hub of Albuquerque. With the addition of a rim, my diagram resembled a wagon wheel, and it effectively illustrated that the scope of this book was bigger than I'd initially guessed.

Within 60 miles of Albuquerque, you'll find six national-forest ranger districts, five national monuments, seven federally designated wilderness areas, a national wildlife refuge, a national preserve, and five state parks. You'll also hit upon equally fascinating but lesser-known tracts under the stewardship of the federal Bureau of Land Management; the New Mexico State Land Office; the Department of Fish, Game and Wildlife; the Department of Energy; and the Middle Rio Grande Conservancy District.

With the hub and rim established, I erased the spokes. The sections they created were useless for any pragmatic arrangement, as few roads serve Albuquerque with the linear efficiency Hannett might have hoped for. But crooked as they are, the primary highways do contribute to a straightforward approach for organizing such widespread hikes. They'll not only point you in the right direction but also reveal something about those who've gone that way before. And though you may end up driving farther than 60 road miles to reach a trailhead (46.5 miles on average), every hike featured in this book is well within the bounds of a reasonable daytrip.

THE DUKE CITY

Named for the Duke of Alburquerque, minus the superfluous *r*, our focal city is fairly easy to spell when you consider its Navajo name: *Bee'eldíildahsinil*. With more than 25 percent of its land protected as public open space, Albuquerque tops the national list of largest city-park systems. In the Duke City section of this book, you'll find quick access to nine invigorating routes. Irrigation ditches, or acequias, and the Rio Grande provide settings for shaded waterside walks, whereas Petroglyph National Monument is so exposed that even the rocks are sunburned. Montessa Park and La Ceja provide opportunities for escape to surreal landscapes on the fringes of Albuquerque and Rio Rancho. Foothills Open Space in the Northeast Heights serves as a gateway to the Sandia Mountains, which rise a mile above this mile-high city.

THE SALT MISSION TRAIL

Take a look at the Sandia Ranger District map and you'll spot 60 hikes in 60 seconds. Extending south from the Sandias, the Manzanita and Manzano ranges continue the possibilities for nearby mountain hikes. Despite their proximity to the urban center of New Mexico, only one road manages to pierce the 60-mile span of these three ranges. The I-40 corridor traverses Tijeras Canyon, which separates the Sandias from the Manzanitas. Once you drive east through the canyon, you face a choice between two historic routes: south on the Salt Mission Trail or north on the Turquoise Trail.

Early Spaniards established Franciscan missions to lord over the Salinas Province and its salt-driven economy. Colonial influences are still apparent in the centuries-old land grants along the scenic highways south of Tijeras. Ruins of the mission at Quarai stand near the last hike in this section, a challenging loop in the Manzano Mountain Wilderness. Both hikes on this side of the Manzanos feature crest views from above 8,700 feet. Closer to Albuquerque, canyons and foothills in the Manzanitas are better suited for quick getaways. The first and nearest hike in this group is one of the southernmost in the Sandia Mountain Wilderness. True, it seems to belong in the next section, but then you'd never find the trailhead if you started north on NM 14, the Turquoise Trail.

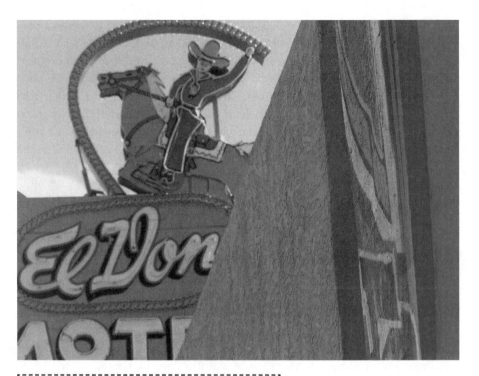

Architectural details on Central Avenue (Historic Route 66)

THE TURQUOISE TRAIL

The east side of the Sandias is gentler and shadier than its stark west face, as you'll notice in this section's first three hikes. Routes at the Golden Open Space and in the Galisteo Basin explore water-sculpted corridors hidden deep in juniper savanna. Another pair of hikes takes you into legendary mining territory: the San Pedro Mountains, where countless men succumbed to gold fever, and Cerrillos Hills, where mystic blue stones are still the object of a thousand-year quest. An unofficial story behind the Turquoise Trail refers to a gaffe in the initial construction of the highway. Road crews allegedly scooped gravel from the wrong mine. The error went largely unrealized until local residents were seen fervently combing the newly graveled road and pocketing their finds. For that brief time, it was quite literally a trail of turquoise.

EL CAMINO REAL

El Camino Real de Tierra Adentro (The Royal Road of the Interior Land) was the primary route between the colonial Spanish capital of Mexico City and the provincial capital of Santa Fe. This 1,600-mile corridor still reflects the diverse heritages of Native America, the Old World, and the modern societies of the United States and Mexico. A 404-mile segment of El Camino Real was designated a National Historic Trail in 2000.

El Camino Real's nearest modern alignment is I-25, and you won't drive more than 50 miles of it to reach the hikes in this northern group. The section begins with Tunnel Spring, our seventh and final hike in the Sandias. Farther north you'll explore three relatively unknown areas (Las Huertas de Placitas, Ball Ranch, and La Cienega) that are rich in archaeological and paleontological features. Getting back to more familiar terrain, you'll visit a national monument and a wilderness area that are famous for rock formations and forest fires, respectively. Also included in this group is La Bajada. Once considered the most perilous hill on the Camino Real, "the descent" now serves as the starting point for a pleasant hike along the Santa Fe River.

THE CITY DIFFERENT

Conceived in response to the City Beautiful movement of the 1900s, this self-inflicted nickname underscores the idea that Santa Fe is, well . . . *different*. In New Mexico's tale of two cities, she plays the eccentric spinster, whereas Albuquerque is the tart with a heart of gold, and together they endure the love–hate relationship of inseparable sisters. In this group you'll find four ways to venture into Santa Fe National Forest. The first two hikes in this group visit Caja del Rio, the volcanic plateau that rises between the Rio Grande and the Santa Fe River. The next three explore different aspects of the Santa Fe Mountains, the southernmost subrange of the Sangre de Cristo Mountains, which in turn represent the southernmost subrange of the Rocky Mountains. Bishop's Lodge and Hyde Park are a popular couple, each just a short drive from the Santa Fe Plaza. Glorieta Canyon Ghost Town and Cowboy Shack are outposts rich in remnants of the Old West.

THE JEMEZ MOUNTAIN TRAIL

Eight of America's 120 National Scenic Byways are in New Mexico, including the Turquoise Trail, El Camino Real, Historic Route 66, and the Jemez Mountain Trail (JMT). The stretch of US 550 from San Ysidro to Cuba accounts for 40 miles of the 132-mile JMT. The Ojito Wilderness, the White Mesa Bike Trails Area, and the San Ysidro Trials Area are the recreational trifecta in the vicinity of San Ysidro. On this convergence of the Rio Grande rift and the Colorado Plateau you'll find slot canyons, sandstone hoodoos, banded mesas, and other classic features that contribute to the irresistible allure of the American Southwest. From San Ysidro, US 550 squeezes between the southernmost uplift in the Rocky Mountains and the volcano fields in the Rio Puerco Basin, where a long stretch of the Continental Divide Trail winds through a rugged land best known as Cabezon Country.

About 60 miles of NM 4, nearly its entire length, have been incorporated into the JMT, and it's as much a scenic drive as an erratic trip through time. It starts at the pastoral 19th-centry villa of San Ysidro, traverses a mountainous landscape reshaped by a massive volcanic eruption 1.2 million years ago, and finally arrives at a corner of the technological frontier known as Los Alamos National Laboratories. Here upon the slopes of a slightly dyspeptic supervolcano, the world's top nuclear eggheads have converged to expand on the pioneering work of J. Bob Oppenheimer, papa of the atomic bomb. Hikes accessed from this stretch of the Jemez Mountain Trail visit a marvelous collection of stone goblins, historic ruins, mountain rivers, cliff dwellings, and the gigantic caldera of the aforementioned volcano.

THE CHIHUAHUA TRAIL

As mentioned earlier, I-25 roughly follows El Camino Real, but then every main road of commerce under the Spanish crown was a *camino real*. The 550-mile segment of El Camino Real from Santa Fe to the capital city of Chihuahua was once distinguished as the Chihuahua Trail. Forged millennia ago as an Indian trade route, the corridor has since rumbled with the traffic of conquistadors, oxcarts, wagon trains, and cattle drives. To reach the distant trailhead in this wildly diverse group, you'll motor it 50 miles south of the last exit to Albuquerque. Features on hikes along the way include a mysterious rock, a sacred hill, and a wooded canyon in the Manzano Mountain Wilderness. To examine a few of the widely varied ecosystems in the Sevilleta National Wildlife Refuge, try Cerro Montoso, Cornerstone Marsh, and San Lorenzo Canyon. At some point along the way, however, you really should attempt the potentially arduous ridgeline ascent in the notorious Sierra Ladrones.

THE MOTHER ROAD

The last group brings us back to Route 66. In his 1939 novel *The Grapes of Wrath,* John Steinbeck dubbed it "the mother road." I-40 now assumes the bulk of its heavy load, but remnants of this song-worthy highway still stand. As you travel to Herrera, you might recognize the Rio Puerco Bridge from its cameo role in the 1940 cinematic adaptation of Steinbeck's book. As with the hikes near Herrera, two excursions well south of I-40 visit lonesome landscapes of rugged beauty. Gorgeously hostile badlands are the big attraction at El Malpais. An exploratory route in the Water Canyon Wildlife Area is just one of 17 hikes new to this edition. To top it all off, the highest and final hike passes through aspen woodland to reach the summit of Mount Taylor.

RECOMMENDED HIKES

TRAILS BY LENGTH IN MILES AND ACCESSIBILITY:

1–3 miles	dogs	mountain bikes
3–6 miles	equestrians	wheelchairs
6–10 miles		

REGION Hike #/Hike name	page	1–3 miles	3–6 miles	6–10 miles	dogs	equestrians	mountain bikes	wheelchairs
THE DUKE CITY								
1 Rio Grande Nature Center	18		▪️		PLR	PR	PR	P
2 The Volcanoes	23		▪️	▪️	L		R	P
3 Piedras Marcadas	28	▪️			LR			
4 Atrisco	33	▪️						
5 Montessa Park	38		▪️		L			
6 Elena Gallegos	42	▪️			L	P	P	P
7 Waterfall Canyon	47	▪️					X	
8 Corrales	52		▪️		L			
9 La Ceja	57	▪️						
THE SALT MISSION TRAIL								
10 Canyon Estates	64		▪️				X	
11 Coyote Trail	69	▪️					R	
12 Sedillo Ridge	73		▪️		LR			
13 Juan Tomas	78		▪️		LR		R	
14 Mars Court	82		▪️	▪️			R	
15 Fourth of July Canyon	87			▪️			X	
16 Box Spring	92			▪️			X	

▪️ = easy   ▪️ = moderate   ▪️ = strenuous

L = leash required	N = nearby trail	X = prohibited
R = recommended trail	P = partially inaccessible	

XV

REGION / Hike #/Hike name	page	1–3 miles	3–6 miles	6–10 miles	dogs	equestrians	mountain bikes	wheelchairs
THE TURQUOISE TRAIL								
17 Mud Spring	100		moderate	strenuous		P	P	
18 Armijo Trail	106		moderate					N
19 Tree Springs	110			moderate			P	
20 Golden	115	easy	moderate		LR			
21 Cerro Columbo	120		strenuous					
22 Cerrillos Hills	124		moderate		LR	R	R	N
23 Cañada de la Cueva	130			moderate				
EL CAMINO REAL								
24 Tunnel Spring	138		strenuous	strenuous			X	
25 Las Huertas	143		moderate		LR			
26 Ball Ranch	148		moderate	moderate	R	R		
27 Kasha-Katuwe	153		strenuous		X	P	X	P
28 Dome Wilderness	158			strenuous			X	
29 La Bajada	164			moderate				
30 La Cienega	169		moderate					
THE CITY DIFFERENT								
31 Twin Hills	176			moderate	R			
32 Buckman	180		moderate	strenuous				
33 Bishop's Lodge	185		strenuous			R		
34 Hyde Park	190		strenuous		L	X	X	
35 Cowboy Shack	194	moderate			R	N	R	
36 Glorieta Canyon	199			strenuous	R	R	R	

‖ = easy   ‖ = moderate   ‖ = strenuous

L = leash required   N = nearby trail   X = prohibited
R = recommended trail   P = partially inaccessible

REGION Hike #/Hike name	page	1–3 miles	3–6 miles	6–10 miles	dogs	equestrians	mountain bikes	wheelchairs
THE JEMEZ MOUNTAIN TRAIL								
37 White Mesa	206		moderate			N	R	
38 Querencia Arroyo	211			moderate			X	
39 San Ysidro	216	easy	moderate					
40 Cabezon Peak	222	strenuous						
41 Deadman Peaks	226	moderate					X	
42 Paliza Canyon	231		easy					
43 Stable Mesa	236			moderate				
44 Valles Caldera	241		easy				X	
45 Falls Trail	247		moderate		X	X	X	N
46 Water Canyon	252		moderate	strenuous	R		X	
THE CHIHUAHUA TRAIL								
47 Hidden Mountain	260	strenuous			R			
48 El Cerro Tomé	265	moderate			X	X	X	P
49 Monte Largo Canyon	270		moderate				X	
50 Cerro Montoso	276		strenuous					
51 Sierra Ladrones	281		strenuous	moderate				
52 Sevilleta NWR	286			moderate	R			P
53 San Lorenzo Canyon	291		moderate		R			
THE MOTHER ROAD								
54 Oh My God	298			moderate				
55 Herrera Mesa	302		moderate					
56 Volcano Hill	307			moderate			N	
57 Mesa Gallina	312			strenuous				
58 Water Canyon Wildlife Area	317		strenuous				X	
59 Sandstone Bluffs	322			moderate	L		X	
60 Gooseberry Spring	327			strenuous	R			

▮ = easy   ▮ = moderate   ▮ = strenuous

L = leash required	N = nearby trail	X = prohibited
R = recommended trail	P = partially inaccessible	

MORE RECOMMENDED HIKES

CATEGORIES:

- ✓ kids
- ✓ summer
- ✓ winter
- ✓ marked trails
- ✓ educational/interpretive
- ✓ sacred sites
- ✓ ghost towns/ruins
- ✓ solitude
- ✓ people-watching

REGION Hike #/Hike name	page	kids	summer	winter	marked trails	educational/interpretive	sacred sites	ghost towns/ruins	solitude	people-watching
THE DUKE CITY										
1 Rio Grande Nature Center	18	✓	✓	✓	✓	✓				✓
2 The Volcanoes	23			✓	✓	✓	✓			
3 Piedras Marcadas	28			✓	✓		✓			
4 Atrisco	33		✓	✓						✓
5 Montessa Park	38			✓						
6 Elena Gallegos	42	✓	✓	✓	✓	✓				✓
7 Waterfall Canyon	47	✓	✓	✓						
8 Corrales	52	✓	✓	✓	✓					✓
9 La Ceja	57			✓						
THE SALT MISSION TRAIL										
10 Canyon Estates	64	✓	✓	✓	✓					
11 Coyote Trail	69		✓	✓						
12 Sedillo Ridge	73	✓	✓	✓					✓	
13 Juan Tomas	78		✓	✓						
14 Mars Court	82		✓	✓	✓					
15 Fourth of July Canyon	87	✓	✓			✓				
16 Box Spring	92	✓	✓			✓				

REGION / Hike #/Hike name	page	kids	summer	winter	marked trails	educational/ interpretive	sacred sites	ghost towns/ ruins	solitude	people- watching
THE TURQUOISE TRAIL										
17 Mud Spring	100	✓	✓	✓	✓			✓		
18 Armijo Trail	106		✓	✓	✓					
19 Tree Springs	110		✓	✓	✓					
20 Golden	115		✓							
21 Cerro Columbo	120		✓					✓	✓	
22 Cerrillos Hills	124	✓		✓	✓	✓		✓		
23 Cañada de la Cueva	130		✓						✓	
EL CAMINO REAL										
24 Tunnel Spring	138		✓	✓						
25 Las Huertas	143		✓							
26 Ball Ranch	148	✓	✓						✓	
27 Kasha-Katuwe	153	✓	✓	✓	✓	✓	✓			✓
28 Dome Wilderness	158		✓						✓	
29 La Bajada	164		✓				✓	✓		
30 La Cienega	169		✓				✓			
THE CITY DIFFERENT										
31 Twin Hills	176			✓						
32 Buckman	180			✓						
33 Bishop's Lodge	185		✓							✓
34 Hyde Park	190	✓	✓		✓	✓				
35 Cowboy Shack	194	✓		✓	✓			✓		
36 Glorieta Canyon	199	✓	✓		✓			✓		
THE JEMEZ MOUNTAIN TRAIL										
37 White Mesa	206			✓	✓					
38 Querencia Arroyo	211		✓						✓	
39 San Ysidro	216		✓						✓	
40 Cabezon Peak	222		✓				✓			
41 Deadman Peaks	226		✓		✓				✓	
42 Paliza Canyon	231	✓	✓							

REGION Hike #/Hike name	page	kids	summer	winter	marked trails	educational/interpretive	sacred sites	ghost towns/ruins	solitude	people-watching
THE JEMEZ MOUNTAIN TRAIL (continued)										
43 Stable Mesa	236		✓					✓		
44 Valles Caldera	241		✓	✓						
45 Falls Trail	247	✓	✓		✓	✓				✓
46 Water Canyon	252		✓							
THE CHIHUAHUA TRAIL										
47 Hidden Mountain	260	✓		✓						
48 El Cerro Tomé	265	✓		✓	✓	✓	✓			✓
49 Monte Largo Canyon	270		✓	✓					✓	
50 Cerro Montoso	276			✓					✓	
51 Sierra Ladrones	281								✓	
52 Sevilleta NWR	286		✓	✓	✓					
53 San Lorenzo Canyon	291	✓		✓						
THE MOTHER ROAD										
54 Oh My God	298	✓		✓					✓	
55 Herrera Mesa	302			✓				✓	✓	
56 Volcano Hill	307			✓				✓	✓	
57 Mesa Gallina	312		✓						✓	
58 Water Canyon Wildlife Area	317		✓							
59 Sandstone Bluffs	322	✓		✓			✓			✓
60 Gooseberry Spring	327	✓	✓	✓	✓		✓			

MORE RECOMMENDED HIKES

CATEGORIES:

- ✓ bird-watching
- ✓ reptiles
- ✓ rock formations
- ✓ water features
- ✓ woodland
- ✓ wildflowers
- ✓ jogging
- ✓ vistas

REGION Hike #/Hike name	page	bird-watching	reptiles	rock formations	water features	woodland	wildflowers	jogging	vistas
THE DUKE CITY									
1 Rio Grande Nature Center	18	✓	✓		✓	✓		✓	
2 The Volcanoes	23		✓	✓					✓
3 Piedras Marcadas	28		✓				✓		
4 Atrisco	33				✓		✓		
5 Montessa Park	38	✓	✓				✓		
6 Elena Gallegos	42	✓			✓		✓	✓	
7 Waterfall Canyon	47	✓		✓	✓	✓	✓		
8 Corrales	52	✓			✓	✓		✓	
9 La Ceja	57		✓						✓
THE SALT MISSION TRAIL									
10 Canyon Estates	64	✓		✓	✓	✓	✓	✓	
11 Coyote Trail	69	✓		✓		✓			
12 Sedillo Ridge	73	✓				✓	✓		
13 Juan Tomas	78	✓				✓	✓		
14 Mars Court	82	✓				✓	✓		✓
15 Fourth of July Canyon	87	✓		✓		✓	✓		✓
16 Box Spring	92	✓	✓	✓		✓	✓		✓

REGION Hike #/Hike name	page	bird-watching	reptiles	rock formations	water features	woodland	wildflowers	jogging	vistas
THE TURQUOISE TRAIL									
17 Mud Spring	100		✓		✓	✓			
18 Armijo Trail	106					✓			
19 Tree Springs	110					✓			✓
20 Golden	115		✓				✓	✓	✓
21 Cerro Columbo	120		✓						✓
22 Cerrillos Hills	124	✓	✓				✓		✓
23 Cañada de la Cueva	130		✓	✓					
EL CAMINO REAL									
24 Tunnel Spring	138	✓				✓	✓		✓
25 Las Huertas	143		✓				✓		
26 Ball Ranch	148		✓	✓					
27 Kasha-Katuwe	153	✓	✓	✓			✓		✓
28 Dome Wilderness	158	✓				✓	✓		✓
29 La Bajada	164		✓		✓		✓		✓
30 La Cienega	169		✓		✓		✓		✓
THE CITY DIFFERENT									
31 Twin Hills	176		✓	✓					✓
32 Buckman	180			✓	✓		✓		✓
33 Bishop's Lodge	185	✓			✓	✓	✓		✓
34 Hyde Park	190	✓			✓	✓	✓		✓
35 Cowboy Shack	194			✓					
36 Glorieta Canyon	199	✓				✓	✓		
THE JEMEZ MOUNTAIN TRAIL									
37 White Mesa	206		✓	✓					✓
38 Querencia Arroyo	211		✓	✓					✓
39 San Ysidro	216		✓	✓					
40 Cabezon Peak	222		✓	✓					✓
41 Deadman Peaks	226		✓	✓			✓		✓
42 Paliza Canyon	231	✓			✓		✓	✓	

REGION Hike #/Hike name	page	bird-watching	reptiles	rock formations	water features	woodland	wildflowers	jogging	vistas
THE JEMEZ MOUNTAIN TRAIL (continued)									
43 Stable Mesa	236	✓		✓		✓	✓		✓
44 Valles Caldera	241	✓				✓	✓		✓
45 Falls Trail	247	✓		✓	✓	✓	✓		✓
46 Water Canyon	252	✓		✓					✓
THE CHIHUAHUA TRAIL									
47 Hidden Mountain	260		✓						✓
48 El Cerro Tomé	265								✓
49 Monte Largo Canyon	270	✓	✓			✓			✓
50 Cerro Montoso	275		✓						✓
51 Sierra Ladrones	281		✓						✓
52 Sevilleta NWR	286	✓					✓		
53 San Lorenzo Canyon	291			✓					
THE MOTHER ROAD									
54 Oh My God	298		✓	✓					✓
55 Herrera Mesa	302			✓					✓
56 Volcano Hill	307								✓
57 Mesa Gallina	312	✓	✓						✓
58 Water Canyon Wildlife Area	317	✓			✓	✓			✓
59 Sandstone Bluffs	322		✓	✓					✓
60 Gooseberry Spring	327	✓				✓	✓		✓

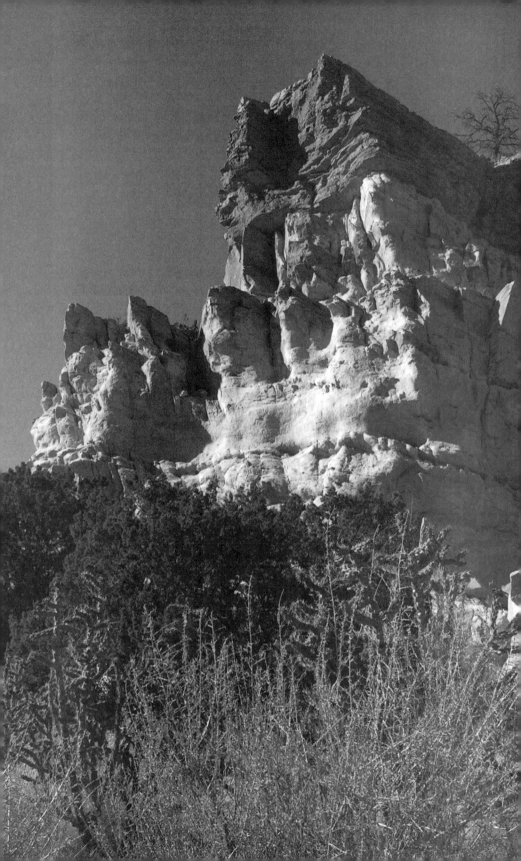

INTRODUCTION

Welcome to *60 Hikes within 60 Miles: Albuquerque*. If you're new to hiking or even if you're a seasoned hiker, take a few minutes to read the following introduction. We explain how this book is organized and how to use it.

HOW TO USE THIS GUIDEBOOK

THE OVERVIEW MAP AND OVERVIEW-MAP KEY

Use the overview map on the inside front cover to find the exact locations of each hike's primary trailhead. Each hike's number appears on the overview map, on the map key facing the overview map, in the table of contents, and in the overview map at the beginning of each regional section. As you flip through the book, a hike's full profile is easy to locate by watching for the hike number at the top of each right-hand page. A map legend that details the symbols found on trail maps appears on the inside back cover.

REGIONAL MAPS

The book is divided into regions, and prefacing each regional section is an overview map of that region. The regional provides more detail than the overview map, bringing you closer to the hike.

TRAIL MAPS

Each hike contains a detailed map that shows the trailhead, the route, significant features, facilities, and topographic landmarks such as creeks, overlooks, and peaks. The author gathered map data by carrying a Garmin eTrex Venture GPS unit while hiking. This data was downloaded into the digital mapping program Topo USA and processed by expert cartographers to produce the highly accurate maps found in this book. Each trailhead's GPS coordinates are included with each hike profile.

ELEVATION PROFILES

Corresponding directly to the trail map, each hike contains a detailed elevation profile. The elevation profile provides a quick look at the trail from the side, enabling you to visualize how the trail rises and falls. Note the number of feet between each tick mark on the vertical axis (the height scale). To avoid making flat hikes look steep and steep hikes appear flat, height scales are used throughout the book to provide an accurate image of the hike's climbing difficulty.

GPS TRAILHEAD COORDINATES

To collect accurate map data, the author hiked each trail with a handheld GPS unit (Garmin eTrex series). Data collected was then downloaded and plotted onto a digital United States Geological Survey (USGS) topo map. In addition to providing a highly specific trail outline, this book also includes the GPS coordinates for each trailhead in latitude–longitude format. These coordinates tell you where you are by locating a point west (latitude) of the 0° meridian line that passes through Greenwich, England, and north or south of the 0° longitude line that belts the Earth, aka the equator.

For readers who own a GPS unit, whether handheld or aboard a vehicle, the latitude–longitude coordinates provided on the first page of each hike may be entered into the GPS unit. Just make sure your GPS unit is set to navigate using WGS84 datum. Now you can navigate directly to the trailhead.

Most trailheads, which begin in parking areas, can be reached by car, but some hikes still require a short walk to reach the trailhead from a parking area. In those cases, a handheld unit is necessary to continue the GPS navigation process. Still, readers can easily access all trailheads in this book by using the directions given, the overview map, and the trail map, which shows at least one major road leading into the area. But for those who enjoy using the latest GPS technology to navigate, the necessary data has been provided.

To learn more about how to enhance your outdoor experiences with GPS technology, refer to *GPS Outdoors: A Practical Guide for Outdoor Enthusiasts (Menasha Ridge Press)*.

HIKE DESCRIPTIONS

Each hike contains seven key items: an "In Brief" description of the trail, a Key At-a-Glance Information box, directions to the trail, trailhead coordinates, a trail map, an elevation profile, and a trail description. Many hikes also include notes on nearby activities. Combined, the maps and information provide a clear method to assess each trail from the comfort of your favorite reading chair.

IN BRIEF

A "taste of the trail." Think of this section as a snapshot focused on the historical landmarks, beautiful vistas, and other sights you may encounter on the hike.

KEY AT-A-GLANCE INFORMATION

The following gives you a quick idea of the statistics and specifics of each hike:

LENGTH This indicates the length of the trail from start to finish. There may be options to shorten or extend the hikes, but the mileage corresponds to the described hike. Consult the hike description to help you decide how to customize the hike for your ability or time constraints.

CONFIGURATION This information tells you what the trail might look like from overhead. Trails can be loops, out-and-backs (trails on which one enters and leaves along the same path), figure-eights, or a combination of shapes.

DIFFICULTY The degree of effort an average hiker should expect on a given hike. For simplicity, the trails are rated as easy, moderate, or strenuous.

SCENERY A short summary of the attractions offered by the hike and what to expect in terms of plant life, wildlife, natural wonders, and historic features.

EXPOSURE A quick check of how much sun you can expect on your shoulders during the hike.

TRAIL TRAFFIC Indicates how busy the trail might be on average. Traffic, of course, varies from day to day and season to season. Weekend days typically see the most visitors. Other trail users whom you may encounter on the trail are also noted here.

SHARED USE Indicates the types and levels of use from nonhikers.

TRAIL SURFACE Indicates whether the trail surface is paved, rocky, gravel, dirt, boardwalk, or a mixture of surfaces.

HIKING TIME The length of time it takes to hike the trail, not counting rest breaks, photo ops, detours, and other distractions. A slow but steady hiker will average 2–3 miles an hour, depending on the terrain.

DRIVING DISTANCE One-way, measured from the "Big I" (the I-40/I-25 exchange).

ACCESS A notation of any fees or permits that may be needed to access the trail or park at the trailhead. Also may include park hours and seasonal closings.

LAND STATUS Indicates which agency manages the land.

MAPS Here you'll find a list of maps that show the topography of the trail, including 7.5-minute USGS topo maps.

FACILITIES What to expect in terms of restrooms, water, shelters, and other amenities at the trailhead or nearby.

LAST-CHANCE FOOD/GAS A bonus category for those who set out not quite fully prepared for the journey.

SPECIAL COMMENTS Additional useful information, such as general trail considerations, warnings/advice, and helpful phone numbers/websites.

DIRECTIONS

Used in conjunction with the overview map, the driving directions will help you locate each trailhead. Once at the trailhead, park only in designated areas.

GPS TRAILHEAD COORDINATES

The trailhead coordinates can be used in addition to the driving directions if you enter the coordinates into your GPS unit before you set out. See page 2 for more information on GPS coordinates.

DESCRIPTION

The trail description is the heart of this book. Here, the author provides a summary of the trail's essence and highlights any special traits the hike has to offer. The route is clearly described, including landmarks, side trips, and possible alternate routes along the way. Ultimately, the hike description will help you choose which hikes are best for you.

NEARBY ACTIVITIES

Look here for information on things to do or points of interest near the trail. These include nearby parks, museums, restaurants, or even a brew pub where you can get a well-deserved beer after a long hike. Note that not every hike has a listing.

WEATHER

My initial field research for this book in 2007 coincided with the onset of an epic heat wave and what seemed like another endless drought. Then the rain came, and no one had guessed that it would bring the 100-year floods. Winter followed suit with record snowfall—26 inches in 24 hours. Spring brought more of it, and Cinco de Mayo just wasn't the same with snow blustering through the fiestas. Tornadoes are a rarity in north-central New Mexico, but a single afternoon storm in June spawned three landspouts near La Bajada. During my second round of field checks in 2011, New Mexico managed to shatter all previous state records for highs, lows, drought, fire, and floods. In short, weather can be unpredictable from year to year or season to season.

With a base elevation of 5,000 feet, Albuquerque usually enjoys a high desert climate. Think of it as the happy medium between the extremes of Denver and Phoenix. Days are generally sunny and warm, but as the sun sets, the temperature falls. The city experiences an average change of 27 degrees from day to night all year. An average year here includes 310 days of sunshine and about 9 inches of rain, with relative humidity normally around 44 percent.

Summer is hot, of course, but low humidity helps keep it cooler than just about anywhere else south of the 36th parallel. And even when daytime temperatures soar into triple digits, you can always count on cool nights. In July and August, afternoon monsoons break the heat with sudden and furious thunderstorms.

Autumn can bring sunshine, thunderstorms, snow, or all of the above at once. Generally, warm temperatures still linger in September and early October, with sweater days firmly established by November.

Winter requires extra layers, though a light jacket often suffices on sunny days. Snow seldom lasts more than a day or two in town. However, deep canyons, north-facing slopes, and elevations above 8,000 feet can take weeks or months to fully defrost.

Spring often begins with high winds that can blow for days. Whether gusting off the West Mesa or howling through Tijeras Canyon, they create miserable conditions for outdoor recreation. On the plus side, it's a sure sign that perfect weather is right around the corner.

Before you go out, check the forecast with the National Weather Service: (505) 821-1111 or **srh.noaa.gov/abq.**

And no matter what they say, be prepared for anything.

ALBUQUERQUE MONTHLY CLIMATE SUMMARY						
	JAN	**FEB**	**MAR**	**APR**	**MAY**	**JUN**
HIGH	47.2°F	53.2°F	60.6°F	70.0°F	79.4°F	89.3°F
LOW	23.4°F	27.8°F	33.0°F	40.8°F	50.1°F	59.2°F
PRECIPITATION	0.37"	0.40"	0.52"	0.54"	0.63"	0.61"
	JUL	**AUG**	**SEP**	**OCT**	**NOV**	**DEC**
HIGH	94°F	93°F	89°F	82°F	73°F	65°F
LOW	75°F	75°F	72°F	62°F	53°F	47°F
PRECIPITATION	1.38"	1.46"	0.96"	0.88"	0.46"	0.46"

WATER

How much is enough? Well, one simple physiological fact should convince you to err on the side of excess when deciding how much water to pack: a hiker working hard in 90-degree heat needs approximately 10 quarts of fluid per day. That's 2.5 gallons—10 quart-sized water bottles or 16 20-ounce ones. In other words, pack along one or two bottles even for short hikes.

Some hikers and backpackers hit the trail prepared to purify water found along the route. This method, while less dangerous than drinking it untreated, comes with risks. Purifiers with ceramic filters are the safest. Many hikers pack along the slightly distasteful tetraglycine–hydroperiodide tablets to purify water (sold under the names Potable Aqua, Coughlan's, and others).

Probably the most common waterborne bug that hikers face is giardia, which may not hit until one to four weeks after ingestion. It will have you living in the bathroom, passing noxious rotten-egg gas, vomiting, and shivering with chills. Other parasites to worry about include E. coli and cryptosporidium, both of which are harder to kill than giardia.

For most people, the pleasures of hiking make carrying water a relatively minor price to pay to remain healthy. If you're tempted to drink found water, do so only if you understand the risks involved. Better yet, hydrate prior to your hike, carry (and drink) 6 ounces of water for every mile you plan to hike, and hydrate after the hike.

THE TEN ESSENTIALS

One of the first rules of hiking is to be prepared for anything. The simplest way to be prepared is to carry the "Ten Essentials." In addition to carrying the items listed below, you need to know how to use them, especially navigation items. Always consider worst-case scenarios like getting lost, hiking back in the dark, broken gear (for example, a broken hip strap on your pack or a water filter getting plugged), twisting an ankle, or a brutal thunderstorm. The items listed below don't cost a lot of money, don't take up much room in a pack, and don't weigh much, but they might just save your life.

1. **Water: durable bottles, and water treatment like iodine or a filter**
2. **Map: preferably a topo map and a trail map with a route description**
3. **Compass: a high-quality compass**
4. **First-aid kit: a high-quality kit including first-aid instructions**
5. **Knife: a multitool device with pliers is best**
6. **Light: flashlight or headlamp with extra bulbs and batteries**
7. **Fire: windproof matches or lighter and fire starter**
8. **Extra food: you should always have food in your pack when you've finished hiking**
9. **Extra clothes: rain protection, warm layers, gloves, warm hat**
10. **Sun protection: sunglasses, lip balm, sunblock, sun hat**

FIRST-AID KIT

A typical first-aid kit may contain more items than you might think necessary. These are just the basics. Prepackaged kits in waterproof bags (Atwater Carey and Adventure Medical make a variety of kits) are available. Even though there are quite a few items listed here, they pack into a small space.

Ace bandages or Spenco joint wraps

Antibiotic ointment (Neosporin or the generic equivalent)

Aspirin, ibuprofen, or acetaminophen

Band-Aids

Benadryl or the generic equivalent, diphenhydramine (in case of allergic reactions)

Butterfly-closure bandages

Epinephrine in a prefilled syringe (for people known to have severe allergic reactions to such things as bee stings)

Gauze (one roll)

Gauze compress pads (a half-dozen 4 x 4–inch pads)

Hydrogen peroxide, Betadine, or iodine

Insect repellent

Matches or pocket lighter

Moleskin/Spenco "Second Skin"

Sunscreen

Whistle (it's more effective in signaling rescuers than your voice)

HIKING WITH CHILDREN

No one is too young for a hike in the outdoors. Be mindful, though. Flat, short, and shaded trails are best with an infant. Toddlers who have not quite mastered walking can still tag along, riding on an adult's back in a child carrier. Use common sense to judge a child's capacity to hike a particular trail, and always count that the child will tire quickly and need to be carried.

When packing for the hike, remember the child's needs as well as your own. Make sure children are adequately clothed for the weather, have proper shoes, and are protected from the sun with sunscreen. Kids dehydrate quickly, so make sure you have plenty of fluid for everyone. Hikes suitable for children are included in the More Recommended Hikes chart on pages xviii–xx.

GENERAL SAFETY

To some inexperienced hikers the deep woods can seem perilous and at times scary. If hiking seems like a hazardous activity, keep in mind that injury, disease, and death are far more likely to result from a sedentary lifestyle—that is, not hiking. But with proper planning and the following tips, your trip can be fun, easy, and, above all else, safe.

- **Always hike with a buddy. While most of these areas are safe, you should have someone else with you while hiking.**

- **Always carry food and water whether you are planning to go overnight or not. Food will give you energy, help keep you warm, and sustain you in an emergency situation until help arrives. You never know if you will have a stream nearby when you become thirsty. Bring potable water or treat water before drinking it from a stream. Boil or filter all found water before drinking it.**

- **Stay on designated trails. Most hikers who get lost do so because they leave the trail. Even on the most clearly marked trails, there is usually a point where you have to stop and consider which direction to head. If you become** disoriented, don't panic. As soon as you think you may be lost, stop, assess your current direction, and then retrace your steps back to the point where you went awry. Using a map, compass, and this book—and keeping in mind what you have passed thus far—reorient yourself, and trust your judgment on which way to continue. If you become absolutely unsure of how to continue, return to your vehicle the way you came in. Should you become completely lost and have no idea of how to return to the trailhead, remaining in place along the trail and waiting for help is most often the best option for adults and always the best option for children.

- Be especially careful when crossing streams. Whether you are fording the stream or crossing on a log, make every step count. If you have any doubt about maintaining your balance on a foot log, go ahead and ford the stream instead. When fording a stream, use a trekking pole or stout stick for balance and face upstream as you cross. If a stream seems too deep to ford, turn back. Whatever is on the other side is not worth risking your life for.

- Standing dead trees and storm-damaged living trees pose a real hazard to hikers and tent campers. When choosing a spot to rest or a backcountry campsite, look up.

- Know the symptoms of heat exhaustion. Excessive sweating, faintness or dizziness, clammy skin, vomiting, and paleness are all common symptoms. If symptoms arise, cool the person off by removing extra clothing, moving him or her to the shade, and giving him or her water.

- Know the symptoms of hypothermia. Shivering and forgetfulness are the two most common indicators of this insidious killer. Hypothermia can occur at any elevation, even in the summer, especially when the hiker is wearing lightweight cotton clothing. If symptoms arise, get the victim shelter, hot liquids, and dry clothes or a dry sleeping bag.

- Take along your brain. A cool, calculating mind is the single most important piece of equipment you'll ever need on the trail. Think before you act. Watch your step. Plan ahead. Avoiding accidents before they happen is the best recipe for a rewarding and relaxing hike.

- Ask questions. Park employees are there to help. It's a lot easier to gain advice beforehand and thereby avoid a mishap than to try to amend an error far away from civilization. Use your head out there.

SAFETY ADVICE FOR HIKERS IN THE SOUTHWEST

The trails are generally safer than the roads you'll drive to reach them, provided of course that you adhere to common sense.

Unfortunately, even experienced hikers suffer an occasional lapse in judgment, as I was reminded recently while hanging upside down by a strap snagged on a dead pine about 80 feet above the floor of Sanchez Canyon. Exactly how I ended up in that awkward position isn't important now. Suffice it to say one of the biggest potential hazards on the trail is gravity. Many hiking injuries result from falling rocks, but even more result from falling hikers. Use caution near cliff edges, whether you're above or beneath them. New Mexico is the fifth-highest state, with five peaks of more than 13,000 feet—so there's no shortage of opportunities for a spectacular fall.

ALTITUDE SICKNESS

Elevations for hikes in this book range from 4,700 to 11,200 feet. A serious case of altitude sickness is unlikely, though lowlanders do occasionally experience shortness of breath, headaches, dizziness, and nausea. Take a day or two to acclimatize before attempting a strenuous hike.

EXPOSURE

Most of these hikes occur in the high desert, where there's precious little shade and less atmosphere to shield you from the sun. Protective clothing and sunscreen are essential, especially for gringos. Also be prepared for sudden drops in temperature. Lost hikers have been known to suffer from heat exhaustion and hypothermia in the same day. Of the two extremes, cold weather is by far the greater danger in New Mexico.

DEHYDRATION

In 1944, several German sailors almost perished from dehydration as they hauled their makeshift raft 20 miles down a dry streambed in the Sonoran Desert. These Nazi POWs had made a potentially fatal mistake in an otherwise flawless escape plan when they assumed that they'd find water in rivers they'd seen on a map. Sure, it sounds hilarious now, but it's not so funny when it happens to you. Always bring enough drinking water for the entire hike, and save your great rafting escape for snowmelt season.

THUNDERSTORMS

Rain is rare, but it can come with a fury. Many of these hikes follow canyon routes and drainages, where flash flooding can be a serious hazard. Areas burned in wildfires and downhill of burn zones are susceptible to flooding. High ridges are just as dangerous when lightning strikes.

Always check the forecast before heading out. Stay aware of cloud conditions, especially during monsoon season (July and August).

HUNTERS

Seasonal hunting is permitted on most public lands. Wear bright colors if hiking in active areas. For more specifics on where and when hunting is permitted, consult the annual game proclamations, which are available free from most sporting-goods retailers and from the New Mexico Department of Game and Fish: (505) 476-8000, **wildlife.state.nm.us.**

ANIMAL AND PLANT HAZARDS

HAZARD TREES

Drought, disease, and insect infestation have taken a toll on New Mexico forests in recent years. Recreation areas occasionally close for hazard-tree removal and cleanup. In wilderness areas, snags (standing dead trees) are often left to fall naturally in order to preserve and protect wilderness character, as required by the Wilderness Act of 1964. Stay alert, especially when entering damaged areas. Risk of death or serious injury increases in windy conditions.

POISON IVY

Recognizing poison ivy and avoiding contact with it is the most effective way to prevent the painful, itchy rashes associated with these plants. Poison ivy ranges from a thick, tree-hugging vine to a shaded groundcover, three leaflets to a leaf. Urushiol, the oil in the sap of this plant, is responsible for the rash. Usually within

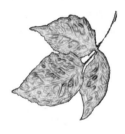

12–14 hours of exposure (but sometimes much later), raised lines and/or blisters will appear, accompanied by a terrible itch. Refrain from scratching, because bacteria under fingernails can cause infection and you will spread the rash to other parts of your body. Wash and dry the rash thoroughly, applying calamine lotion or another product to help dry the rash. If itching or blistering is severe, seek medical attention. To avoid spreading the rash to others, wash not only any exposed parts of your body but also oil-contaminated clothes, gear, and pets.

YUCCA AND CACTI

Steer clear of spiny plants. A casual bump against a yucca hurts worse than a flu shot. Cactus needles easily penetrate canvas shoes. Sturdy footwear is essential. For more-drastic encounters, use tweezers to pluck thick needles, then remove the finer ones with careful applications of adhesive tape or school glue.

PLAGUE AND HANTAVIRUS

Bubonic plague can be transmitted from infected rodents to humans via fleas. Pets that are allowed to roam may become infected or carry infected fleas, leading to plague transmission to people. Incidents are rare but can be fatal if untreated. From 1949 to 2009, a total of 262 human plague cases, 34 fatal, were reported in New Mexico.

Deer mice are the primary carriers of the viruses that cause hantavirus pulmonary syndrome, a rare but often fatal infection. Rodents shed the virus in their urine, droppings, and saliva. The virus is mainly transmitted to people when they breathe in contaminated air. From 1993 to 2011, 87 cases, 35 fatal, were reported in New Mexico.

Hikers should take precautions to reduce the likelihood of their exposure to infectious materials. Avoid coming into contact with rodents and rodent burrows, or disturbing dens such as pack-rat nests. Also avoid confined spaces such as caves and abandoned structures that contain evidence of rodent activity. Always keep kids and pets a safe distance from wild animals.

For more information, check with the New Mexico Department of Health at **www.health.state.nm.us.**

MOSQUITOES

West Nile Virus is a mosquito-borne disease. Though rare, cases have been reported in New Mexico every year since 2003. Infections in humans occur seasonally, with the peak of cases in late summer and early fall. At this time of year—especially at dusk and dawn, when mosquitoes are most active—you may want to wear protective clothing, such as long sleeves, long pants, and socks. Loose-fitting, light-colored clothing is best. Spray clothing with insect repellent. Remember to follow the instructions on the repellent and to take extra care with children when using a repellent with DEET.

SCORPIONS

You probably won't find any scorpions unless you look at night. As many desert ravers have learned, scorpions glow under black light. Though a sting from most scorpions is painful, none of the dangerous species, such as the bark scorpion, commonly range within 60 miles of Albuquerque. (The last scorpion-related death in the U.S. was reported from Arizona in 1968.) If camping, shake out your shoes, sleeping bags, and any clothes left on the ground. If stung, gently cleanse and elevate the wound, and apply a cold compress to reduce swelling.

TICKS

Ticks like to hang out in the brush that grows along trails. Though they're rare in this region, you should be tick-aware during all months of the year. Ticks need a host to feast on in order to reproduce. The ticks that alight on you while hiking will be very small, sometimes so tiny that you won't be able to spot them. Primarily of two varieties, deer ticks and dog ticks, these arthropods (not insects) need a few hours of actual attachment before they can transmit any disease they may harbor. Ticks may settle in shoes, socks, hats, and they may take several hours to actually latch on. The best strategy is to visually check every half-hour or so while hiking, do a thorough check before you get in your car, and then, when you take a posthike shower, do an even more thorough check of your entire body. Ticks that haven't attached are easily removed but not easily killed. If you pick off a tick in the woods, just toss it aside. If you find one on your body at home, dispatch it and then send it down the toilet. For ticks that have embedded, removal with tweezers is best.

SNAKES

The most important preventative measure is to watch your step. Like most hikers in snake country, I've developed a habit of continuously scanning the ground ahead. However, one thing I learned while standing nose-to-nose with a viper in the forest: rattlesnakes can climb trees. Don't hike during times of peak rattle-

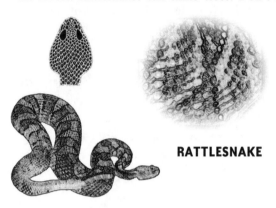

RATTLESNAKE

snake activity, which is usually at night. Wear high-top hiking boots and long pants for additional protection. If bitten, gently cleanse the area and apply a clean dressing. If bitten on the arm or hand, splint the limb. Do not use pressure dressings or tourniquets or make incisions. Remain calm and seek transport to a medical facility. If you need to walk to reach help, do so as soon as possible. Severe reactions from a venomous snakebite may not occur for several hours. Rattlesnakes rarely strike hikers, and when they do it's usually a dry bite. They don't want to kill you. They just want you to leave them alone.

LIVESTOCK

Cows encountered on the trail are generally skittish, but there are a few exceptions. For example, bovine thugs near the Ojito Wilderness have proved themselves more hostile than any I ever faced in the bullring. And though my stint as a matador was ill-advised and short-lived, I can offer this sage advice: if it doesn't run away, steer clear.

BEARS AND MOUNTAIN LIONS

In May 2007, a 200-pound black bear wandered into a medical office in Rio Rancho. Three months later, a 100-pound mountain lion broke into a jewelry store on the Santa Fe Plaza. Yes, New Mexico is still quite wild, but chances are you won't see any either of these animals on the trail. Still, to be on the safe side, there are a few things you should know, just in case.

BLACK BEARS Unlike unpredictable and fearsome grizzly bears, black bears are North America's smallest bear (although still weighing in at 300 to 400 pounds!) and are more interested in your food than anything else. It is extremely rare for a black bear to act aggressively toward humans, and it is almost always due to human provocation. That's not to say that black bears can't be destructive. They will go to great lengths to secure a free meal—everything from tearing the door off a car to raiding a carelessly maintained camp. If any of these hikes are planned as overnighters, it is no longer a viable option to hang your food, as bears have learned to undo your handiwork. Instead, bear-proof food canisters are recommended.

If you do see a bear on the trail or in your camp, it is best to back away slowly while shouting loudly and making noise to scare off the animal. Never try to wrestle food away from a bear, and never get between a mother and her cub!

MOUNTAIN LIONS   Mountain lions are the largest cats found in North America, but your chances of seeing one are extremely small (most hikers are content to simply look for the cat's four-toed print on the trail). Sometimes called cougars or pumas, they are shy, solitary creatures that hunt (mostly deer) alone and are masters at camouflage with their tawny coats and preference for wooded cover. They can grow up to 8 feet in length, including their distinctively long tails. In the unlikely instance that you should come across a mountain lion, you should make eye contact, try to appear larger by spreading your arms, and make noise. Do not run from a mountain lion as this may trigger its natural instinct to chase you.

Here are a few helpful guidelines for handling potential mountain lion encounters:

- **Keep kids close to you. Observed in captivity, mountain lions seem especially drawn to small children.**
- **Do not run from a mountain lion. Running may stimulate the animal's instinct to chase.**
- **Don't approach a mountain lion—give him room to get away.**
- **Try to make yourself look larger by raising your arms and/or opening your jacket if you're wearing one.**
- **Do not crouch or kneel. These movements could make you look smaller and more like the mountain lion's prey.**
- **Try to convince the mountain lion you are dangerous—not its prey. Without crouching, gather nearby stones or branches and toss them at the animal. Slowly wave your arms above your head and speak in a firm voice.**
- **If all fails and you are attacked, fight back. People have successfully fought off attacking mountain lions with rocks and sticks. Try to remain facing the animal, and fend off its attempts to bite your head or neck—the lion's typical aim.**

That may sound a bit alarmist in nature to some people, but it's always best to be prepared just in case. That said, you probably will never see a mountain lion on any of these hikes.

DOGS

A more common hazard than any of the above animals is another hiker's unrestrained dog. Pets are allowed on most public lands, but taking one along is rarely recommended. Encounters between domestic and wild animals rarely end well for anyone. Coyotes, porcupines, and skunks can be especially hazardous to dogs. If you do bring your dog, note that canine fecal coliform is one of the biggest problems facing local water supplies. Collect your pet's waste and dispose of it properly to keep these bacteria from being washed into our aquifers.

INVASIVE SPECIES

An invasive species is any non-native animal or plant that has the ability to spread and cause damage to the environment. To help prevent the spread of hitchhiking invasive species, clean your boots, clothing, and other gear before and after each hike. For more info, visit **invasivespeciesinfo.gov.**

TOPO MAPS

The maps in this book have been produced with great care and, used with the hiking directions, will direct you to the trails and help you stay on course. However, you will find superior detail and valuable information in the USGS's 7.5-minute series topographic maps. One well-known free topo service on the Web is **Microsoft Research Maps (msrmaps.com)**. Online services such as **Trails.com** charge annual fees for additional features such as shaded relief, which makes the topography stand out more. If you expect to print out many topo maps each year, it might be worth paying for such extras. The downside to USGS topos is that most are outdated, having been created 20–30 years ago. But they still provide excellent topographic detail.

Digital topographic-map programs, such as DeLorme's TopoUSA, enable you to review topo maps of the entire United States on your computer. You can download data gathered while hiking with a GPS unit onto the software and plot your own hikes.

If you're new to hiking, you might be wondering, "What's a topographic map?" In short, a topo indicates not only linear distance but elevation as well, using contour lines. Contour lines spread across the map like dozens of intricate spiderwebs. Each line represents a particular elevation, and at the base of each topo, a contour's interval designation is given. If the contour interval is 20 feet, then the distance between each contour line is 20 feet. Follow five contour lines up on the same map, and the elevation has increased by 100 feet.

Let's assume that the 7.5-minute series topo reads "Contour Interval 40 feet" and that the short trail we'll be hiking is 2 inches long on the map and crosses five contour lines from beginning to end. What do we know? Well, because the linear scale of this series is 2,000 feet to the inch (roughly 2.75 inches representing 1 mile), we know our trail is approximately .8 miles long (2 inches equals 2,000 feet). But we also know we'll be climbing or descending 200 vertical feet because there are five contour lines and each is 40 feet. And the elevation designations written on occasional contour lines will tell us if we're heading up or down.

You'll find topos at major universities, in many outdoor shops, and in some public libraries; you might try photocopying the ones you need to avoid the cost of buying them. But if you want your own and can't find them locally, visit the USGS website, **topomaps.usgs.gov.**

TRAIL ETIQUETTE

Whether you're on a city, county, state, or national-park trail, always remember that great care and resources (from nature as well as from your tax dollars) have gone into creating these trails. Treat the trail, wildlife, and fellow hikers with respect.

- **Hike on open trails only. Respect trail and road closures (ask if not sure), avoid possible trespassing on private land, and obtain all permits and authorization as required. Also, leave gates as you found them or as marked.**

- **Leave only footprints. Be sensitive to the ground beneath you. This also means staying on the existing trail and not blazing any new trails. Be sure to pack out what you pack in. No one likes to see the trash someone else has left behind.**

- **Never spook animals. An unannounced approach, a sudden movement, or a loud noise startles most animals. A surprised animal can be dangerous to you, to others, and to themselves. Give them plenty of space.**

- **Plan ahead. Know your equipment, your ability, and the area in which you are hiking, and prepare accordingly. Be self-sufficient at all times; carry necessary supplies for changes in weather or other conditions. A well-executed trip is a satisfaction to you and to others.**

- **Be courteous to other hikers, bikers, equestrians, and others you encounter on the trails.**

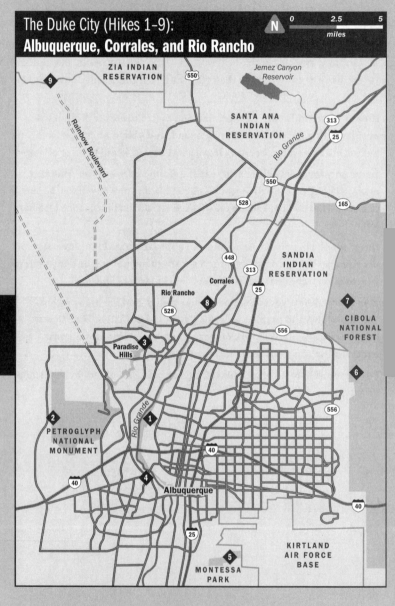

The Duke City (Hikes 1–9):
Albuquerque, Corrales, and Rio Rancho

N 0   2.5   5
miles

ZIA INDIAN
RESERVATION

550

Jemez Canyon
Reservoir

SANTA ANA
INDIAN
RESERVATION

313

25

Rio Grande

550

528

165

Rainbow Boulevard

448

313

SANDIA
INDIAN
RESERVATION

Corrales

25

Rio Rancho

528

7

556

CIBOLA
NATIONAL
FOREST

Paradise
Hills

3

6

Rio Grande

1

556

PETROGLYPH
NATIONAL
MONUMENT

2

40

40

4

40

Albuquerque

25

MONTESSA
PARK

5

KIRTLAND
AIR FORCE
BASE

9

THE DUKE CITY
(ALBUQUERQUE, CORRALES, AND RIO RANCHO)

RIO GRANDE NATURE CENTER– PUEBLO MONTAÑO

KEY AT-A-GLANCE INFORMATION

LENGTH: 5.5 miles on interconnected loops

DIFFICULTY: Easy

SCENERY: Riparian habitat, cottonwood forest, ponds, wetlands, sculpture garden

EXPOSURE: Mostly shaded

TRAIL TRAFFIC: Popular

SHARED USE: High (no dogs or bikes on Nature Center trails; pets must be leashed on Open Space trails)

TRAIL SURFACE: Packed dirt, gravel, pavement

HIKING TIME: 1–3 hours

DRIVING DISTANCE: 4 miles

ACCESS: Nature Center: 10 a.m.– 5 p.m. daily, except Thanksgiving, Christmas, and New Year's days; trails: April–October, 7 a.m.–9 p.m., and November–March, 7 a.m.–7 p.m.

LAND STATUS: State park; Albuquerque Open Space

MAPS: Albuquerque Bicycle Map, free at most local bike shops and Albuquerque Open Space; (505) 768-2680 or cabq.gov/gis/bike map.html; USGS Los Griegos

FACILITIES: Wildlife blinds, picnic areas, visitor center, wheelchair-accessible restrooms

SPECIAL COMMENTS: See note at the end of the Description.

GPS TRAILHEAD COORDINATES

| Latitude | 35° 07' 46" |
| Longitude | 106° 40' 56" |

IN BRIEF

Cottonwood-shaded interpretive trails to the banks of the Rio Grande offer a quick escape from the urban desert and a thorough introduction to the state's most vital ecosystem. From here, hikes can be extended along newer trails in adjacent Aldo Leopold Forest and across the river at Pueblo Montaño.

DESCRIPTION

The Rio Grande heads from the San Juan Mountains in southwestern Colorado to the Gulf of Mexico. At 1,885 miles, it's the third-longest river in the United States. The 175-mile stretch from Cochiti Dam to Elephant Butte is known as the Middle Rio Grande. Here the river supports a cottonwood forest often referred to simply as "the bosque" (BOHS-kay, or sometimes: BAH-skee). At the heart of the Middle Rio Grande bosque is the Rio Grande Valley State Park, a narrow, 4,300-acre multiuse area that extends along the river from Sandia Pueblo to Isleta Pueblo (Albuquerque's northern and southern neighbors, respectively). And at the heart of the RGVSP is the Rio Grande Nature Center, a 270-acre preserve managed by New Mexico State Parks.

Rio Grande Nature Center is a popular spot for wildlife viewing. One of the bigger draws is

Directions

From I-40 West, take Exit 157A to Rio Grande Boulevard. Drive north 1.4 miles and turn left onto Candelaria Road. Go west 0.6 mile and turn right at the park entrance. Note that if you park your car inside, the 5 p.m. gate closure can force you to rush an otherwise leisurely hike. To avoid the worry (and the $3 parking fee), go back one block and park on Trellis Drive.

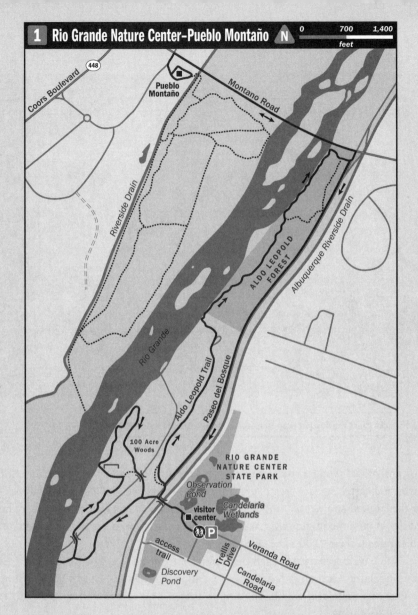

448

Coors Boulevard

Pueblo
Montaño

Montano Road

Riverside Drain

ALDO LEOPOLD FOREST

Albuquerque Riverside Drain

Rio Grande

Aldo Leopold Trail

Paseo del Bosque

100 Acre
Woods

RIO GRANDE
NATURE CENTER
STATE PARK

Observation
Pond

Candelaria
Wetlands

visitor
center

access
trail

Veranda Road

Trellis Drive

Candelaria
Road

Discovery
Pond

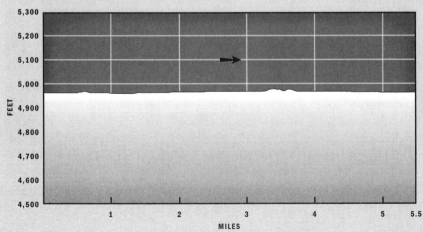

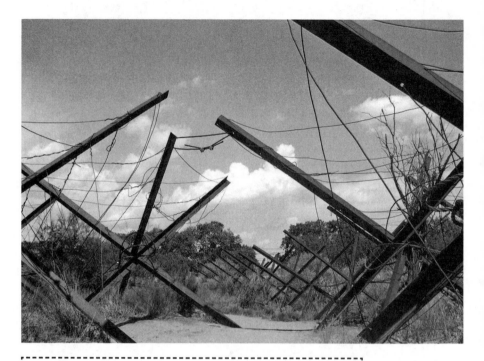

Jetty jacks guard the Bosque Loop trailhead at the Rio Grande Nature Center.

a reconstructed wetland on the northeast side of Rio Grande Nature Center. The ponds and cattail swamp attract thousands of Canada geese and sandhill cranes during the late fall and winter, and about as many bird-watchers show up to ogle them. But if you miss the migratory season, there's plenty more to see here, including two short trails in their "100 Acre Woods."

You have two ways to reach the trailhead. If the parking lot gate is closed, take the Candelaria Access Trail, a narrow corridor that begins at the yellow pylons at the end of Candelaria Road. Turn right at the far end and follow the path to a wooden footbridge.

Otherwise, start down the path on the west side of the parking lot. The left fork leads straight to the footbridge. The right one detours into what appears to be a half-buried drainage pipe. This is the entrance to the visitor center. Inside, you'll find natural history exhibits, a gift shop, restrooms, and a glass-walled library overlooking a wildlife pond. Exit through the back door and proceed to the aforementioned footbridge.

The bridge spans the Albuquerque Riverside Drain. Stairs ahead and a ramp to the right climb the levee. Both the drain and levee are part of an elaborate flood-control and irrigation system in the Rio Grande Valley. The trail atop the levee is Paseo del Bosque. This paved 16-mile recreation route crosses the city without traffic interruption from Alameda Bridge to the Rio Bravo Bridge, making it suitable for strollers, wheelchairs, bicycles, skates, dogs, and horses.

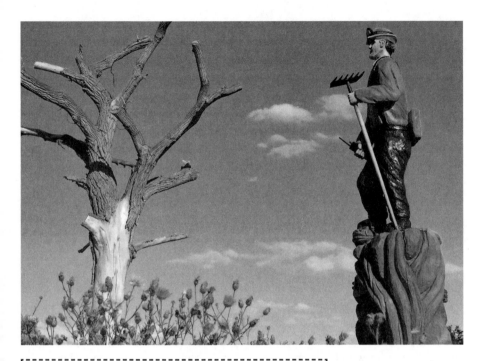

Chainsaw sculpture depicts a hero of the bosque at Pueblo Montaño.

The ramp leads to the Aldo Leopold trailhead, described following; the Bosque Loop begins opposite the stairs. The trail leads through a gap in a tangle of flood-control fences, or jetty jacks, which resemble anti-tank obstacles. The U.S. Army Corps of Engineers installed more than 32,000 of these giant iron crosses throughout the Middle Rio Grande bosque to protect the levee from flood debris. Upriver damming has since rendered them obsolete (although they did prove useful for a few scenes in the 2009 movie *Terminator Salvation*). The Corps also installed the Silvery Minnow Channel, which crosses Bosque Loop Trail twice. During high flows in the Rio Grande, the channel fills with slower moving water to provide habitat for this federally endangered species.

The trail is well groomed, clearly marked, and edged with fallen cottonwood limbs. A sign at the junction ahead presents a choice of staying on 0.7-mile Bosque Loop Trail or picking up the 0.6-mile River Loop Trail. Both lead to clearings on the east bank of the Rio Grande. Vegetation grows thick elsewhere along the river's edge, where native species contend with invasive ones—such as the thorny Russian olive and tamarisk, a salt cedar imported to control riverbank erosion. Once blamed for guzzling the river, cottonwoods faced annihilation in 1969 when the Bureau of Reclamation proposed clearing them from the bosque in an effort to provide more water to farmlands. They later determined that the tamarisk was by far the heavier drinker. Adding to the native trees' disadvantages is the beavers' appetite for local wood, as evidenced in the hefty cottonwoods they topple throughout the bosque.

Aldo Leopold Forest covers 53 acres extending from the north boundary of the Nature Center to the southeast side of the Montaño Bridge. The trail here is also named for the local hero. Aldo Leopold, often cited as "the father of modern wildlife ecology," served as the Secretary of Albuquerque's Chamber of Commerce in 1918 and championed what would later become the Rio Grande Valley State Park. His efforts also eventually led to the creation of the Rio Grande Zoological Park, Botanical Gardens, and the Rio Grande Nature Center. This trail is paved for the first half-mile. It falls short of a river view, but a sandy 100-yard extension reaches the riverbank. A few dirt paths split off from there and stray through the bosque. Webbing the wooded corridor between the river and the levee, these shaded interior trails offer an opportunity for miles of further exploration with no chance of getting lost. Bosque rehabilitation projects and the establishment of a formal trail in 2009 make it all the easier to navigate. The north end of Aldo Leopold Trail returns you to Paseo del Bosque near Montaño Bridge, about a mile north of the Nature Center. The walk to Pueblo Montaño is 0.6 mile. Use the protected pedestrian/bicycle lane to cross the Rio Grande, and enjoy the viewing platforms along the way.

Pueblo Montaño, on the southwest side of Montaño Bridge, is an Open Space project that rose from the ashes of the 2003 bosque fire. The blaze burned more than 250 acres of woodland on both sides of the river. Chainsaw artists have since transformed the thick trunks of scorched trees into fictive images and sculptural memorials to lost wildlife. One towering work depicts a firefighter standing on the head of a slain dragon. In another, the amputated Y of charred tree limbs evolved into the wings of a bald eagle. And beneath carved owls and crows perched on high sits a howling coyote, because no Southwestern art collection would be complete without one. A 0.15-mile loop through the sculpture garden is ADA-compliant. You could easily wander another 10 miles along natural-surface trails north and south of the bridge. Keep in mind that the walk from Pueblo Montaño to the Nature Center parking lot (via Montaño Bridge and Paseo del Bosque) is about 2 miles.

Note: The Nature Center often hosts special events and guided tours. Call (505) 344-7240 or visit **rgnc.org**.

NEARBY ACTIVITIES

Extend your hike from Pueblo Montaño to the **Albuquerque Open Space Visitor Center:** Cross beneath Montaño Bridge and walk 1 mile northeast on the dirt road along Riverside Drain. Turn left to cross the bridge and follow the concrete channel 0.3 mile north to the visitor center, which features outdoor viewing platforms, an art gallery, and interpretive exhibits. Hours are Tuesday–Sunday, 9 a.m.–5 p.m. Call the Open Space Visitor Center at (505) 897-8831 or visit **cabq.gov/openspace/visitorcenter.html** for more information.

PETROGLYPH NATIONAL MONUMENT:
The Volcanoes

IN BRIEF

Walk the flanks of four scoria cones and look for lizards in the lava rock. The Albuquerque Volcanoes also boast the West Side's best views of both the city and the Sandia Mountains.

DESCRIPTION

Try counting every volcano within 60 miles of Albuquerque, and you should come up with a tally in the neighborhood of 270. They range in size from scorched dents in the earth to the towering peak of Mount Taylor.

Ten volcanoes reside within Albuquerque's city limits, with five blistering the otherwise flat western horizon. Compared to the Sandia granite that dominates the eastern vista, the spatter cones are mere babes, born in the final throes of a fissure eruption just 140,000 years ago.

Lava spilled primarily east into the Rio Grande Valley. Concealed beneath the sand and sage of Albuquerque's West Mesa, a lava crust (basalt caprock) rests upon older layers of sediments. Thousands of years of erosion undermined the eastern edges of the caprock, causing it to break apart and collapse. The result is an exposed volcanic escarpment that appears from a distance as a fairly uniform black cliff.

Pueblo Indians have long considered this a sacred landscape. Later cultures developed their own interpretations, with each new generation

Directions

From I-40 West, take Exit 149 and go 4.8 miles north on Atrisco Vista Boulevard. Turn right on the access road and follow it east 0.3 mile to the parking lot. The trailhead is near the southeastern corner of the lot.

KEY AT-A-GLANCE INFORMATION

LENGTH: 1.0-, 2.0-, and 6.3-mile loop options

DIFFICULTY: Easy–moderate

SCENERY: Cinder cones, city views, birds, and reptiles

EXPOSURE: Full sun

TRAIL TRAFFIC: Popular

SHARED USE: Moderate (mountain bikers, equestrians; dogs must be leashed; no motorized vehicles)

TRAIL SURFACE: Packed dirt, sand, loose rock

HIKING TIME: 20 minutes–3 hours

DRIVING DISTANCE: 15 miles

ACCESS: Daily, 9 a.m.–5 p.m.

LAND STATUS: National Park Service; Albuquerque Open Space

MAPS: Trail map at nps.gov/petr; USGS The Volcanoes

FACILITIES: Shade shelters, interpretive signage, no water, limited wheelchair access to trails, wheelchair-accessible restrooms

SPECIAL COMMENTS: See note at end of Hike 3 (page 32) for information about the Petroglyph National Monument Visitor Center.

GPS TRAILHEAD COORDINATES

Latitude   35° 07' 50"
Longitude   106° 46' 50"

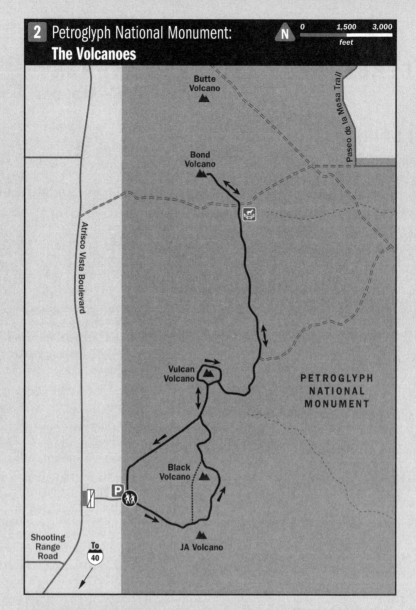

N

0   1,500   3,000
feet

Butte
Volcano

Bond
Volcano

Paseo de la Mesa Trail

Atrisco Vista Boulevard

Vulcan
Volcano

PETROGLYPH
NATIONAL
MONUMENT

Black
Volcano

P

Shooting
Range
Road

To
40

JA Volcano

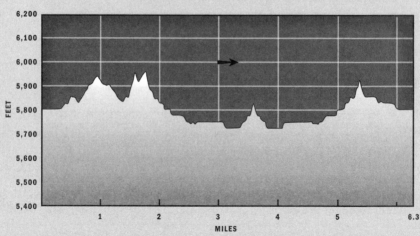

6,200

6,100

6,000

5,900

5,800

5,700

5,600

5,500

5,400

FEET

1   2   3   4   5   6.3

MILES

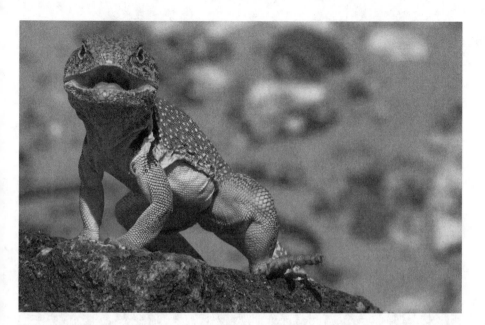

Collared lizard

finding unique ways to express its fondness for the volcanoes. The U.S. Air Force hasn't bombed them in more than 60 years, and in 2007 the U.S. Army Corps of Engineers announced plans to retrieve all the ordnances out there that have, so far, failed to detonate.

On a quiet morning in 1947, Albuquerque residents seemed to gain a new appreciation for their volcanoes when they woke to find thick black smoke billowing from the biggest cone. Citywide panic naturally ensued. A brave crew eventually assessed the fuming crater and returned to announce that the smoke was coming from strategically placed car tires, soaked in gasoline and set ablaze. The prank would be repeated over successive years with considerably less impact.

In 2002 the volcanoes park area received a few new amenities, including shade shelters and interpretive signage. But the biggest improvements came with relocating the parking lot. Visitors can no longer drive to the base of the big volcano, and many seem unwilling to attempt the 2-mile trek on foot. As a result, vegetation stands a healthy chance of reclaiming a surplus of roads and trails.

Navigating the wide-open space in the volcanoes area is easy. You'd have to go completely blind to get lost out here; however, it takes a sharp eye to discern designated trails from discontinued ones. Sometimes the best you can do is just make a good-faith effort to stay on the right ones. Also, although climbing to the top of the volcanoes is not expressly prohibited, it is considered an act of desecration to many Pueblo peoples.

Most volcano visitors tend to dash to the scenic overlook at JA Volcano for a gawk before rushing back to the interstate. This 1-mile out-and-back takes about

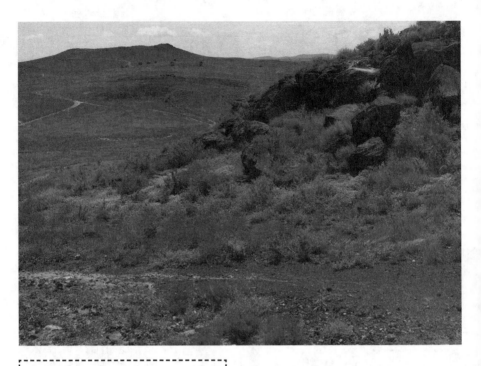

View south from the slopes of Vulcan Volcano

20 minutes. Those traveling at a more leisurely pace might consider the longer options outlined following.

Start the hike from the gate at the southeast corner of the parking lot, take a moment to read the interpretive displays under the nearby shelter and at the trailhead, and then proceed out to JA Volcano. An arrow sign helps you stay on the right track at the intersection with a discontinued road to the southwest escarpment. Continue straight past the shelter ahead to the one at the overlook.

JA Volcano gets its name from a pair of initials painted long ago on its eastern face. They've since faded, but those who know where to look claim the letters are still visible from 8 miles away. These tend be the same people who claim to see gases rising from the cones and insist that the city's Technicolor sunsets are due to the filtering effect of volcanic vapors.

From the overlook, turn left and head north on the main trail. It skirts around east sides of Black and Cinder volcanoes—or what's left of them. Some Burqueños still remember when six robust cones stood out here, before miners cut Black down to a stump and reduced Cinder to a pit.

About 1.4 miles into the hike, you'll arrive at the junction with the return path at the base of Vulcan Volcano. Named for the Roman god of fire, this cone is the biggest in the group. The old parking area was here, which helps explain the remnants of roads and footpaths blazed in at least seven directions. Stick to the main path going up the south side of the cone. About a third of the way up the slope, the trail curves to the left and crosses over a saddle between the main volcano and a baby cone. Continuing clockwise to the north, it passes by a half-domed outcrop. From here the path tends to fade as it rounds the steepest flank. Stick to the base of Vulcan until you reach the hollowed-out area of a former quarry. From here you can finish the loop and head back to the parking lot via the old access road, which runs southwest to a fence, and then straight south. The Vulcan loop totals 2 miles and takes about an hour.

To visit Bond Volcano, follow the road south-southeast from the Vulcan quarry. Refrain from taking any shortcuts, as you may disturb birds and snakes nesting in the grassy areas. The trail soon curves left and goes roughly north about 1.2 miles to the remains of an old corral at the junction of five roads. Take the road heading northwest about 0.25 mile to Bond's southern flank. There you'll find a cave that sometimes smells ripe with musk, depending on the season.

The best time of year to visit the volcanoes is debatable. Certainly the cooler weather in fall and spring makes hiking more pleasant. Fresh snow on the West Mesa has its own mystical allure. But my favorite time is in the fierce heat of summer, on days following heavy rain. The crowds are thin and the craters are thick with insects. These combined factors tend to draw out resident wildlife. Collared lizards do push-ups on skillet-hot basalt. (*Warning:* They bite.) Blister beetles fat as lug nuts display shiny black carapaces with brilliant red pinstripes. (*Warning:* Do not touch. They're called blister bugs for a reason). And though I have yet to greet any of the three species of rattlesnake, I've met numerous nonvenomous cousins and several horned lizards on the road to Bond Volcano.

Return to Vulcan the same way you came. From there you can return to the parking lot via the old access road. If you're parched at this point, the nearest refreshment stand is at the shooting range (see below).

NEARBY ACTIVITIES

Shooting Range Park is a public facility for target practice and skeet shooting. So whether you're packing a rifle, pistol, or muzzleloader, this is the place to pull the trigger. Open Wednesday–Sunday, 9 a.m.–5 p.m.. Fees start at $4.50. No credit cards accepted. To get there from the Volcanoes area, turn left (south) onto Atrisco Vista Boulevard and go 0.4 mile to Shooting Range Road. Turn right (west) and follow the signs 3 miles to the park. For more information, call (505) 836-8785 or visit **cabq.gov/openspace/shootingrange.html**.

Paseo de la Mesa Trail is open to bicyclists, walkers, persons in wheelchairs, inline skaters, and equestrians. Highlights include a 4.2-mile paved trail uninterrupted by roadways, side paths to geologic windows, probable encounters with West Mesa wildlife, and 360-degree views encompassing mountain ranges. For an exhilarating downhill ride, start at the dirt access lot off Atrisco Vista, near Paseo del Norte, and finish at the paved lot off 81st Street near Unser Boulevard. Overall, it's a 400-foot drop in elevation, with some steep sections and sharp curves. For more information, call Albuquerque Open Space at (505) 452-5200 or visit **cabq.gov/openspace/PaseodelaMesa.html**.

3   PETROGLYPH NATIONAL MONUMENT:
Piedras Marcadas

 **KEY AT-A-GLANCE
INFORMATION**

LENGTH: 1.8 miles of interconnected loops

DIFFICULTY: Easy

SCENERY: Ancient etchings on volcanic rock; city views

EXPOSURE: No shade

TRAIL TRAFFIC: Popular

SHARED USE: Low (dogs must be leashed; no motorized vehicles)

TRAIL SURFACE: Sand

HIKING TIME: 1 hour

DRIVING DISTANCE: 12 miles

ACCESS: Year-round, dawn–dusk

LAND STATUS: National Park Service; Albuquerque Open Space

MAPS: Basic trail map posted at trailhead and available at visitor centers; USGS Los Griegos

FACILITIES: Picnic shelter, playground

SPECIAL COMMENTS: For more information, visit the Petroglyph National Monument Visitor Center online at nps.gov/petr or check out the Open Space Visitor Center at cabq.gov/openspace/visitor center.html. See note at the end of the Description for more details.

GPS TRAILHEAD
COORDINATES

Latitude   35° 11' 19"

Longitude   106° 41' 09"

IN BRIEF

Hidden in West Side suburbia, the northernmost outpost of this national monument contains an estimated 5,000 petroglyphs. Hunts for images carved into the basalt lava escarpment of Piedras Marcadas Canyon never fail to yield fascinating finds.

DESCRIPTION

Albuquerque's escarpment is a product of the volcanoes described in the previous hike. This 17-mile ribbon of basalt lava winds along the base of the West Mesa, forming points, alcoves, and canyons. The flat surfaces of boulders found here are shiny and smooth, with a sheen known as "desert varnish." People figured out long ago that by pecking through this patina, they could create pictures that were, if nothing else, durable. The oldest of their squiggly lines date back to around 1000 BC.

Most works seen in Piedras Marcadas ("marked rocks") Canyon feature the elaborate designs from what was likely the largest pueblo in the Rio Grande Valley during the Pueblo IV period (AD 1300–1600). The pueblo flourished with more than 1,000 rooms before expeditionary forces under Francisco Vasquez de Coronado arrived. Though largely unexcavated

----

Directions ——————————————————➤

From I-40 West, take Exit 155 and go 5.8 miles north on Coors Boulevard. Turn left on Paseo del Norte and go west 1.2 miles. (Alternate directions: From I-25 North, take Exit 232 on Paseo del Norte and go west 5.9 miles.) Turn right on Golf Course Road and go 0.6 mile north. Turn left on Jill Patricia Street. The parking lot entrance is about 100 yards ahead on the right. The trail begins on the sidewalk on the west side at the sign for Piedras Marcadas.

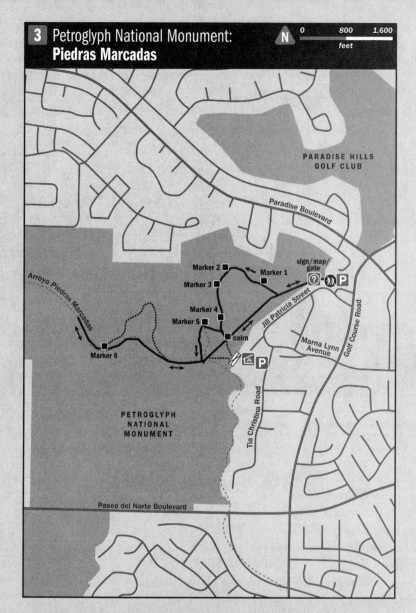

N

0   800   1,600
feet

PARADISE HILLS
GOLF CLUB

Paradise Boulevard

Marker 2

Marker 3

Marker 1

sign/map/
gate

Arroyo Piedras Marcadas

Jill Patricia Street

Marker 4

Marker 5

cairn

Golf Course Road

Marna Lynn
Avenue

Marker 6

P

Tia Christina Road

PETROGLYPH
NATIONAL
MONUMENT

Paseo del Norte Boulevard

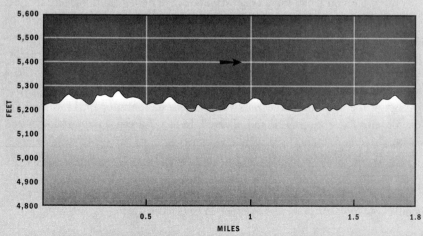

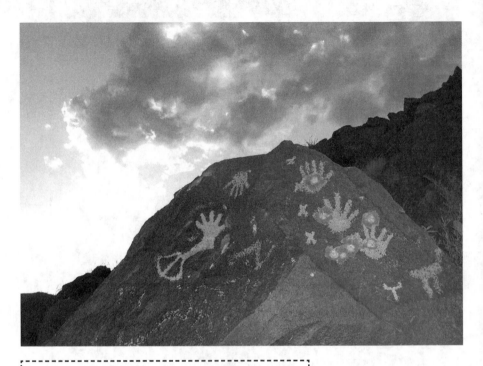

Fifteenth-century petroglyphs bear 20th-century bullet wounds.

today, the Piedras Marcadas Pueblo ruins are at the Open Space Visitor Center. (See Special Comments.)

The canyon contains about a fourth of the monument's petroglyphs, yet only 3 percent of the 124,000 annual visitors venture into this area. Suburban sprawl is the chief deterrent. Residential developments over the past decade have nearly sealed off this area of the park, which you'll no doubt notice as you begin your hike up a concrete alley between two houses wedged into a corner behind a Valvoline station.

It's not what you'd call the classic Attenborough expedition. Instead, Piedras Marcadas Canyon might be best appreciated as a study in contrasts. For better or worse, few places in America present such an immediate juxtaposition of ancient and modern worlds. And though you'll be reminded in every piece of tourist literature, it bears repeating: the land is a living shrine that continues to have a sacred role in contemporary Pueblo cultures.

A sign at the top end of the walkway shows a basic trail map. However, the canyon contains far more trails than indicated. In fact, for every mile of designated trails within the monument, local wanderers have blazed 5 miles of "social trails."

From the sign, follow the trail to your left past a barrier gate. Bypass any little shortcuts angling toward the south side of the escarpment. At the Y ahead, turn right on a wide path. **Marker 1,** a subtle gray post about knee-high, is just around the bend. Now look up at the escarpment to find faces staring back at you.

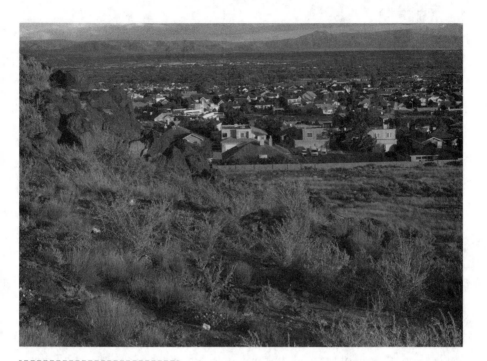

A cross-town view to the Sandias

First-time visitors share a tendency to climb up for a closer look. Park regulations aside, your time is better spent at the petroglyphs ahead, which are not only closer to the trail but also represent finer craftsmanship in terms of detail and definition. The most-revered designs include full-bodied kachina iconography and crosses and cattle brands from the Spanish colonial era.

As you follow the trail deeper into the alcove, the views and sounds of the city diminish, and it's easy to forget for a moment that just outside the walls of this basalt fortress, the suburban hordes are mustering in golf carts and SUVs. **Markers 2** and **3** are set off the main trail. Side trails allow for a closer look at nearby petroglyphs. Also keep an eye out for petroglyphs between markers. Half the fun is finding one without the assistance of trail markers.

After Marker 3, you will cross a dry wash and head downhill. The trail points directly toward a prominent cluster of buildings about 8 miles to the southeast. The tall one is the Bank of Albuquerque Tower on the downtown Civic Plaza. Also dead ahead, **Marker 4** indicates the location of five handprints, three of which are riddled with bullet holes. Kirtland Air Force Base, now largely contained within Albuquerque's southeastern quadrant, used these and other petroglyphs for target practice in the 1950s. (Others say it was the National Guard in the 1970s, but so far neither has claimed credit for the skilled marksmanship.)

Turnoffs for the trail into the second alcove, where you'll find **Marker 5,** start about 80 feet ahead on the right. Access to this smaller trail is sometimes obscured under dense vegetation. If you stumble across a large cairn, you've gone too far. Go back and follow the trail nearest the escarpment wall. The trail heading out of the alcove is easy to lose, but it runs parallel to the wash and stays close to the escarpment. Once out of the alcove, you'll find a perpendicular trail. Turn right and follow it around the basalt outcropping.

Unlike the trails in previous alcoves, this one bends in only slightly en route to the next marker on the far side. However, at least one park official has hinted that the path skirting the base of the escarpment is the best of the social trails. This detour into the canyon's deepest alcove meets up with the main trail at **Marker 6** and adds less than 0.25 mile to the overall hike.

If you continue straight ahead, the trail soon becomes more of a trench, with devil's claw growing from the edges as though reaching for a handout. Park maps show this trail ending about 200 feet past Marker 6, but there it arrives at another trail. To the right it climbs through a gap in the escarpment. From there the canyon widens, exposing developments along Paradise Boulevard to the north.

To return to the parking lot, follow the trail that crosses in front of the last alcove. Or, if you packed a lunch and the kids, visit the sheltered picnic table and playground 250 yards east of the outcropping.

Despite the commercial and residential encroachments, the canyon still echoes with the call of the wild. Just wait until sunset, when coyotes set off howling from the mesa's edge. Sure, it's a Southwestern cliché, but it still sounds wonderful, even if they are just coming to dine on house pets.

Note: The **Petroglyph National Monument Visitor Center, Las Imágenes,** is best reached en route from I-40 west. Take Exit 155 and go 1.8 miles north on Coors Boulevard. Turn left on Western Trail, and go west about 1 mile. Open all year, 8 a.m.–5 p.m.; closed Thanksgiving, Christmas, and New Year's days. Call (505) 899-0205 or visit **nps.gov/petr** for more information. The **Open Space Visitor Center** is also en route from I-40 at 6500 Coors Blvd., on the right about 2 miles north of Western Trail. Open Tuesday–Saturday, 9 a.m.–5 p.m.; call (505) 897-8831 or visit **cabq.gov/openspace/visitorcenter.html.**

ARENAL AND ATRISCO DITCH TRAILS

IN BRIEF

Walk along a centuries-old system of working irrigation ditches for a unique cultural study of one of Albuquerque's first neighborhoods and a memorable lesson in cynology.

DESCRIPTION

The mystery legend and Los Ranchos resident Tony Hillerman was known to muse at length on his serene walks along the ditches around his neighborhood, particularly in colder months, when flocks of sandhill cranes descend upon harvested fields. By no coincidence, recent years have seen a surge in the popularity of ditch-bank walks in the North Valley, with the trend spreading all the way up to the foothill arroyos. Fortunately, there's no shortage of waterways in the Rio Grande Valley.

Formed in 1925 to control flooding and reclaim farmland, the Middle Rio Grande Conservancy District now operates more than 1,200 miles of canals, laterals, and drains. The irrigation system helps sustain 30,000 acres of bosque and delivers water to 70,000 acres of cropland in a greenbelt that stretches 150 miles from Cochiti to the Bosque del Apache National Wildlife Refuge.

In 2007 the district put out an open call for recreational-trail proposals for its short-lived Ditches with Trails effort. The first studies on formal ditch-trail corridors occurred

KEY AT-A-GLANCE INFORMATION

LENGTH: 3-mile loop

DIFFICULTY: Easy

SCENERY: Irrigation canals; old-growth cottonwoods; a residential area with both urban and agrarian characteristics; and dogs—lots of dogs

EXPOSURE: Half-shaded

TRAIL TRAFFIC: Heavy

SHARED USE: Moderate (bicycles, joggers, equestrians; restricted motorized-vehicle access on ditch trails)

TRAIL SURFACE: Mostly dirt, some pavement

HIKING TIME: 1–2 hours

DRIVING DISTANCE: 4 miles

ACCESS: Not recommended after dark

LAND STATUS: Middle Rio Grande Conservancy District; City of Albuquerque

MAPS: USGS Albuquerque West

FACILITIES: None

SPECIAL COMMENTS: Goatheads (*Tribulus terrestris*), common on ditch trails, can damage bike tires and bare paws. Also beware of loose dogs. Walk softly and carry a big stick.

Directions

From I-40, take Exit 157A and go 0.7 mile south on Rio Grande Boulevard. Turn right on Central Avenue and go 1.1 mile. Turn left on Atrisco Drive (the third left after the bridge). Continue south one block on Atrisco Drive, then turn right and park at Atrisco Park.

GPS TRAILHEAD COORDINATES

Latitude   35° 04' 57"

Longitude   106° 41' 03"

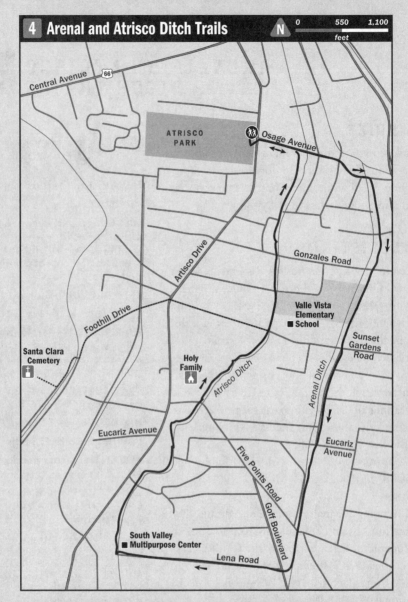

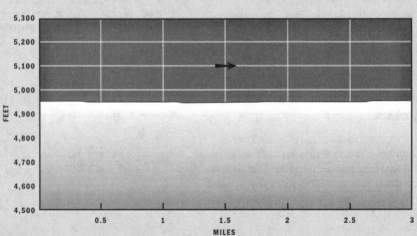

along the Arenal and Atrisco acequias in the Atrisco neighborhood of Albuquerque's South Valley.

Many of the ditches predate the Spanish settlers, who first arrived with Juan de Oñate's 1598 expedition. According to one version of local history, Nahuatl Indians later referred to the area of settlements on the west bank of the Rio Grande as *Atlixo*, meaning "across the water." The earliest known record of its name comes from a 1662 government document that describes the valley of Atrisco as "the best site in all New Mexico."

In 1692 the Spanish crown awarded the 41,000-acre Atrisco Land Grant to Fernando Durán y Chávez for his services in the reconquest of New Mexico. It would be the first of 300 such grants in the province. By 1896, heirs of the grant successfully petitioned to incorporate additional lands, expanding the Atrisco Land Grant to nearly 83,000 acres.

The South Valley maintained its agrarian character well into the 20th century. Its small farm economy boomed during World War II but began to falter in the following decades. The Atrisco neighborhood, with its proximity to Route 66 (Central Avenue), was among the first to experience the ensuing pressures for rapid development and the consequences of it. And despite efforts of many Atrisqueños to maintain tradition, development continues at pace that sometimes seems reckless.

Start the hike by exiting the parking lot the same way you drove in. Cross Atrisco Drive and proceed east on Osage Avenue. The first ditch, Atrisco Acequia, crosses under this street near the end of the first block. You'll follow it on the return segment of this loop. Note the house with the green tin roof on your right so you'll know where to turn when you get back to this point.

Stay on Osage Avenue another three short blocks. Just past Stella Drive you'll see the second ditch, Arenal Acequia. Turn right and follow it south. After a couple of cross streets, you'll see the Valle Vista Elementary schoolyard on the right.

Continue south, crossing Sunset Gardens Road and then Eucariz Avenue. Along the way, residential properties alternate with Atrisco's few remaining agricultural fields. Yard animals include sheep, goats, horses, llamas, and gamecocks. (The centuries-old tradition of cockfighting was finally outlawed in New Mexico in 2007.)

About 100 yards or so past Five Points Road, a diagonal cross street, you'll see a second diagonal street. Look to the right for the street signs marking the junction of Goff Boulevard and Lena Road.

Take Lena Road west about 0.4 mile to its end. There on the right is the South Valley Multipurpose Center. Completed in 2011, this community complex includes an audiovisual room devoted to the collection of the oral and written histories of long-term residents of this 300-year-old town.

The Atrisco Acequia runs along the west side of the complex. Turn right and follow this winding ditch north. You'll see the Holy Family Church before

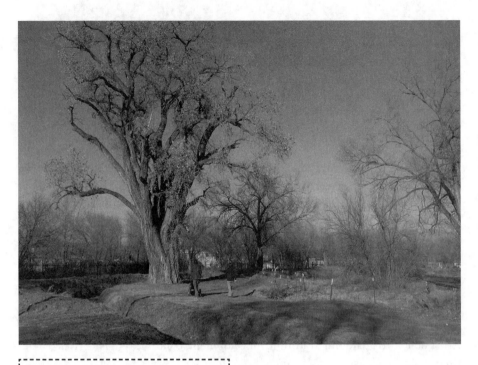

Venerable cottonwood on the Atrisco Acequia

you reach Five Points Road. Be careful at the crossing—there's a blind curve on your right.

Optional detour: The next intersection, Sunset Gardens Road, presents an opportunity for a side trip to the historic Santa Clara Cemetery. Be warned, however, that the streets are a bit narrow for a comfortable stroll. If you're up for the challenge, turn left and cross Atrisco Drive, then proceed southwest on Foothill Drive to the Arenal Main Canal, which runs along the base of the escarpment. Go south one block and look for the angelic murals on the walls and gate on the right. A small graveyard extends up the face of the escarpment. Walk up to the mesa rim to see the rest of the handcrafted markers and folk monuments in this rustic cemetery. You'll also get an excellent view over the neighborhood. Return to the Atrisco Acequia the way you came, and proceed north. This detour adds about 1.3 miles to the hike.

The path continues past the other side of the schoolyard and back up to Osage Avenue. You won't see a road sign from the ditch trail, so keep an eye out on your left for the house with the green tin roof. The road in front of it is where you turn left for Atrisco Park. If you encounter a metal guardrail across the ditch, you've gone a block too far.

There are plenty more canals and drains to explore throughout the South Valley, but moving between them isn't always as easy as a walk down Lena Road.

Rights-of-way are few, and private-property boundaries should be strictly observed. A simple guideline to remember: when in doubt, stay out.

NEARBY ACTIVITIES

Visit the art museum at the **National Hispanic Cultural Center** (NHCC), take a guided tour of its attractive campus, and enjoy lunch at La Fonda del Bosque, rated by *Hispanic Magazine* as one of the 50 best Hispanic restaurants in the country. To get there from Atrisco Park, go 1.25 miles south on Atrisco Drive. Turn left on Bridge Boulevard and go 2 miles east to cross the Barelas Bridge. The first right after the bridge leads into the NHCC parking lot. For hours, fees, and event schedules, call (505) 246-2261 or visit **nationalhispaniccenter.org**.

For a wine-country alternative to the South Valley's marginalized aesthetic, consider a ditchbank hike from **Los Ranchos de Albuquerque**. From I-40, take Exit 157A and go 4 miles north on Rio Grande Boulevard. Turn right and park at Harnett Park. Locate the irrigation ditch behind the playground and follow it south 0.5 mile to the northwest corner of Los Poblanos Fields, a 138-acre Open Space Farmland with miles of ditch trails.

5 MONTESSA PARK

KEY AT-A-GLANCE INFORMATION

LENGTH: 4.4-mile loop

DIFFICULTY: Easy

SCENERY: Desert wildlife, abandoned railroad tracks, aircraft, postmodern landscaping

EXPOSURE: Minimal shade

TRAIL TRAFFIC: Low

SHARED USE: Moderate (Frisbee golfers, motorized vehicles)

TRAIL SURFACE: Gravel, sand

HIKING TIME: 2–3 hours

DRIVING DISTANCE: 11 miles

ACCESS: Daylight hours

LAND STATUS: Albuquerque Open Space

MAPS: USGS Albuquerque East and Albuquerque West

FACILITIES: Off-leash dog park, disc-golf course

SPECIAL COMMENTS: Heed military boundary notices; trespassing convictions carry a potential 6-month jail term and a $5,000 fine.

GPS TRAILHEAD COORDINATES

Latitude   35° 01' 05"

Longitude   106° 35' 57"

IN BRIEF

For those who enjoy hiking unusual environments, this route uses an abandoned railroad spur and a major arroyo for a mostly flat hike through roller-coaster terrain. Despite its reputation for high-flying motorbikes and low-flying aircraft, this semiurban area along the lower Tijeras Arroyo is often quieter than most city parks.

DESCRIPTION

The Tijeras ("scissors") Arroyo, Bernalillo County's largest, is a conduit for runoff from the mountains to the east, draining into the Rio Grande to the west. To the south is Mesa del Sol, site of imminent residential developments. And to the immediate north are the runways of Kirtland Air Force Base and the Albuquerque International Sunport, the state's primary airport. The arroyo floodplain spans more than 1,000 feet, with embankments on either side rising up to 300 feet.

Erosion of the embankments has created steep, hilly terrain well suited for the antics of vehicular daredevils. Accordingly, the 577-acre Montessa Park, along the lower arroyo, is currently the only area in the Open Space system available for off-road driving. Dirt bikes, quads, and other all-terrain vehicles have ripped a hundred trails in and around the park. It's

-----

Directions _____

From I-25 South, take Exit 220 and go 0.4 mile west on Rio Bravo Boulevard. Turn left onto Broadway Boulevard and go 1.8 miles south. Turn left on Bobby Foster Road and cross over I-25. Turn left on Los Picaros Road and follow it 3 miles. Park near the green gate on the left side of the road.

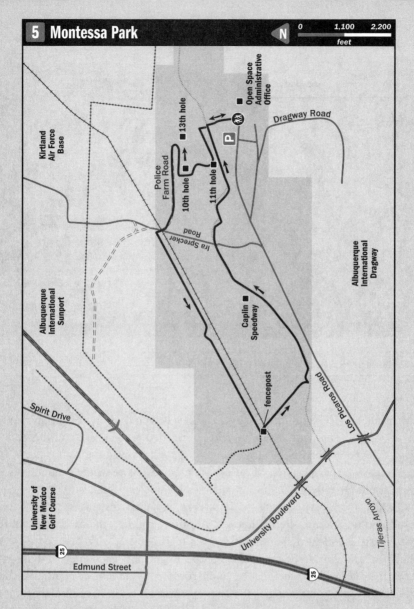

N

0   1,100   2,200
feet

Open Space
Administrative
Office

Dragway Road

13th hole

P

Police
Farm Road

10th hole

11th hole

Kirtland
Air Force
Base

Ira Sprecker
Road

Albuquerque
International
Sunport

Caplin
Speedway

Albuquerque
International
Dragway

Los Picaros Road

fencepost

Spirit Drive

University of
New Mexico
Golf Course

25

University Boulevard

Tijeras Arroyo

25

Edmund Street

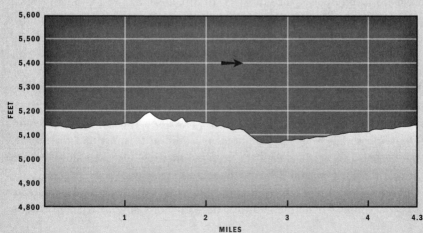

5,600

5,500

5,400

5,300

5,200

5,100

5,000

4,900

4,800

FEET

1   2   3   4   4.3

MILES

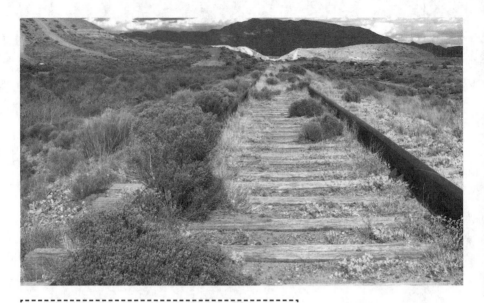

Abandoned tracks seem to aim straight for South Sandia Peak.

a sacrificial land; without it, these ersatz Knievels would surely tear up more property elsewhere. The park also long held a tarnished reputation as an illegal dump site, but cleanup efforts in 2011 have significantly improved the landscape.

From some perspectives, Montessa Park seems a place where communion with nature could get ugly. Neighboring facilities include the Bio-Disease Management Unit, which monitors the state for outbreaks of hantavirus, rabbit fever, bubonic plague, and other critter-borne illnesses. Another neighbor, the Zia Pistol and Rifle Club, boasts a 600-yard shooting range for high-powered rifle competitions. You might hear the crackle of their M-16s. You might also encounter "T-hunters"—they're the ones with devices that resemble rooftop TV antennae. Transmitter hunting, or radio direction finding, is the ham operator's version of geocaching, and this area seems to be a popular place for it. And, of course, there's the occasional Air Force jet screaming overhead. Time this hike with reveille or retreat and you might hear a chorus of coyotes responding to a bugle call.

From other perspectives, Montessa Park is a fascinating study on the urban–wildlife interface at the southern fringe of the state's biggest city.

Begin the hike by exploring the grounds of the Brent Baca Memorial Disc Golf Course, accessed by slipping through the pedestrian gateway to the right of the green gate. If you have time and a Frisbee, toss a few rounds. This challenging 7,805-foot course has four par-four holes in addition to short tees for novices. Maps and scorecards are in a mailbox near the first tee. Or just follow the path straight past the 15th tee and down to a concrete spillway.

The return leg of this hike runs about 1.5 miles up the arroyo streambed to return to this point, so note conditions beneath the spillway. If there's water, you'll need to consider alternate return routes. Also note the depth of the channel: 15–20 feet in places. Debris wrapped around tree trunks growing above the rim should give you a good idea of what to expect in the event of a flash flood.

After crossing the spillway, make your way to the 10th hole in the northwestern corner of the course. The easiest route involves turning right by the stacks of metal frames that compose the hazard on the 11th hole.

Behind a solitary tree on the 10th hole, a doubletrack runs north. Follow it to its end, then turn right at the fence ahead. The road widens into a dry wash. Once you reach the end of the fence on your left, you're in undesignated motocross country. Stay alert. Airborne bikes don't brake for anything.

The railroad tracks lie to the north on the far side of the nearest hill. The easiest way to reach them is by taking the dirt road northwest (it shows up on some maps as Police Farm Road, named for the City Police Prison and Farm that was located here in the 1950s). The road crosses the tracks just before reaching Ira Sprecker Road. For a slightly more challenging approach to the railroad tracks, follow a motocross trail straight up the hill, and then scramble down into the cut on the other side.

Cross Ira Sprecker Road and follow the railroad tracks southwest. You'll pass north of the Harvey Caplin Memorial Speedway, a 0.2-mile dirt oval track used primarily for kart racing.

A gap in the tracks ahead indicates where flash flooding washed out a trestle. Pick up the tracks on the other side of the wash. About 0.5 mile farther is a lone fencepost wrapped in barbed wire.

Optional detour: From the fencepost, a sandy track climbs 0.4 mile northwest, gaining 150 feet, to a bumpy doubletrack that follows the airport perimeter fence. A nearby hilltop is a good spot to watch inbound aircraft and get a view of the arroyo basin. (*Note:* If the streambed seemed muddy earlier, now is the time to scout out alternate routes. A few options should come into plain view, keeping in mind that the easiest points to cross the arroyo are at Ira Sprecker Road and the spillway at the 15th tee.)

Continuing the loop from the fencepost, head southeast on a prominent trail straight down to the arroyo. You'll cross under two sets of power lines. Hawks and falcons often perch on the utility poles.

The descent from the road to the streambed is easy, but as you walk upstream, the walls are higher, and you'll soon notice limited opportunities to exit. River rock adds color, with greenstone, red jasper, and glassy chunks of obsidian. Fossils found in Tijeras Arroyo include ancient species of land tortoise, camel, llama, and mammoth.

Follow this winding corridor 1.4 miles to Ira Sprecker Road. Cross the road, and continue upstream. When you reach the spillway, climb up, and turn right. Follow the path back to the parking area at the green gate.

If returning at dusk, watch for great horned owls; you may find one perched above the tire swing in the old cottonwood by the gate.

6 ELENA GALLEGOS PICNIC AREA

KEY AT-A-GLANCE INFORMATION

LENGTH: 1.4-mile balloon, with longer options

DIFFICULTY: Easy

SCENERY: Open foothills, continuous mountain views

EXPOSURE: Minimal shade

TRAIL TRAFFIC: Popular

SHARED USE: Moderate (mountain bikers and equestrians permitted on one short trail segment; dogs must be leashed)

TRAIL SURFACE: Pavement, fine gravel

HIKING TIME: 1 hour

DRIVING DISTANCE: 17 miles

ACCESS: April–October, 7 a.m.–9 p.m., and November–March, 7 a.m.–7 p.m.; $1 per car weekdays, $2 weekends; free with Open Space annual pass

LAND STATUS: Albuquerque Open Space

MAPS: cabq.gov/openspace/pdf/elena.pdf; Sandia Ranger District; USGS Sandia Crest

FACILITIES: Interpretive trail, picnic areas, group reservation areas with barbecue grills, restrooms. Drinking water near parking areas is shut off in winter months but available at information center year-round.

GPS TRAILHEAD COORDINATES

Latitude   35° 9' 57"

Longitude   106° 28' 22"

IN BRIEF

Artistic enhancements along an all-access interpretive trail and the old nature loop provide a stylish introduction to the cultural history and abundant wildlife in the Sandia Mountain foothills.

DESCRIPTION

What is the Elena Gallegos? The short answer defines it as a 1694 Spanish land grant that stretched from the Sandia Mountains to the Rio Grande. However, interpretations of its original boundaries have entered disputes in matters ranging from President Lincoln's 1864 land patent to the T'uf Shur Bien Preservation Trust Area Act of 2003.

Although New Mexico governance passed from Spain to Mexico (1821) to the United States (1848) to the Confederacy (1862, albeit briefly) before New Mexico achieved statehood (1912), the Elena Gallegos Land Grant remained in the possession of one family. State claims and realty demands have since carved up the estate beyond recognition. From this vast parcel, once estimated at 35,084 acres, all that officially bears the name of Elena Gallegos today is an 11-acre picnic area in Albert

----

Directions

From I-40, take Exit 167 and go 6 miles north on Tramway Boulevard. (Or from I-25, take Exit 234 and go 7.5 miles east and then south on Tramway Boulevard.) Turn east on Simms Park Road and go 1.5 miles to the fee station at Elena Gallegos Picnic Area/Albert G. Simms Park. Take a hard left around the station, toward the Kiwanis Reservation Area. At the end of this 0.3-mile drive, just past the reservation area, is the Cottonwood Springs Trail parking area.

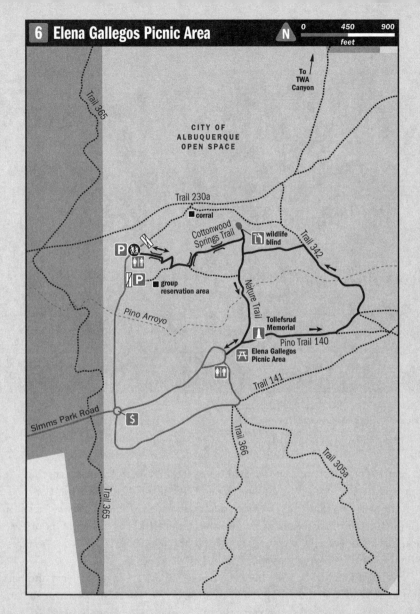

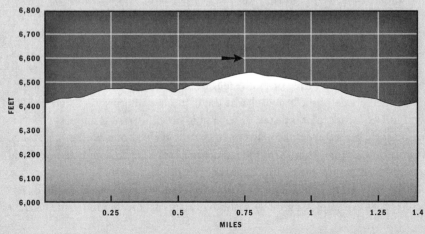

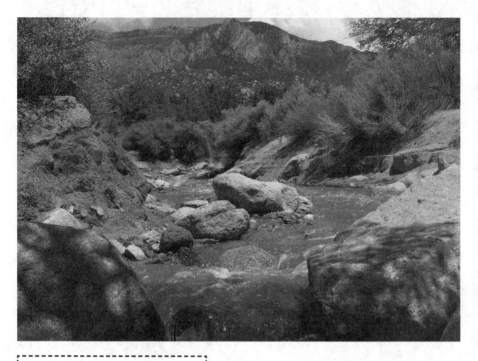

Pino Arroyo in a good monsoon season

G. Simms Park. But most people who are familiar with this 640-acre city park refer to it by the more lyrical name, Elena Gallegos. (The park's information center is tiny but worth a stop for more details about the Elena Gallegos Picnic Area and the extraordinary woman behind the name. It keeps the same hours as the park, but it's open only when a park official happens to be there. Your best chance at finding one present is between 9 a.m. and 4:30 p.m.)

Situated in a buffer zone between pricey suburban developments and Sandia Mountain Wilderness, the popular recreation area often rumbles with equestrians and mountain bikes. By contrast, the 0.25-mile **Cottonwood Springs Trail** leads through a relatively quiet corner of the park. Created in response to the Americans with Disabilities Act and dedicated in April 2000, the trail has since been nurtured into a secret garden of sorts.

A broad cement walkway leads to a wooden bridge over a (usually) dry wash. Thick stands of juniper thrive on both sides despite the scarcity of water. A latilla shelter on the far side of the bridge shades the first of six interpretive stations. Each is a work of art, with sculptural steel and ceramic tiles illustrating snippets of information on local geology, cultural history, and ecology. The one on the first bridge highlights a few animals that share the Sandia habitat. A more complete list would include 200 bird, 34 mammal, and 23 snake and lizard species.

At the intersection ahead, a right turn would take you to the Kiwanis Reservation Area, worth exploring later. For now, turn left and continue to the next

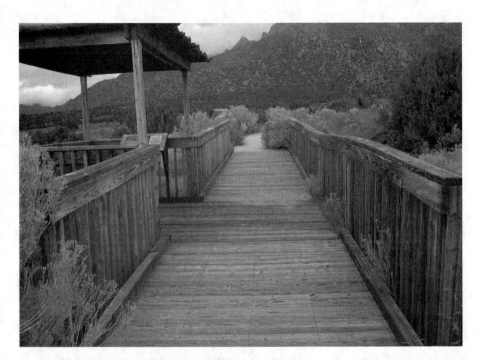

A bridge and shelter on Cottonwood Springs Trail

bridge. Halfway across, another interpretive station sums up 12,000 years of local human habitation in 66 words. As you cross the bridge, a corral comes into better view, a remnant of the last days of ranching in the Sandia foothills. Directly behind it, the mountains gain 4,000 feet in less than 3 miles.

The paved walkway ends at a wire fence surrounding a protected wildlife area. To the left, a bridge extends to a shaded wildlife blind overlooking a cattail pond. The Kiwanis Club of Albuquerque installed a plastic lining in 1992 to extend the seasonal life of a spring-fed watering hole for deer, mountain lions, and other creatures you probably won't see here. Note, however, that frogs seem to emerge from the signage. These and other relief designs in the tiles are textural enhancements for visitors with visual limitations.

Cottonwood Spring Trail ends here, but the hike continues. Cross back over the bridge and go straight up the **Nature Trail,** a 0.8-mile loop that begins as a gravel path along the fence. At the top of the hill, a post points the way to Domingo Baca Canyon. That path is part of your return route, so continue straight past it. A slight descent ahead takes you down into the Pino Arroyo. In the monsoon season, you may need to detour upstream for an easier crossing point.

The grounds on the south side of the arroyo are by far the most popular, as evidenced by the increasing number of worn footpaths. You may find yourself at a loss when you reach the point where the trail splits in seven or eight directions.

At least three lead to the main parking lot, about 40 yards to your right. It's worth the short detour for commanding views of the city.

The Nature Trail turns east, overlapping **Pino Trail (140)**. This segment begins as pebbled asphalt aggregate but soon gives way to crusher fines as it approaches the Philip B. Tollefsrud Memorial, which is often misidentified as the Five Stones of Elena Gallegos. The first of these prominent boulders is inlaid with 38 copper rods, one for each year in the short life of the conservationist Phil Tollefsrud. The remaining four bear symbols to represent the aspects of nature he treasured.

Pino Trail continues through the memorial and gains nearly 2,800 feet in elevation in 4.7 miles before ending at the Crest Trail (130). For this hike, however, it's only another 200 yards or so before you switch to **Trail 342**. You'll find it at the fence posts ahead. Turn left, following a sign indicating the direction of the Nature Trail. This is the only segment of the Nature Trail that permits bicycles and horses, so keep your head up for high-speed riders. Smaller paths appear on either side, but stay on this broad trail as it curves back around to the Pino Arroyo.

Trail 342 connects Pino Trail to the Domingo Baca Route (230). The latter leads into the aforementioned canyon, now better known as TWA Canyon for the airliner that crashed there in 1955. The 7-mile round-trip hike to the crash site is one of the most arduous in the Sandias, and yet visitors enticed by the spectacle of plane wreckage have made it among the most popular.

The trail soon crests at a hilltop, providing one of the most expansive views in the park. Aging signage and more fence posts on the left indicate your next turn. Follow the Nature Trail alongside the protected wildlife area. On hot days, a stand of mature cottonwoods seems to beckon from beyond the fence. Fortunately, the next shade shelter is just around the corner; a right turn at the end of this brief segment leads you back to the wildlife blind.

Follow the paved trail back to your car by taking the right fork ahead—or detour straight into the Kiwanis Reservation Area for a quick inspection of its handsome facilities. Exit through the parking lot and turn right on the road. Cottonwood Springs Trail parking area is right around the corner. Approach quietly and you may likely spot more wildlife here than anywhere on the trail.

Note: A trail map can be acquired from the fee station, or you can download it online. For information on guided hikes, educational programs, and volunteer opportunities offered throughout the year, call Albuquerque's Open Space Division at (505) 452-5210 or visit **cabq.gov/openspace/elenagallegos.html**.

NEARBY ACTIVITIES

Route 66 Open Space is a 60-acre site in Tijeras Canyon that connects to the Four Hills/Manzano Open Space. Mature cottonwoods shade a perennial stream locally known as Beaver Creek, and scenic outcroppings dominate the arid uplands. Parking and access are on the south side of historic Route 66 (NM 333), about 1 mile east of Tramway Boulevard. For more information, call Albuquerque Open Space at (505) 452-5200 or visit **cabq.gov/openspace**.

WATERFALL CANYON 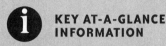 7

IN BRIEF

It begins on one of the most popular trails in the Sandias and ends in a relatively unknown niche of paradise. The connecting segment is occasionally unforgiving, but almost always worth the effort.

DESCRIPTION

How many waterfalls can you find in Waterfall Canyon? A visitor from the Pacific Northwest might see one, whereas a native New Mexican could find seven or more. Water covers a scant 0.2 percent of our state, making it the driest in the nation. That's why in New Mexico, trickles can be rivers, ponds count as lakes, and the glass is always half-full. It's just a matter of perception.

The hike to what we call "waterfalls" begins at the Piedra Lisa parking area. Walk about 0.4 mile north on FR 333D. A prominent wooden post there on the right marks the Piedra Lisa trailhead. Continue another 0.3 mile north-northeast on this broad trail, following it over a low ridge and down to the floor of a shaded canyon. There you'll arrive at another post marking Piedra Lisa Trail. Just beyond it is the first of two arroyos flowing from Juan Tabo Canyon, which is perhaps better described as two separate canyons. The south branch of Juan Tabo Canyon is also known as Waterfall Canyon. The destination of this hike is a mere

KEY AT-A-GLANCE INFORMATION

LENGTH: 2.8-mile out-and-back; longer options

DIFFICULTY: Moderate, seasonally difficult

SCENERY: Wooded canyons, granite formations, waterfalls

EXPOSURE: Mostly shaded

TRAIL TRAFFIC: Moderate

SHARED USE: Low (closed to all vehicles)

TRAIL SURFACE: Dirt, rock

HIKING TIME: 2–4 hours

DRIVING DISTANCE: 15 miles

ACCESS: Year-round; $3 parking fee

LAND STATUS: Cibola National Forest–Sandia Mountain Wilderness

MAPS: Sandia Ranger District; USGS Sandia Crest

FACILITIES: None (restrooms at nearby Juan Tabo Picnic Area)

SPECIAL COMMENTS: Mountain lion tracks are common in Waterfall Canyon. Keep little hikers close at hand.

Directions ⟶

From I-25 North, take Exit 234 and turn right on Tramway Boulevard. Go 4 miles east to FR 333. Turn left and go 2.2 miles northwest to the Piedra Lisa parking area. Note the last 0.4 mile (FR 333D) is not paved and can be icy in winter.

GPS TRAILHEAD COORDINATES

Latitude   35° 13' 23"

Longitude   106° 29' 00"

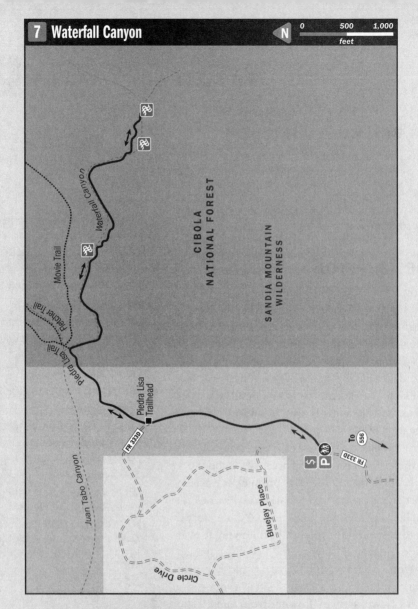

N

0   500   1,000
feet

CIBOLA
NATIONAL FOREST

SANDIA MOUNTAIN
WILDERNESS

Waterfall Canyon

Movie Trail

Fletcher Trail

Piedra Lisa Trail

Juan Tabo Canyon

Piedra Lisa
Trailhead

FR 333D

Circle Drive

Bluejay Place

FR 333D

To 556

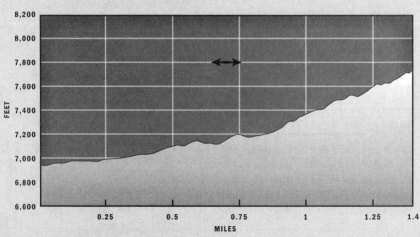

8,200

8,000

7,800

7,600

7,400

FEET

7,200

7,000

6,800

6,600

0.25   0.5   0.75   1   1.25   1.4

MILES

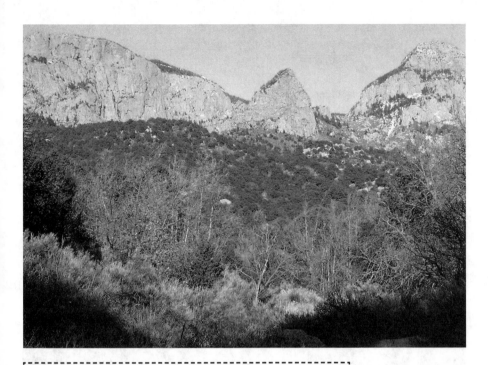

Legends of the Sandias (left to right): the Shield, the Prow, and the Needle

0.7 mile upstream, but there are a few things you should know before embarking on that leg of the journey.

Waterfall Canyon is notorious for scrub—the tangled, thorny, and sometimes ornery kind. Wear long sleeves and pants, or you'll end up looking like the victim of vicious kitten attacks. Your best strategy for finding a way through it is to watch for cut branches. Occasionally an anonymous saint hacks out a route (and does an admirable job), but it is not officially maintained, and brush grows back quickly. You may find a clear path all the way through, or you may find yourself bushwhacking through willow and wild rose for the next 3 hours. In a wet summer, the upper falls might be unreachable. You could wait till winter, of course, but then be prepared for snow and ice.

Few parts along this route involve scrambling; none presents any serious hazard. If you find yourself facing dangerous exposure, go back and find another way. Some paths climb the canyon walls to avoid thicker vegetation below. Problem is, they often end high on a ledge. Generally it's easier to stick to paths running closest to the stream, if not the streambed itself.

With all that in mind, turn right at the post and head upstream about a quarter-mile. This short segment is usually clear, since it's a fairly popular side trip for Piedra Lisa pedestrians. The 15-foot cascade often resembles a rooster tail as it splashes down through the rocks. The surrounding shady nook makes a fine destination for casual strollers.

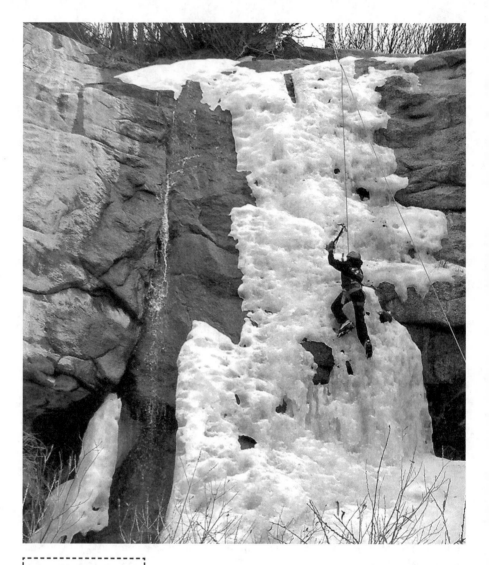

The upper falls, thawing

To find bigger falls, pick a nearby route up the south side of the canyon. Several options should be obvious. Whichever way you choose, pay careful attention to details because it'll be more difficult to spot on the way back. This part is the most challenging climb in the hike, but again, there's no reason to engage significant exposure. (Then again, if you're looking for that kind of excitement, you'll find sufficiently dangerous climbing routes closer to the falls.) Just keep in mind that smooth Sandia granite is surprisingly slippery when wet. Consider "Piedra Lisa" a warning sign: it means "smooth rock."

About 0.2 mile past the first waterfall, the canyon takes a sharp turn south. You may find it easier to stay close to the wall on the right side of the stream,

stairstepping up to a flattop outcrop. Another 100 yards or so ahead, start looking for a path climbing from the left side of modest waterfall. It's a relatively easy
way around the 25-foot falls located around the next bend, and it'll lead you to
the base of 70-foot falls in a majestic amphitheater. (In dry seasons, the detour
around the 25-foot falls isn't necessary—you can just follow the streambed to the
upper falls.) Northern exposure keeps these falls frozen through most of winter,
making it a popular spot for ice climbers. In summer, it can slow to a trickle, but
the scenery is still usually worth the effort it takes to get there.

NEARBY ACTIVITIES

If you get only as far as the first waterfall, you still have plenty of other options
to make the most out of your time here.

Piedra Lisa Trail, one of the most popular on this side of the Sandias, continues north, rising 1,200 feet in 1.4 miles to peak on Rincon Ridge. A signpost
there marks the intersection with the Rincon spur.

The area north of Waterfall Canyon and east of Piedra Lisa Trail is closed
annually to protect certain rare species of birds. Notices are posted accordingly. The
closure is in effect from March 1 to August 15 and affects the following trails:

Fletcher Trail begins in the second dip on Piedra Lisa Trail. Turn right in the
northern arroyo for a 2-mile trek up "Upper" Juan Tabo Canyon. Though unmain-
tained, Fletcher Trail gets enough traffic to keep its definition all the way to the
base of UNM Spire.

Movie Trail climbs the ridge between Upper Juan Tabo Canyon and Waterfall
Canyon. It starts on the left side of the latter, about 20 yards east of Piedra Lisa
Trail, and climbs 1,400 feet in 1.7 miles to the base of the Prow. Unlike Fletcher
and Piedra Lisa, this trail tends to get murky in spots. Some trivia to consider dur-
ing a hike here: Movie Trail was created for the filming of *Lonely Are the Brave*,
which was based on *The Brave Cowboy,* the second novel by Edward Abbey, a
University of New Mexico graduate. Abbey's best-known efforts include the novel
The Monkey Wrench Gang and the nonfiction work *Desert Solitaire.*

8   CORRALES ACEQUIAS AND BOSQUE PRESERVE

KEY AT-A-GLANCE INFORMATION

LENGTH: 7.4-mile loop

DIFFICULTY: Easy

SCENERY: Vineyards, historic buildings, deciduous forest, mountain views

EXPOSURE: Half-shaded

TRAIL TRAFFIC: Popular

SHARED USE: Moderate (mountain bikers, equestrians; popular with dog owners; restricted motorized-vehicle access)

TRAIL SURFACE: Dirt, some asphalt

HIKING TIME: 4 hours, longer with optional detours

DRIVING DISTANCE: 13 miles

ACCESS: Daily, 5 a.m.–10 p.m.

LAND STATUS: Village of Corrales; Middle Rio Grande Conservancy District

MAPS: USGS Alameda and Bernalillo

FACILITIES: Restrooms inside and soft-drink vending machines outside the rec center

SPECIAL COMMENTS: Village Hall at 4324 Corrales Road (0.3 mile past Jones Road) has brochures for touring Corrales. Interpretive information is also posted on their outdoor display boards. For more information, visit the Village of Corrales website, corrales-nm.org, and the Corrales Historical Society website, corraleshistory.org.

GPS TRAILHEAD COORDINATES

Latitude   35° 13' 18"

Longitude   106° 37' 23"

IN BRIEF

Follow the waterways around the village of Corrales for a display of eclectic architecture from the past and present. Groves of cottonwood and Siberian elm and plentiful waterfowl also highlight the route. You may also spot riparian creatures such as beavers, muskrats, and pocket gophers.

DESCRIPTION

Each spring the villagers of Corrales come together to apply adobe mud to the walls of the Old Church and attend to other restoration chores in an event celebrated as "Mud Day." Yet personal experience tells me every day is Mud Day in this charming village. For some reason, I can never seem to escape without mud caked on my boots, bike, and truck. And this isn't just any kind of mud—it dries into some kind of titanium-grade adobe. I snapped the tip off a tire iron trying to pry it off my mountain bike.

Perhaps in a similar manner, the settlers of Corrales discovered how such mud might enhance the durability of their buildings. Some of these structures, most notably the Old San Ysidro Church, highlight the first half of this route.

Acequias (3.3 miles): Begin by crossing the soccer field behind the rec center. The line of

Directions

From I-25 North, take Exit 233 at Alameda Boulevard (NM 528). Turn left (west) on Alameda Boulevard, and go 4.2 miles. Turn right (north) on Corrales Road (NM 448—notorious for speed traps), and drive 2 miles. Turn left on Jones Road (immediately after Territorial Plaza). Go 0.2 mile and park near the Corrales Recreation Center.

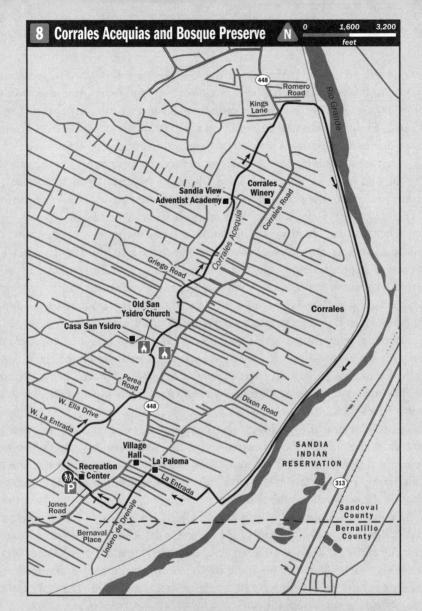

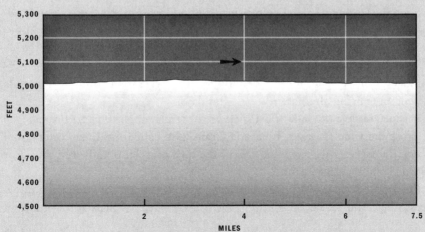

trees on the far side indicates where the Corrales Lateral flows. This prominent acequia, or irrigation ditch, has been channeling water to local farm fields since the early 18th century. The system has since been enhanced. Currently about 17 miles of canals and ditches course through Corrales. The ditch rider, or system administrator, maintains the flow of water from early May through early November.

Service roads run along both sides of the acequia. Turn right after the gate and take the one with the least mud. Dams allow for frequent crossings in case you change your mind. You can simply follow the ditch for the first 3 miles of the loop or take a few detours for a closer look at nearby historic buildings.

Often you can identify an architectural style by the roof alone. Red tiles suggest Spanish Revival. Rounded corners are indicative of the Pueblo style. Flat roofs with stepped parapets and exposed vigas (ceiling beams) indicate Spanish-Pueblo Revival, more popularly known as Santa Fe style, which in turn developed into a craze for incorporating multiple styles into a single structure for no apparent reason. You'll find numerous examples of that in Corrales.

About a mile into the hike, when you reach the end of a long coyote fence, you'll see the new San Ysidro Church over on Corrales Road on the right. Ahead on the left are the pitched tin roofs of the Old San Ysidro Church's twin bell towers. The towers function as buttresses to support the old adobe walls, which are nearly 3 feet thick.

The Gutiérrez-Minge House, also known as Casa San Ysidro, is across the street from the old church. This extension of the Albuquerque Museum features a replica of a 19th-century rancho and offers tours for a small fee. To visit the San Ysidro complex, turn left at the next crossroad, Old Church Road. This detour adds less than 0.4 mile to the hike.

To keep track of your pace, note that Old Church Road is 1.2 miles into the hike. Stella Lane marks the end of the second mile. Ahead you'll pass by Sandia View Adventist Academy on the left and, soon after, the Corrales Winery on the right (see Nearby Activities for more information). At the end of the third mile, you arrive at the intersection of Kings Lane and Corrales Road. The latter is often busy, so use care in crossing it.

Soon the Corrales Lateral merges into the Sandoval Lateral. Turn right, heading toward the mountains. The mature Rio Grande Valley cottonwoods closer ahead mark the western edge of the Corrales Bosque Preserve.

There is a small parking area on the near side of a green pipe gate. The Sandoval Lateral turns right and flows south. Shady service roads running alongside it present an enticing alternate route on hot days.

Bosque Preserve (3.1 miles): To stick with the planned route, go through the gate, cross the wide Corrales Riverside Drain (also called the Clear Ditch), and climb up the levee. Turn right and follow the high road (also known as the Clear Ditch road and the dike road).

But before setting off in that direction, note two footpaths continuing down the east side of the levee. Both lead to the Rio Grande, less than 500 feet ahead.

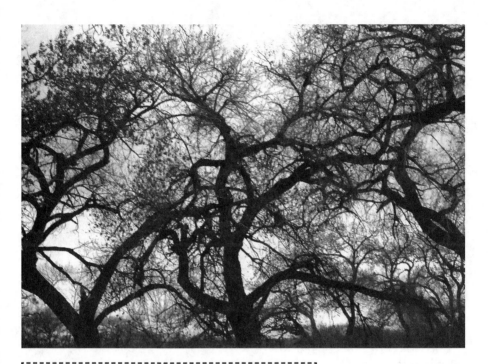

A wintry silhouette of cottonwood in the Corrales Bosque Preserve

These, too, are shaded alternatives to the planned route and are part of an informal path system that spiderwebs between the road and the river throughout the cool deciduous woods.

The paths often break up or disappear under weeds and fallen trees, but this dense floodplain habitat makes for a more interesting hike than does the linear dike road. Though rare, black bears occasionally raid nearby apple orchards and leave evidence along these trails. Getting lost may look effortless in places; just remember to keep the river on your left and the levee on your right. Detours along these trails can add a few hundred feet or a couple of miles to the hike, depending on how much you want to explore the bosque.

Of course, the dike road has the advantage of being remarkably easy to follow, and its elevation affords more expansive views. Overlooking the bosque, the drain, and nearby farm fields, you're more likely to spot wildlife, such as cottontails, porcupines, and any one of approximately 180 bird species—from ruby-crowned kinglets to yellow-rumped warblers. Hawks, owls, herons, and woodpeckers are also common in the area.

Opportunities to cross back over the riverside drain are few. About 1.5 miles downstream from your first crossing, the river and the road bend westward. Another mile past the bend, you'll see a single-lane bridge that leads to Dixon Road. Continue on the dike road another 0.6 mile, rounding a slight bend, to a wooden bridge. Cross that one and turn right on the lower embankment. You'll

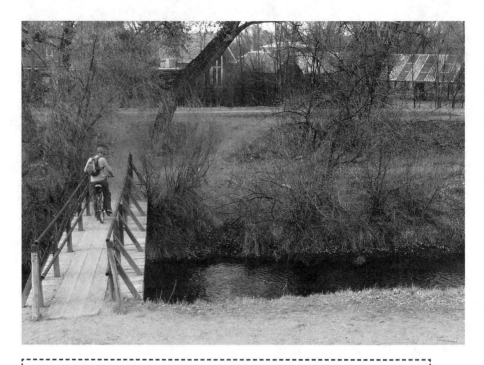

Cross the wooden bridge over the Riverside Drain to reach the access gate on East La Entrada.

see a board over the ditch. Cross it and turn left. About 200 yards ahead, turn right and exit through the green gate.

Bosque access gate to Rec Center (1 mile): You're now on East La Entrada Road. It goes straight to Corrales Road, which is not what you'd call pedestrian-friendly. So instead, go one block west, just past La Paloma Greenhouse, and turn left on a ditchbank road marked LINDERO DEL DRENAJE. Follow it south about 0.25 mile, then turn right at the fourth crossroad, Bernaval Place (paved, but missing signage). About 200 feet ahead it ends at a T-junction with Priestly Place. Turn left and follow it around to the right, where it becomes Coroval Road. Follow that to its end at Corrales Road; Territorial Plaza is across the street. To the immediate right is Jones Road. Follow it back to the rec center.

NEARBY ACTIVITIES

Corrales Winery is open for free tours and wine tastings Wednesday–Saturday, noon–5 p.m. Its entrance is on Corrales Road, 2.2 miles north of Jones Road. Call (505) 898-5165 or visit **corraleswinery.com** for more information.

LA CEJA DE RIO RANCHO 9

IN BRIEF

From the far corner of the West Mesa, the view plunges to a sculpted landscape below. Admire it from above with a hike along the rim, or descend into the labyrinth of ridges and ravines to explore it up close.

DESCRIPTION

The Albuquerque Basin spans west to the Rio Puerco and east to the Sandia foothills, a distance of 20–30 miles. It's one of the largest and deepest basins of that fracture in the Earth's crust known as the Rio Grande Rift. The original basin is more than 5 miles deep but has since filled in with sediments eroding from the surrounding mountains.

The Llano de Albuquerque, better known as the West Mesa and less well known as Ceja Mesa, is a remnant of the broad floor of the western basin between the Rio Grande and the Rio Puerco. It now stands more than 400 feet above the present floodplain of the Rio Grande and more than 500 feet above the Rio Puerco Valley. How it achieved this impressive stature is not entirely clear. Whether the

Key At-A-Glance Information

i KEY AT-A-GLANCE INFORMATION

LENGTH: 1.1-mile balloon, longer out-and-back options

DIFFICULTY: Easy

SCENERY: Barrancas (eroded cliffs), diverse wildflowers and cacti

EXPOSURE: Shade along the streambeds

TRAIL TRAFFIC: Low

SHARED USE: Moderate (target shooting and motor vehicles on the rim; mountain biking)

TRAIL SURFACE: Dirt road, sandy ridges and draws

HIKING TIME: 1 hour (or more)

DRIVING DISTANCE: 30 miles

ACCESS: Daylight hours; State Trust Land Recreational Permit required

LAND STATUS: State trust land

MAPS: USGS Sky Village NE (Cerro Conejo)

FACILITIES: None

Directions

From I-25 North, take Exit 232 at Paseo del Norte. Go 5.2 miles west. Turn right onto Eagle Ranch road and go 0.2 mile north. Turn left onto Paradise Boulevard and go 2 northwest to Lyon Boulevard. Turn right and go 2 miles north to Unser Boulevard. Continue straight another 7.8 miles north to King Boulevard. Turn left and go 2.3 miles west to Rainbow Boulevard, a dirt road just past the cattle guard. Turn right and follow Rainbow Boulevard 6.5 miles northwest to its end. The last 0.4 mile gets a little rough, but most cars should be OK in dry conditions.

GPS TRAILHEAD COORDINATES

Latitude   35° 24' 00"
Longitude   106° 47' 00"

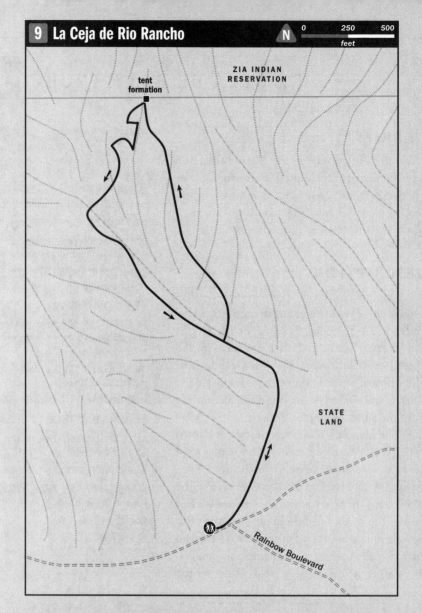

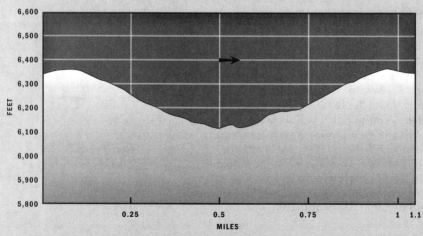

llano (YAH-no, and meaning "plain") uplifted or the surrounding valley sank, it happened in a geologic rush about 600,000 years ago, long before the Albuquerque Volcanoes first pimpled its eastern edge.

The llano rises gently from the east but comes to an abrupt end at the northern and western rim. Here's where you'll find the barrancas—the cliffs and steep slopes below that are cut into an endless labyrinth of ridges and drains. On the northern rim, the scarp arches up to a precipice known as La Ceja (SAY-ha, and meaning "eyebrow"). Similarly, the 70-mile-long west-facing escarpment of Ceja Mesa is sometimes referred to as Ceja del Rio Puerco. (In common local usage, I've never heard anyone outside my circle of map-freak associates use the word *ceja* to refer to anything but eyebrows. Hence, if you stop to ask for directions to La Ceja, you'll likely get an arched eyebrow in reply.)

Rio Rancho occupies the northern part of the Llano de Albuquerque, with the bulk of development concentrated well to the southeast of La Ceja. For now, the western half is relatively empty. Various local peoples have long used this outland to conduct elaborate funeral rites for their elderly possessions. Old cars, sofas, and major household appliances are sacrificially burned and/or tossed from cliffs, then ceremoniously adorned with bullet holes. The decades-old rituals continue even as the modern developments of Rio Rancho creep ever closer to the outer fringes of the mesa.

To the north of western Rio Rancho lies the Zia Reservation. Sandwiched between the impending crunch of residential developments and the vast pueblo land are seven contiguous sections of state land. Sections are generally designated as 1-square-mile parcels. At La Ceja, however, the rim of the llano defines the southern Zia boundary, effectively shaping six of the state-land sections into a row of broken teeth.

The hike at La Ceja isn't so much about following a certain route but rather knowing where you should and should not go. Problem is, if boundary notices ever *were* posted, they're gone now. To stay in fair play, you need to be aware of a few landmarks.

For the most part, the barrancas are on Zia land, meaning that hikers keen on thoroughly exploring them first need to obtain permission from the Pueblo administration. However, Section 36 is an unbroken tooth; that is, it extends beyond the rim, creating a more convenient opportunity for impromptu exploration. At about 200 acres, the state's portion of barrancas may seem a mere puddle in the ocean. Rest assured: it's enough to get in over your head if you're not careful.

Rainbow Boulevard ends at a crossroads near the center of Section 36. The barrancas are not visible from here—sand dunes and juniper block the view. The rim is just a few yards ahead. Follow the trail of shotgun shells to a point where cars and appliances spill down into a heap reminiscent of bone piles at the bottom of a buffalo jump. It's a tragic sight, but it's generally confined to the area around this dirt-road junction.

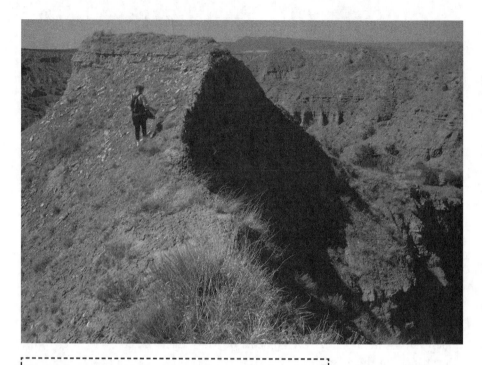

To avoid trespassing on Zia land, do not hike beyond this formation.

Before deciding whether to embark on a rim hike (outlined following) or to venture down into the barrancas, assess the landscape. The steep slopes and serpentine draws don't seem traversable, but they are easier to negotiate than they initially appear. The rumpled terrain fills in the valley from the West Mesa to the gypsum slope of White Mesa, which shines like a glacier, about 9 miles to the north-northeast.

The barrancas are shaped from malleable sediments, mainly silt and coarse-grained sand, with bits of red granite, obsidian, quartz, sandstone, and petrified wood in the mix. Exposed pockets of smooth pebbles and cobbles resemble colorful abstract mosaics throughout the gullies below.

For a **hike in the barrancas**, turn right at the rim and follow it about 300 yards to the northeast. There a ridge branches out and gradually descends to the northwest. Follow it out about 100 yards to a fork. Stay to the right and continue another 0.25 mile to a formation that resembles a pitched roof or a large pup tent. (See photo above.) Getting around it on this narrow ridge may prove difficult, which is just as well because it approximates a point on the otherwise invisible state land–Zia boundary. (In other words, stay south of the tent formation.)

From here, turn left and negotiate your way down to the streambed. Use a diagonal approach on the steep slopes for more secure footing, and use a feeder wash to avoid the otherwise vertical bank at the bottom. Turn left and follow the sinuous main channel upstream about 200 yards to a dead end. Climb up the embankment, and then turn left at the crest of the ridge. Follow the ridge uphill, and in less than 0.25 mile you should be back on the rim. Now that you know how easy it is to get in and out of the barrancas, you can explore them further at your leisure.

Of course, a descent into these twisted gullies is not a requirement for a fine hike at La Ceja—you can just as well enjoy a **hike along the rim.** Starting your walk from the end of Rainbow Boulevard, you have miles to wander in either direction before you run out of state land. You can also wander down a single-lane dirt road that's set back 10–100 feet from the rim. It often forks, so when in doubt, follow the branch that stays closest to the rim. It also gets too sandy and steep around La Ceja for most cars, but you might encounter an off-highway vehicle or two.

If you're facing the barrancas, the road to the right curves to the northeast as it drops from La Ceja. After about 2.5 miles, it takes a sharp turn to the southeast at a mesa corner. From here, a 1.4-mile stretch of east-facing scarp marks the eastern boundary of state land.

The road to the left undulates upward to Cerro Conejo (SAIR-oh koh-NAY-ho, "Rabbit Hill"), about 3 road-miles west. Peaking at 6,615 feet, it approximates the point where the southwest corner of the Zia Reservation meets the northwest corner of state land. Bones found near Cerro Conejo belonged to land mammals that inhabited the area 9–16 million years ago.

On one walk along the rim, I crossed fresh cat tracks but couldn't be sure whether they were from a mountain lion or just a really big bobcat. (Months later I found a pair of similar tracks along the streambed below.) Fuchsia petals emerged from hedgehog cacti. Piñon seemed to flourish despite devastating bark-beetle outbreaks elsewhere in the state. Glittering sands whipped off the mesa as winds gusted up to 40 mph, and in a sure sign of springtime at La Ceja, semiautomatic weaponry crackled behind a not-too-distant hill while a pair of quail scrambled for cover.

NEARBY ACTIVITIES

Coronado State Monument features the ruins of the Tiwa pueblo of Kuaua. The expedition of Spanish conquistador Francisco Vásquez de Coronado encountered the pueblo in 1540. Access the visitor center via Kuaua Road, on the north side of US 550, on the west bank of the Rio Grande in Bernalillo. Hours: Wednesday–Monday, 8:30 a.m.–5 p.m. (505) 867-5351; **nmmonuments.org.**

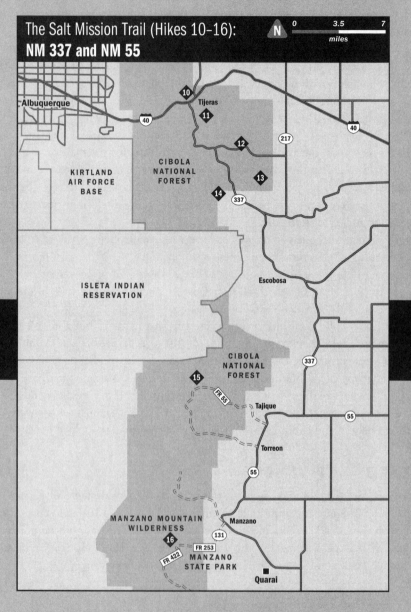

The Salt Mission Trail (Hikes 10–16): NM 337 and NM 55

N

0   3.5   7
miles

Albuquerque

Tijeras

40

40

217

KIRTLAND
AIR FORCE
BASE

CIBOLA
NATIONAL
FOREST

337

ISLETA INDIAN
RESERVATION

Escobosa

CIBOLA
NATIONAL
FOREST

337

FR 55

Tajique

55

Torreon

55

MANZANO MOUNTAIN
WILDERNESS

Manzano

131

FR 253

FR 422

MANZANO
STATE PARK

Quarai

THE SALT MISSION TRAIL
(NM 337 AND NM 55)

10   CANYON ESTATES-FAULTY TRAILS

KEY AT-A-GLANCE INFORMATION

LENGTH: 5.7-mile balloon

DIFFICULTY: Moderate

SCENERY: Travertine grotto, waterfall, seasonal wildflowers, wooded canyons

EXPOSURE: Mostly shaded

TRAIL TRAFFIC: Popular

SHARED USE: Low (closed to equestrians and all vehicles)

TRAIL SURFACE: Packed dirt, rock

HIKING TIME: 2–3 hours

DRIVING DISTANCE: 15 miles

ACCESS: Trailhead area open 6 a.m.–10 p.m., year-round

LAND STATUS: Cibola National Forest–Sandia Mountain Wilderness

MAPS: Sandia Ranger District; USGS Tijeras

FACILITIES: None

LAST-CHANCE FOOD/GAS: All services at Exit 167 (Tramway Boulevard and Central Avenue)

GPS TRAILHEAD COORDINATES

Latitude   35° 05' 23"

Longitude   106° 23' 29"

IN BRIEF

Well-marked trails just minutes east of Albuquerque are perfect for casual hikes most of the year. A short stroll up Hondo Canyon leads to a waterfall spilling over a travertine formation. Continue up the Crest Trail to join the Faulty trails for a pennant-shaped loop on gentle terrain through cool pine wilderness.

DESCRIPTION

It's a fact that complicates the organizational scheme of this book: Nearly every hike somehow connects to at least one of the many convoluted routes of old 66. Likewise, the Hondo Canyon's proximity to post-1936 Route 66 is hard to miss. What's more, this hike begins on the Crest Trail (130), which in some ways is similar to the mother road. To riff on Steinbeck: hikers come into 130 from the tributary trails, from the canyon corridors, and the rutted forest roads. They beat paths directly from nearby parking lots and their own backyards in their flight to 130, the mother trail.

In short, hike any Sandia Mountain pathway long enough, and you'll eventually arrive on 130. The Crest Trail runs 26 miles to span the length of the range. It's the connecting leg between Cañoncito Trail and Bart's Trail in Hike 17, and it's the extension from Tree Springs Trail to the upper tramway terminal in

----

Directions ———————————————➤

From I-40 East, take Exit 175 and aim for Tijeras, but turn left before you reach the traffic light at the bottom of the ramp. Drive north under the interstate and bear right on Arrowhead Trail ahead. Follow it 0.6 mile to its end at the Canyon Estates trailhead. The hike begins on the west side of the parking circle.

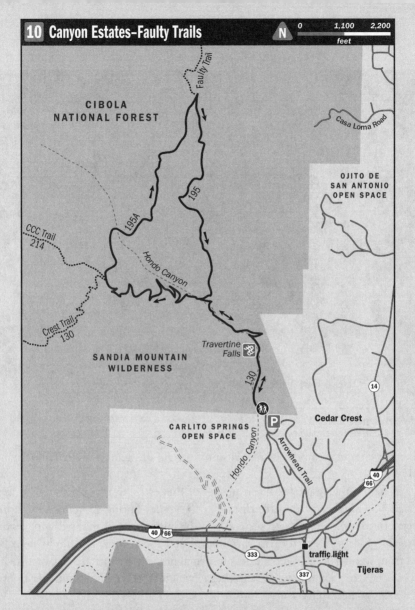

N

| 0 | 1,100 | 2,200 |

feet

CIBOLA
NATIONAL FOREST

Faulty Trail

Casa Loma Road

OJITO DE
SAN ANTONIO
OPEN SPACE

195

195A

CCC Trail
214

Hondo Canyon

Crest Trail
130

SANDIA MOUNTAIN
WILDERNESS

Travertine
Falls

130

14

Cedar Crest

CARLITO SPRINGS
OPEN SPACE

P

Hondo Canyon

Arrowhead Trail

40
66

40 66

333

337

traffic light

Tijeras

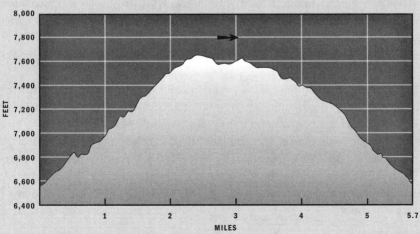

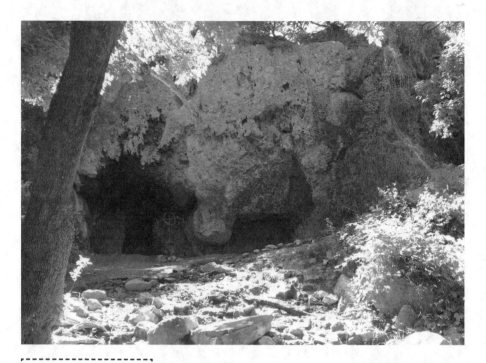

Travertine grotto and falls

Hike 19; its northernmost end makes up the bulk of the hike from Tunnel Spring in Hike 24.

A map on a signboard illustrates all of that at the Canyon Estates trailhead. A sign posted ahead indicates distances to Sandia Spring (5 miles) and Sandia Crest (16 miles). The three trails used on this hike are well marked with wooden posts and blazes at every turn; carefully placed rocks, logs, and limbs help keep you from wandering down countless informal paths and shortcuts between switchbacks. The extra maintenance simplifies navigation. You can help further by sticking to designated trails.

The hike begins alongside a mostly dry creek, which you'll cross a few times throughout the route. The lower trail lacks shade, but tree cover increases intermittently as you gain elevation. It also passes in the shadow of a stone cliff that seems ideal for impromptu climbing practice, provided you don't cause any rocks to fall on hikers below.

Less than 0.4 mile up the trail, a post marks the 100-yard spur to the travertine falls. A popular destination among mini-hikers, the falls are situated in an alcove. By late spring, it becomes a cool green oasis, thanks in large part to box elder and its little twin, poison ivy. The falls are usually just a trickle, but through eons of depositing dissolved limestone, they've created impressive travertine grottoes. A cruciform etched at the cave entrance appears to be the handiwork of modern teen goths, though local lore suggests that it's a centuries-old display of Franciscan devotion.

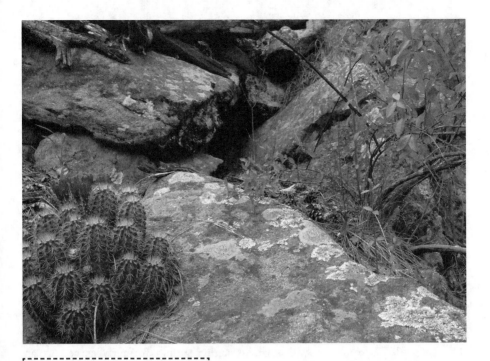

Landscape detail along the Faulty Trail

From the falls, return to the Crest Trail and continue uphill on the designated switchback. A vista opens to the south, across Tijeras Canyon, to reveal the industrial side of the Manzanita Mountains. Although it may not be the view you'd hope for in a national forest, the factory and quarries you see there meet up to 80 percent of Albuquerque's demand for cement. This mountainside blight passes out of view as you approach the top of the waterfall. Farther ahead on the right, several worn paths lead down to the shaded stream that feeds the falls. Stick to the main trail, following rectangular blazes in the trees.

One mile into the hike, you will arrive at the junction with Faulty Trail (195), so named because it roughly follows a fracture in the Earth's crust known as the Flatiron Fault. You'll use this trail on the return route, so stay on 130 for now. The south end of Upper Faulty Trail is another 0.5 mile up, but multiple switchbacks more than double the hiking distance. With an elevation gain of 600 feet, this segment is the most strenuous mile in the hike.

When you reach the clearing at the top, take a breather. A nearby marker indicates that the Crest Trail continues to the west. It turns north to meet Embudito Trail (192) at a junction 4.1 miles ahead. Also, although there's no indication of it here at the clearing, the seldom-used CCC Trail (214) starts nearby to the northwest on a more direct 1.8-mile route to the same junction. From there, a short spur leads to South Sandia Peak. Anyone bent on bagging it can set off in either direction, but take a detailed map and be advised of the 1,200-foot elevation gain.

To stick with this more relaxing route, head north past the enormous cairn on Upper Faulty Trail. This 1.3-mile segment gently undulates between 7,540 and 7,650 feet, where ponderosa, oak, and Rocky Mountain juniper flourish. Much of this trail is a quiet walk on a bed of pine needles.

The post marking the junction with Faulty Trail stands 3.5 miles into the hike. You can pad on a few easy miles by continuing north along the shaded Faulty Trail and returning to this point at your leisure, or you can pull a U-turn now to head south on Faulty Trail, back down to the Crest Trail. This segment is not quite as flat as the one above. Turn a rocky corner ahead, and you'll find yourself even with the tops of trees growing from the canyon below. The trail drops to the bottom and quickly climbs out the other side. The mile that follows is a fairly tame descent that ends with a stunning view over Hondo Canyon. If the reason for the name hasn't already become apparent, it should be now—*hondo* is Spanish for "deep." The remaining bit of Faulty Trail proves to be the most challenging. It's steep, with plenty of loose rock to test your balance. Take it slowly. When you reach the Crest Trail below, turn left and backtrack 1 mile to the trailhead.

NEARBY ACTIVITIES

The gated 177-acre site now known as **Carlito Springs** formerly served as an ancestral Puebloan camp, a stagecoach stop, a Union veteran's homestead, and a tuberculosis sanatorium. It features spring-fed ponds, lush riparian habitats, and ornamental gardens and orchards planted by previous owners. On-site buildings include a historic house made of travertine and a stone cabin dating to 1894. To get there, drive back toward Tijeras and turn right (west) at the traffic light onto NM 333 (Historic Route 66). Drive about 0.5 mile and turn right (north) onto Carlito Springs Road. Follow the road less than 1 mile to Carlito Springs. Site development is an ongoing project for Bernalillo County Open Space, so check with them before you go by calling (505) 314-0400 or logging on to **bernco.gov/ openspace.**

COYOTE TRAIL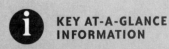

IN BRIEF

Multiple designated trails, informal paths, and forest roads add up to innumerable hiking routes through this quickly accessible area of Cibola National Forest. This unofficial route is a helpful primer in making the most of a popular mixed-use area.

DESCRIPTION

The southern tip of the Sandia Ranger District, which extends into the Manzanita Mountains, contains an extensive network of roads and trails. Map them all and you end up with what resembles a textbook illustration of varicose veins. Few of these skidmarks would exists today in such robust form were it not for the persistence and moxie of motorized nature enthusiasts.

In 2009, in response to concerns over the growing abundance of motor traffic in the forest, the Sandia Ranger District released a Travel Management Plan that essentially designates 42 miles of singletrack trail for motorcycle use and adds 13 miles for ATVs and full-sized vehicles. A supplementary Motor Vehicle Use Map (MVUM) clearly identifies these routes by omitting all nonmotorized trails. For those who enjoy throttling through woodlands, the MVUM is an invaluable document, and unlike the outdated hiking map, it's free.

Directions ⟶

From I-40 East, take Exit 175 south to Tijeras. Go south 1.3 miles (or 0.8 mile past the ranger station) on NM 337. Turn left on Chamisoso Canyon Road (FR 462) and go 0.7 mile east. Park in the lot on the left.

KEY AT-A-GLANCE INFORMATION

LENGTH: 2.9 miles

DIFFICULTY: Easy

SCENERY: Rolling hills, wooded trails, open meadows

EXPOSURE: Some tree cover

TRAIL TRAFFIC: Moderate

SHARED USE: Moderate (mountain bikers, equestrians, limited motorized-vehicle access, hunting, primitive and motorized dispersed camping)

TRAIL SURFACE: Dirt

HIKING TIME: 1 hour

DRIVING DISTANCE: 17 miles

ACCESS: Year-round

LAND STATUS: Cibola National Forest

MAPS: Sandia Ranger District; USGS Sedillo

FACILITIES: Restrooms, picnic shelters, fire pits

LAST-CHANCE FOOD/GAS: All services at Exit 167 (Tramway Boulevard and Central Avenue); dining in Tijeras

GPS TRAILHEAD COORDINATES

Latitude   35° 03' 56"

Longitude   106° 22' 07"

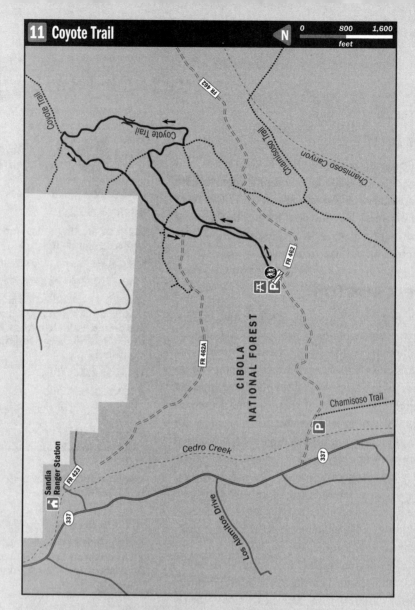

0   800   1,600
feet
N

Coyote Trail

Coyote Trail

Coyote Trail

FR 462

Chamisoso Trail

Chamisoso Canyon

FR 462

FR 462A

CIBOLA
NATIONAL FOREST

Chamisoso Trail

P

Cedro Creek

337

Sandia
Ranger Station

FR 423

337

Los Alamitos Drive

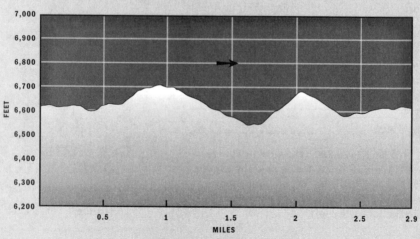

7,000
6,900
6,800
6,700
6,600
6,500
6,400
6,300
6,200

FEET

0.5   1   1.5   2   2.5   2.9

MILES

It's also a fine resource for those looking for a path without petrol fumes: just choose any trail that does *not* appear on the map.

The District also constructed a new staging area for motorized expeditions. Named for a trail that does not appear on the MVUM, the Coyote Trailhead facility opened with ample parking and signage to assist motorists, particularly those with trailers and/or oversized vehicles. However, as of December 2010, no signage at the Coyote Trailhead facility indicated where Coyote Trail actually begins.

Don't be dissuaded if this end of the forest doesn't sound completely pedestrian-tolerant. You still have every right and plenty of reasons to hike here. Completing the old Coyote Trail, along with a return via FR 462, would amount to a hike in the neighborhood of 7 miles. Our unofficial route is considerably shorter, and perhaps should be nicknamed "Coyote Pup." The shortcut is along one of the many well-defined trails that does not appear on either map.

Wooded canyons and open meadows are similar to those elsewhere in the area. There's also the usual abundance of limestone pavements riddled with marine fossils. But you're less likely to encounter motorists here, since FR 462 and Chamisoso Trail are favored cruising strips.

Vistas from ridges are lovely, even if occasionally tempered by traffic noise. The nearby Salt Mission Trail is popular with bikers, and the thundering flatulence of Harleys with short pipes can resonate to the mountaintops. Still, it seems like an even trade-off on days when you need quick access to a national forest. And when you're strolling down a quiet canyon, it's easy to forget how close you are to the roads you drove to get there.

If you're prone to straying off the beaten track and wandering down unmapped trails, you'll love exploring this area. Just be sure to note the towers standing atop the 7,767-foot summit of Cedro Peak, 1.3 miles southeast of the Coyote trailhead. Visible for miles, they make a useful reference point if you happen to you lose your bearings.

The hike begins with a 0.2-mile walk up the main road to a locked gate. To the right is a wooden post that marks Coyote Trail (46) and welcomes mountain bikers, equestrians, motorcycles, and (lowest on this totem pole) hikers. The trail parallels the forest road for about 0.2 mile. Bear left at the unmarked fork along the way, then right at the next unmarked fork. The trail soon climbs and narrows, then hooks south to a junction.

The old map shows Coyote Trail continuing another 3 miles or so, while both the MVUM and trail signage indicate that you're now at the junction of Trails 05619 and 05620. Turn left on 05619 (formerly 46) and follow it as it hooks north to run alongside a small arroyo for the next half-mile, crossing a narrow wooden bridge along the way.

From the lowest point on this segment, 05619 continues northeast alongside another arroyo. At the same point, two trails converge from the west. One follows the arroyo downstream. It ends at the forest boundary in less than 0.25 mile, but rock features along the way make it worth the short detour down and back. The

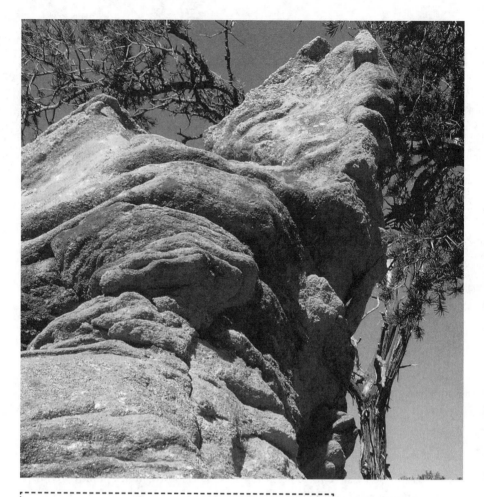

Short detours down unmapped trails often lead to memorable places.

other trail climbs southwest about 0.3 mile to peak at an unmarked junction on a ridge, then descends another 0.3 mile to put you back on FR 462A. Turn left and follow this graded road 0.4 mile back to the parking lot.

NEARBY ACTIVITIES

Visit the **Tijeras Pueblo Archaeological Site** for self-guided tours of the 14th-century ruins. Excavations from 1948 to 1976 uncovered 200 rooms, though it appears that all but a few have been reburied. The 0.3-mile interpretive trail is nonetheless pleasant and informative. Entered into the National Register of Historic Places in 2005, the site is behind the Sandia Ranger Station in Tijeras. Call (505) 281-3304 or visit **fs.usda.gov/cibola.**

SEDILLO RIDGE AND SABINO CANYON

IN BRIEF

Two east mountain sites provide a range of hiking options over meadows, forested hills, and a historic site.

DESCRIPTION

Since the Sandia Ranger District surrendered the bulk of its holdings south of I-40 to motorcyclists and other off-road warriors, Sedillo Ridge and nearby Sabino Canyon stand out as small hiking havens in an otherwise mechanized wilderness. Both are properties in the Bernalillo County Open Space inventory. The ruins of the Reidmont Fur Farm arguably make Sabino Canyon the bigger draw. However, its trail system seems too easy to stand as a hike on its own. So we bumped it down to Nearby Activities (page 75) and made Sedillo Ridge the featured hike. Both routes appear on the map; however, the elevation profile refers to the hike at Sedillo Ridge only.

Sedillo Ridge is one of the wilder sites in the BernCo inventory, and at 500-plus acres, it offers plenty of space and trails to roam. The hilly terrain ranges between 7,200 and 7,750 feet. Piñon–juniper dominates the landscape, and it can grow fairly dense. Like Sabino Canyon, the site was still under development at the end of 2010, but the trail system is well established and receives moderate use from hikers, mountain bikers, and

Directions

From I-40 West, take Exit 175 to Tijeras. Go 5 miles south on NM 337. Turn left on Juan Tomas Road and go 2.5 miles east. Park in the area on the right, across from the trailhead signed "05027." Note that the last mile can get a bit rugged after inclement weather.

KEY AT-A-GLANCE INFORMATION

LENGTH: 5 miles

DIFFICULTY: Moderate

SCENERY: Woodland, meadows, nearby 20th-century ruins

EXPOSURE: Half-shaded

TRAIL TRAFFIC: Moderate

SHARED USE: Moderate (mountain bikers; dogs must be leashed; no motorized vehicles)

TRAIL SURFACE: Packed dirt

HIKING TIME: 2 hours

DRIVING DISTANCE: 22 miles

ACCESS: Year-round

LAND STATUS: Bernalillo County Open Space; Cibola National Forest–Sandia Mountain Wilderness

MAPS: USGS Sedillo

FACILITIES: Interpretive signage

LAST-CHANCE FOOD/GAS: All services at Exit 167 (Tramway Boulevard and Central Avenue); restaurants in Tijeras

SPECIAL COMMENTS: Sedillo Ridge Open Space is a work in progress. For updates, call Bernalillo County Open Space at (505) 314-0400 or visit bernco.gov/openspace.

GPS TRAILHEAD COORDINATES

Latitude   35° 02' 05"

Longitude   106° 19' 13"

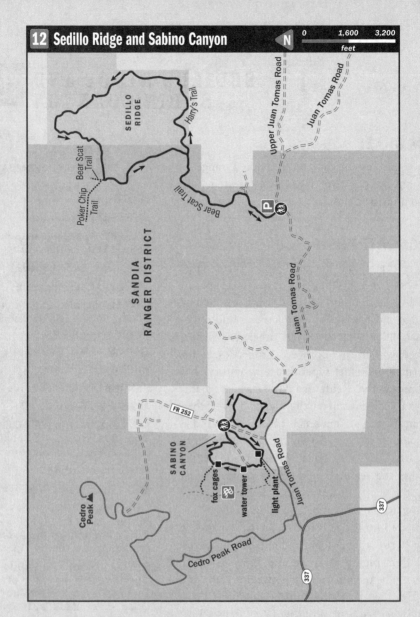

N

0   1,600   3,200
feet

SEDILLO RIDGE

Harry's Trail

Upper Juan Tomas Road

Juan Tomas Road

Bear Scat Trail

Bear Scat Trail

Poker Chip Trail

P

SANDIA RANGER DISTRICT

Juan Tomas Road

FR 252

SABINO CANYON

Juan Tomas Road

fox cages

water tower

light plant

Cedro Peak

Cedro Peak Road

337

337

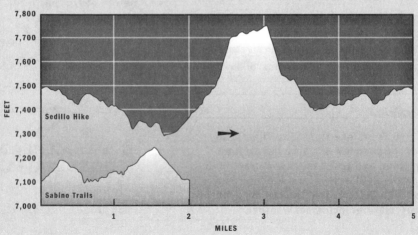

FEET

7,800
7,700
7,600
7,500
7,400
7,300
7,200
7,100
7,000

Sedillo Hike

Sabino Trails

1   2   3   4   5

MILES

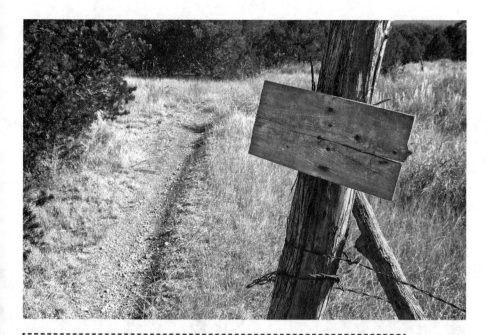

Signs posted in the area aren't always helpful, but the trails are easy enough to follow.

equestrians. It also seems fairly popular with rattlesnakes in the summer, so watch your step.

The hike begins on Forest Service property at the Bear Scat trailhead (signed "05027" at the trailhead and on the Sandia Ranger District Motor Vehicle Use Map; signed BEAR SCAT along the trail). Hike north on this motorcycle track about a mile to the signed junction with Harry's Trail. Turn right and follow Harry's Trail to the southwest corner of Sedillo Ridge Open Space. The wooded trail descends 100 feet in about a quarter-mile to cross a meadow in Juan Tomas Canyon.

Over the next mile, it rounds a ridge and turns north to cross another meadow. Pass through a gate to unmarked junction and continue north. The trail gets steep and rocky as it climbs 200 feet over the next quarter mile.

Keep an eye out for a left turn marked with a tombstone-shaped rock near the top. If you start downhill along the main trail, you've gone too far. It's easy to miss, but once you pick it up you'll have no problem staying on track. Over the next half-mile it turns south, then bears west to follow an old fenceline back down into the upper reaches of Juan Tomas Canyon. There you'll find the a sign for Bear Scat Trail. Turn left and follow it south 2.7 miles back to the parking area.

NEARBY ACTIVITIES

This short stroll takes you back a hundred years to the Reidmont Fur Farm, an enterprise that was, for better or worse, destined for failure. Stables and cages in

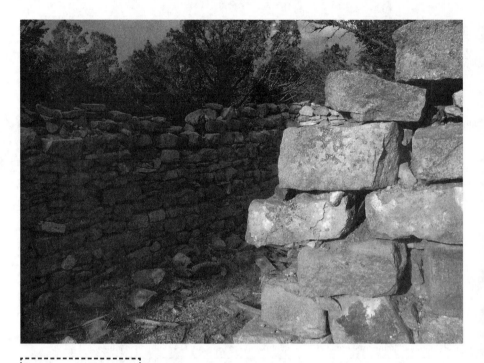

Ruins of the light plant

ruins add a melancholic twist to the otherwise serene site. Adjacent national forest adds miles of options to this relatively short route.

For the definitive guide to this area, see *Sabino Canyon: A History,* from the East Mountain Historical Society (**eastmountainhistory.org**). For a quick recap, read on: About a mile south of Cedro Peak, Cibola National Forest surrounds an island of Open Space. Both share a seamless patchwork of piñon–juniper forest and upland meadows. Evidence of human habitation in the area dates back to 5500 BC. From the early 17th century to the late 19th century, farmers cultivated the land for pinto beans and potatoes, but the site is best known for a short-lived attempt to capitalize on the fur craze of the flapper era. In the late 1920s, Austrian immigrant Alexander Riedling built the Riedmont Fur Farm, complete with hundreds of silver foxes, minks, and rabbits. But the fur market soon tanked with the onset of the Depression, and Riedling died on the farm a few years later.

In October 1999, Bernalillo County purchased the 117-acre parcel. Recreational developments, including an information board and 2 miles of trail development, took a mere 11 years to approve and install, during which time this Open Space property was rarely open. At last check (October 2010), it was closed (again) for tree thinning and other maintenance projects. Signs stood blank among the ruins, presumably awaiting interpretation, but the new singletrack trails looked fabulous.

The hike here is more of a casual stroll along well-defined trails. If you don't have time for the full figure-eight, skip the 0.9-mile East Trail. This loop begins with a short stem across a shallow drainage and up to the edge of the treeline. From there turn left and continue a mild climb along the wooded path. The loop portion encircles a meadow with blue grama, pine dropseed, and other grass species, but the trail stays under just enough tree cover for the illusion of a forest hike until it returns to the stem that leads back to the parking area.

Across the road from the parking area, the hike begins on a gravel road but soon diverts south on the West Trail. After about a quarter-mile, it takes a wide detour around the light plant. (This stone ruin is easier to view from a path that starts near the farmhouse.) The trail soon turns north to visit the remaining structures, which soon come into view.

Once you reach the fox cages in the northwest corner of the property, you might consider a short, scenic foray into the adjacent national forest. Look for a break in the fence behind the cages. You should be able to pick up a trace of an old road heading west. It'll lead you to a shallow drainage in less than 5 minutes (or twice that long when vegetation grows dense, as it commonly does in late summer). Once in the drainage, turn left and follow it downstream. It soon channels deeper and drops over a couple of modest falls. These stony sites are serene enough for a picnic, or at least a moment of quiet contemplation. Sit still long enough and something will likely fly, crawl, or slither by. Mule deer, black bear, piñon deermouse, black-tailed jackrabbit, porcupine, diamondback rattlesnakes, and the canyon wren are listed as local residents.

When you're ready, continue down the streambed another quarter-mile or so. A faded road leading out on your left climbs back up to rejoin the West Trail. If you miss that exit, don't worry. You'll soon reach Juan Tomas Road, 0.2 mile east of the junction with FR 252. Turn left on this graded road. The parking area is 0.25 mile up on the right.

13 JUAN TOMAS OPEN SPACE

KEY AT-A-GLANCE INFORMATION

LENGTH: 3.5 miles

DIFFICULTY: Easy–moderate

SCENERY: Forested hills and canyon, meadow

EXPOSURE: Moderate shade

TRAIL TRAFFIC: Moderate

SHARED USE: Low (mountain bikers; dogs must be leashed; no motorized vehicles)

TRAIL SURFACE: Dirt

HIKING TIME: 1–2 hours

DRIVING DISTANCE: 26 miles

ACCESS: Year-round

LAND STATUS: Albuquerque Open Space

MAPS: USGS Sedillo

FACILITIES: Restrooms and drinking water at Oak Flat Picnic Area. Open for day use May–October; on Oak Flat Road, 2 miles west of the Juan Tomas trailhead

LAST-CHANCE FOOD/GAS: All services at Exit 167 (Tramway Boulevard and Central Avenue); restaurants in Tijeras

GPS TRAILHEAD COORDINATES

Latitude   35° 00' 05"

Longitude   106° 17' 51"

IN BRIEF

Managed by the City of Albuquerque, recently rehabilitated land in the East Mountains is now an ideal spot for casual hiking, mountain biking, bird-watching, and (timed right) cross-country skiing.

DESCRIPTION

This Open Space area takes its name from the village of Juan Tomas, about 2 miles due north of the trailhead. Settled around 1860, the village grew modestly on logging and farming until water shortages led to its abandonment in the early 1960s. Few buildings remain, including its church, which is now a private residence.

In 1983 the City of Albuquerque acquired 1,290 acres from the U.S. Forest Service (USFS) to create Juan Tomas Open Space. Development began 14 years later to make the area suitable for recreational use, including projects to reduce forest-fire hazards and repair damage caused by decades of off-road driving. Progress thus far has been commendable, thanks in large part to cooperation from local communities.

An informal network of trails crisscrosses the property, with some connecting to the Oak Flat Picnic Area and USFS trails. Like the previous hiking areas at Sedillo Ridge, Juan Tomas adjoins the Sandia Ranger District of Cibola National Forest, yet it stands apart with

Directions

From I-40 West, take Exit 175 to Tijeras. Go 8.7 miles south on NM 337. Turn left on Oak Flat Road and go 2.7 miles east. Park in the area on the left, across from the junction with Anaya Road.

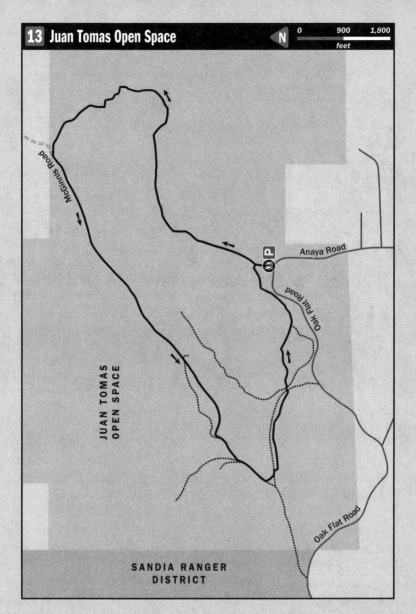

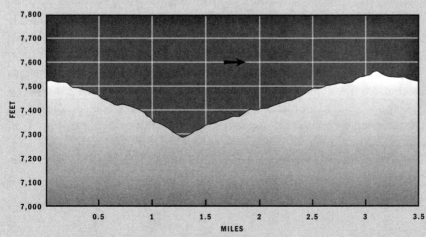

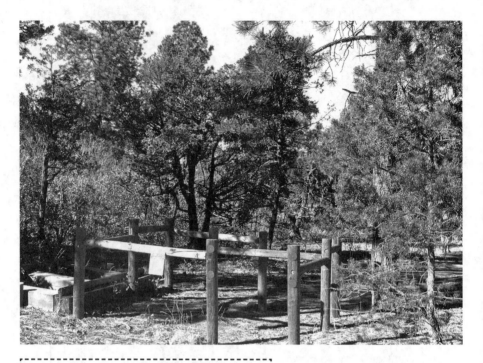

Equestrian and pedestrian access gates at the trailhead

quietude. True, mountain bikes do occasionally careen through the woods here. Can't blame them—miles of smooth singletrack over gently rolling hills make Juan Tomas irresistible to beginner and moderate riders.

With elevations ranging from 7,300 to 7,760 feet, Juan Tomas features Rocky Mountain juniper, alligator juniper, piñon, and ponderosa, interspersed with scattered stands of ponderosa, Gambel oak thickets, and open meadows. Local inhabitants include mule deer, wild turkey, and elk.

The hike begins at equestrian- and pedestrian-access gates at the edge of a gravel parking area. Heading north, you'll soon pass an OPEN SPACE sign and a T-junction (your return route) on your left. The trail is straight, flat, and sparsely shaded for the first half-mile or so. As you begin a downhill bend east, you'll catch a glimpse of Sandia Peak standing about 18 miles northwest.

Over the next mile, the trail continues descending and curves northwest into denser tree cover, following a drainage most of the way down. Alternating between double- and singletrack, it eventually arrives at the edge of a meadow. Just ahead, another OPEN SPACE sign stands at an elevation 200 feet lower than where you began.

From here the trail curves southwest and joins another stretch of double-track (formerly McGuinness Road) on a modest climb up a 1.5-mile canyon. As it becomes steeper and rockier, look on your left for a broad trail. (It still shows as

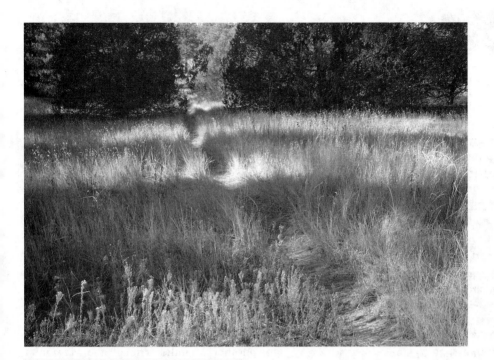

Partially shaded singletrack on the canyon floor

a Forest Service road on some maps; but if you see signs for the Open Space–Forest Service boundary, you passed it about a quarter-mile back.)

Head east on the broad trail about 0.3 mile until it splits into four trails. If you have time for a detour, the path on your left heads north into denser woods. To stick to this route, take the uphill singletrack going east. This half-mile segment twists over a shaded hillside and arrives at a signed fork. Follow the arrow pointing right to return to the parking area.

NEARBY ACTIVITIES

Carolino Canyon Reservation Area straddles the Salt Mission Trail (NM 337) just 0.3 mile south of Oak Flat Road. This 40-acre Open Space property can accommodate up to 250 people. Facilities include two picnic areas, shelters, fireplace, grills, restrooms, water, electricity, a wheelchair-accessible paved nature trail, and a playing field for volleyball, tetherball, or horseshoes. The facility is available by reservation from May through September. Fees range from $50 to $325. Contact the Albuquerque Open Space Division: (505) 452-5217; **cabq.gov/open space/carolino.html.**

14   MARS COURT

KEY AT-A-GLANCE INFORMATION

LENGTH: 4.7- to 8.2-mile loop options

DIFFICULTY: Moderate, with some strenuous climbs

SCENERY: Forested ridges, meadows, abundant birdlife, wildflowers

EXPOSURE: Half-shaded

TRAIL TRAFFIC: Light–moderate

SHARED USE: Moderate (mountain bikers, joggers, equestrians; limited motor-vehicle access)

TRAIL SURFACE: Dirt roads, rocky trails

HIKING TIME: 3–5 hours

DRIVING DISTANCE: 25 miles

ACCESS: Year-round

LAND STATUS: Cibola National Forest

MAPS: Sandia Ranger District; USGS Escabosa

FACILITIES: Maps posted on trail

LAST-CHANCE FOOD/GAS: Small grocery and cafe on NM 337, 0.8 mile south of Raven Road; nearest gas station on NM 14 in Cedar Crest, about 4 miles north of Tijeras

SPECIAL COMMENTS: Sandia Ranger Station is on the left side of NM 337, 0.5 mile south of I-40. Consider stopping in for maps and updates on current trail conditions.

GPS TRAILHEAD COORDINATES

Latitude   34° 59' 02"

Longitude   106° 20' 59"

IN BRIEF

Tucked away in a far corner of the Manzanita Mountains, a well-marked network of single-track and former logging roads winds across canyon meadows and forested ridges. Though the trails are easily accessible from a residential area, views from high points give the illusion of deep wilderness surroundings.

DESCRIPTION

For those driving south on the Salt Mission Trail, Mars Court is a final chance to hike in the Sandia Ranger District. Pass it by, and you won't be able to access Cibola National Forest for another 25 miles. Though the Manzanita and Manzano mountains appear to be in a continuous north–south trending range, the Manzanitas are a separate subrange. For hiking purposes, the two ranges may as well be 20 miles apart, with Isleta Pueblo accounting for most of the buffer zone between them.

Contiguous military properties further restrict access to most of the Manzanitas. In the not-too-distant past, hikers in nearby Otero Canyon regularly strolled past NO TRESPASSING signs inexplicably posted deep in the woods. In recent years, however, the U.S. Department of Defense upgraded the signs with unsubtle warnings regarding live ammunition. Hikers who ignored the new postings wound

----

Directions

From I-40 East, take Exit 175 south to Tijeras. Go 8.8 miles south on NM 337. Turn right on Raven Road and follow it 1.6 miles. Turn right on Mars Court. Drive about 200 feet, through the open gateway, and park along the loop before the second gate. The trailhead is next to the first gate.

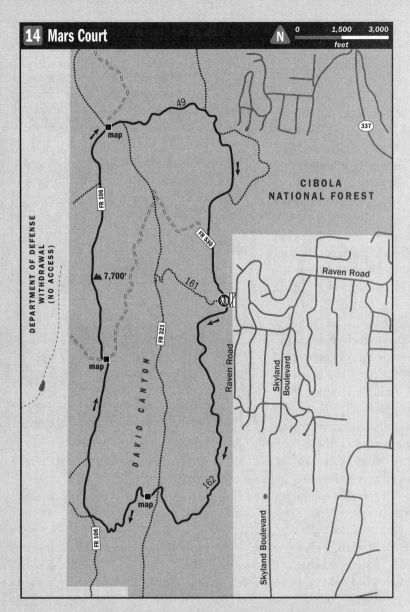

N

0   1,500   3,000
feet

CIBOLA
NATIONAL FOREST

337

49

FR 106

FR 530

map

map

map

DEPARTMENT OF DEFENSE
WITHDRAWAL
(NO ACCESS)

▲ 7,700'

161

162

FR 321

D A V I D   C A N Y O N

FR 106

Raven Road

Raven Road

Skyland
Boulevard

Skyland Boulevard

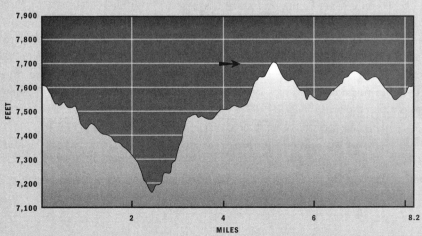

FEET

7,900
7,800
7,700
7,600
7,500
7,400
7,300
7,200
7,100

2   4   6   8.2

MILES

up in court, facing potential six-month jail terms and $5,000 fines. In the ensuing battle for Otero Canyon, the U.S. Air Force seems unlikely to surrender to local hiking activists.

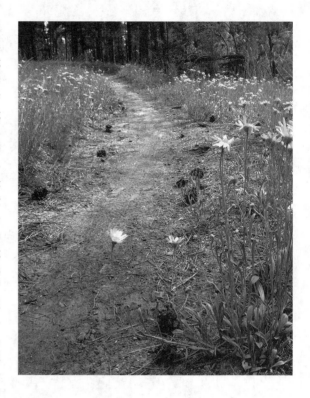

Otero Canyon was the primary destination for hikers and mountain bikers at this end of the Sandia Ranger District, but motorized vehicles tended to dominate the tangle of roads leading from Mars Court. "Drunks in trucks stuck in the mud" is how one longtime local resident described the scenery back then. Since then, rehabilitation projects and unusually merciful travel-management decisions keep motor-vehicle access to a minimum, and myriad roads blazed through the woods have been modified to a simplified trail system.

That same local resident describes the scenery now as consisting of "more birds and wildflowers" than she can name. And she could name quite a few, including Mexican squawroot, silvery lupine, the ubiquitous Indian paintbrush, and several types of fern and yucca growing side-by-side. Gray flycatcher, black-throated gray warbler, and vesper sparrow thrive in the Manzanitas but are rare in the neighboring Sandias. Wild turkeys, recently introduced to the Manzanos, now occasionally turn up in the Manzanitas.

The 14-mile Mars Court trail system is basically confined along a stretch of David Canyon about 3 miles long and less than 1 mile wide. Military property flanks the west side, the expanding Tranquillo Pine residential developments encroach on the east, and the Isleta Reservation cuts off the southern end of the canyon. Yet a hike here approximates the wilderness experience of any backcountry forest—minus the long drive up rugged access roads. More bears than hikers wander the area, judging by tracks along the trail.

This hike relies primarily on Trail 162, a stretch of FR 106, Trail 49, and a bit of FR 530 for an 8.2-mile loop. As the map indicates, several shorter and longer variations are possible. On that note, compare the map in this book with the Sandia Ranger District map, the USGS Escabosa map, and maps posted along the trail, and you may soon notice several discrepancies. What's more, none of the above thoroughly depict what's actually on the ground, but that shouldn't be a problem.

Trails 161 and 162 both begin at their respective markers next to the first gate. Trail 161 takes a more direct route into the upper canyon, whereas 162 gradually sinks to the south. Follow 162 as it starts out as a narrow, rocky single-track. It becomes more defined as it enters denser woods. A lush mix of pine and broadleaf shade the path. A break in the trees before the first steep decline offers a glimpse of the forested mountains to the south.

A couple of paths split off at the edge of the cutting-unit boundary, but the main trail is clear. Strategically placed rocks and branches help keep you from straying in the wrong direction, and a post marked "T 162" appears within the first mile. Just ahead, a fading road approaches from the right, and it seems you've reached the canyon floor. Not quite—after a short climb, the trail descends for another mile to the south-southwest, passing a second marker, and then drops for 0.25 mile to the northwest. The canyon floor comes into view as you approach the final switchback. This long, grassy meadow seems more of a narrow valley than a canyon in the traditional Southwestern sense.

A map posted at the crossroads ahead illustrates your route options from here. At last check, it was faded beyond legibility, but keep this in mind: you're 2.4 miles into the hike, and so far it's been easy. But you've lost more than 450 feet in elevation. So no matter which way you go from here, you've got some climbing ahead of you.

FR 321 (FR 335 on other maps) runs the length of the floor, north to south. It's an obvious road that shows signs of frequent motor-vehicle use, despite its deliberate omission from the Motor Vehicle Use Map. (Feel free to report any motorized vehicles you see in this vicinity to the Sandia Ranger District.) A left turn here would take you 1 mile down to the Isleta boundary. It's a pleasant detour along a distinct road that becomes more shaded as the canyon sinks deeper. A fence and signage leave little doubt as to where you must turn around.

To shorten this hike and skip its steepest climbs, turn right on FR 321 and hike north about 1.6 miles to Trail 161. Take another right turn there, and it's a steep 0.7-mile push back to the gate. Or go north 2 miles to FR 530, then turn right for a more gradual mile-long ascent to the gate. Or go north 2.5 miles to rejoin this hike at the western end of Trail 49.

This hike continues on Trail 162, now named Turkey Trot. It's a 0.8-mile climb to the west rim of David Canyon, about 300 feet above your current elevation. This final segment of 162 is rocky and strenuous but scenic and well shaded. A marker at the top tells you when you've reached FR 106.

The junction of Trail 162 and FR 106 offers limited choices. A detour to the left ends 0.5 mile down at a multitude of signs reading DANGER: UNMARKED UNEXPLODED ORDNANCE AREA and PELIGRO: AREA DE BOMBAS INEXPLOTA-DAS. (It goes on like that.) So unless you need to practice Spanish for military situations, turn right on FR 106 and follow it north. As long as you don't stray down any roads on your left, you won't detect a hint of the U.S. Air Force installation to the immediate west.

The next junction, FR 530, is 1.3 miles ahead. An oversized panel here bears the cryptic message LEAVING WILDING AREA on one side and ENTERING WILD-ING AREA on the other. A road barrier and another marker with a trail map also stand nearby. Again, you can turn right for shortcut options. Or to stick to this hike, turn left, and then make a quick right up a steep, rocky road. This ridgeline route is only half the climb of Turkey Trot but somehow takes twice the effort.

The view is your incentive. Aside from a few rooftops poking through the crowns on the east side of David Canyon, it's an uninterrupted vista of forested mountains and canyons on all horizons. Clear across the Isleta Reservation, the twin peaks of Guadalupe and Mosca stand 12 miles to the south-southwest. (You can visit Mosca Peak on the next hike, Fourth of July Canyon–Cerro Blanco.) Just 8 miles to the northwest and covering the next 180 square miles, Albuquerque is nowhere to be seen.

The road tops out at 7,700 feet and then gradually descends 1 mile to the next posted map. From this junction, FR 106 and Trail 236, head north to con-nect with trails originating from the Otero Canyon trailhead. To stay on this hike, turn right on FR 321. A singletrack soon splits off to the right, only to rejoin 321 near the head of Trail 49 about 0.25 mile downhill.

You could stay on 321, drop back down into David Canyon, and then climb out the other side on 530. Or to stay on this hike, hook around the head of the canyon by starting east on Trail 49. The latter option involves less climbing, but it's about 0.5 mile longer. Also known as the Cajun Pine, Trail 49 is the least developed in the Mars Court network, so you'll need to pay special attention to the trail. Forks are unmarked; when in doubt, go right. The narrow trail winds through scrub in a burn zone, where clearings afford final glimpses of mountains to the south.

The 1.7-mile Cajun Pine ends at FR 530. Turn left on this prominent road and go uphill 0.4 mile back to the parking area. Or if you need to put in a few more miles, cross the road and start on a new trail, Cajun Turk. Its destination is as much a mystery to me as the rationale that goes into naming these trails.

NEARBY ACTIVITIES

Big Block Climbing Area presents an array of bouldering problems and sport climb-ing on limestone cliffs. The block itself is big enough for three routes rating around 5.7. The main wall has at least five established routes. Parking for Big Block is unmarked. Look for a trailhead between the guardrail and the road cut on the south side of NM 337 between Mile Markers 25 and 24. The trail to the area is short but steep, and it crosses a small stream populated with goldfish.

FOURTH OF JULY CANYON– CERRO BLANCO

15

IN BRIEF

Crowds turn out each autumn to gawk at leaves, but you can find solitude here throughout most of the year. Meander along established trails from a popular picnic area to the crest of the Manzano Mountains. Clearings on the ridgeline reveal vistas that seem to stretch halfway to the next state.

DESCRIPTION

New Mexico is blessed with two Fourth of July canyons. One is on the border of Colfax and Taos counties, while the more famous one is in Torrance County. Each fall, hikers mob the latter's trails to witness a pyrotechnic display of foliage. This Fourth of July Canyon contains concentrations of bigtooth and Rocky Mountain maples to rival any autumnal clump in New England.

If the crowds are too dense, take heart in the fact that most will turn back within the first mile and won't return for another year because what they don't seem to understand is that the trails are just as colorful in other seasons.

Spring and summer bring neotropical migrants—Central and South American birds

---

Directions

From I-40, take Exit 175 to Tijeras. Follow NM 337 south 29 miles to the T-junction with NM 55. Turn right, going west 3.2 miles on NM 55 to Tajique. Turn right on FR 55 (also marked as A013) and follow the signs to the Fourth of July Campground, 7 miles up the dirt-and-gravel road. Turn right through the gate, and park in the hiker parking area. Note that the gate is locked November–March. If arriving then, park at the gate and walk up toward the campground. The trailhead is on the left, about 400 feet past the gate.

KEY AT-A-GLANCE INFORMATION

LENGTH: 6.4-mile loop and spur

DIFFICULTY: Moderate

SCENERY: Seasonal wildflowers and foliage, wooded canyons, eastern and western vistas

EXPOSURE: Mostly shaded

TRAIL TRAFFIC: Popular

SHARED USED: Low (livestock; limited equestrian and mountain bike access; no motor vehicles)

TRAIL SURFACE: Gravel forest roads, dirt trails

HIKING TIME: 3–4 hours

DRIVING DISTANCE: 54 miles

ACCESS: Year-round

LAND STATUS: Cibola National Forest

MAPS: Mountainair Ranger District–Manzano Division; Manzano Mountain Wilderness–North Half; USGS Bosque Peak

FACILITIES: Campsites (April–October), picnic area, and restrooms (no water). All are wheelchair-accessible.

LAST-CHANCE FOOD/GAS: Ray's One Stop in Tajique

SPECIAL COMMENTS: For forest-road and trail conditions, visit the Sandia Ranger Station on the east side of NM 337 in Tijeras.

GPS TRAILHEAD COORDINATES

Latitude   34° 47' 24"

Longitude   106° 22' 46"

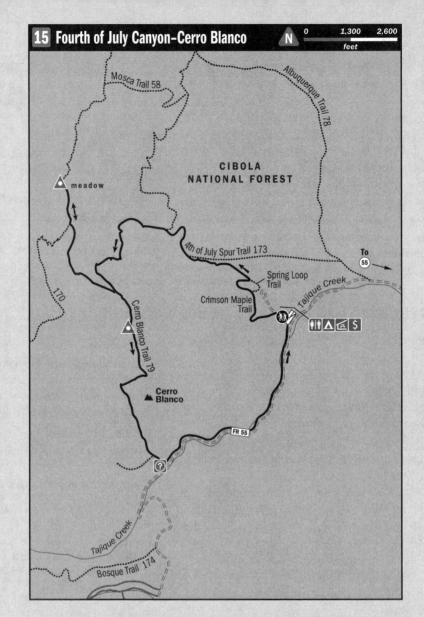

Mosca Trail 58

Albuquerque Trail 78

CIBOLA
NATIONAL FOREST

meadow

4th of July Spur Trail 173

To
55

Spring Loop
Trail

Crimson Maple
Trail

Tajique Creek

170

Cerro Blanco Trail 79

Cerro
Blanco

FR 55

Tajique Creek

Bosque Trail 174

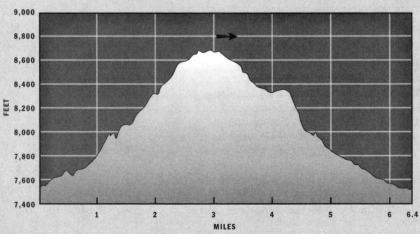

9,000
8,800
8,600
8,400
8,200
8,000
7,800
7,600
7,400

FEET

1   2   3   4   5   6   6.4

MILES

of brilliant plumage, such as orange-crowned warblers. Dense clusters of seep-spring monkeyflowers bloom from March to October. Like snapdragons, they can be manipulated to resemble their namesake. A healthy population of Abert's squirrels stays active year-round. Named after the U.S. Army lieutenant who cataloged them during a New Mexico expedition in the 1840s, these tassel-eared arboreal rodents were released into the Manzano Mountains in 1929 and have thrived here since.

Hikers can choose from multiple loop options to explore the area. No two maps agree exactly on where all these trails go. So although the route described below is fairly simple, keep in mind that, like many Forest Service trails, the designated ways are subject to alteration.

Start your hike with a detour along Crimson Maple Trail. Whether you parked at the gate or in the hiker parking area, the trailhead begins a short way up the gravel road, at the picnic area on the near side of the first restrooms. A prominent sign along the way maps out the trails in the campground area. Just beyond that, another sign indicates where to turn left for Crimson Maple Trail.

A green box at the northwest corner of the picnic area contains brochures with interpretive text corresponding to the 11 numbered stations ahead. Unless you're already well versed in the history and ecology of the Manzano Mountains, this enlightening detour is worth the extra 15 minutes.

Follow numbered signs 1–8 to the end of Crimson Maple Trail, then turn right on Spring Loop Trail for signs 9–11. Pick up the **Fourth of July Trail (173)** on the other side of the loop and turn left toward a sheltered bulletin board. If this is your first expedition into the Manzanos, take a moment to review the comprehensive display of data, rules, ethics, maps, hazards, and warnings.

After passing through a gate, note the wooden sign pointing ways and distances to nearby trails. Similar signs have been positioned along trails throughout the Manzanos. However, black bears seem bent on destroying them, so don't be surprised if any are missing or defaced beyond legibility.

The next sign indicates the trailhead on the right for the Fourth of July Trail Spur, a 1-mile link to the Albuquerque Trail (78). Continue straight and cross through a pedestrian gateway ahead.

The trail splits around the Upper Fourth of July Spring within the next 500 feet. A sign seems to be missing here. Some hikers slog straight up the streambed, but a drier trail climbs to the right. Massive alligator junipers tower over the trail as it nears an elevation of 8,000 feet. Yucca and cacti persist on the south-facing slopes, while old-growth maples prefer the damp canyon below.

The trail drops back down just upstream of a round trough. Signage in view ahead marks the eastern edge of the Manzano Mountain Wilderness, as indicated by the icons that forbid bicycles and mopeds beyond this point. (For reference, a sharp right here would put you on a 3.5-mile course back to FR 55 via the Albuquerque Trail.)

Continue straight to the end of the Fourth of July Trail, 0.6 mile ahead. Pine needles soften the path as it climbs up steadily into mixed-conifer forest. Icy

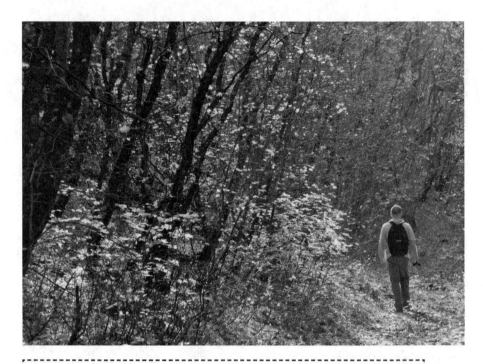

An attractive detour runs west from the junction near the Cerro Blanco trailhead on FR 55.

patches can linger here for weeks after an early-autumn snow. As the trail seems to level out, crossing through rocky outcroppings, the crest comes into view above. These absorbent limestone bands allow rainwater to sink into the mountain and seep out through the canyons below to support the diverse vegetation.

Signage at the T-junction with **Cerro Blanco Trail (79)** indicates that FR 55 is 1 mile to your left, the Crest Trail is 0.5 mile to your right, and the Fourth of July Campground is 1.5 miles back the way you came. But if you followed this hiking route, including the nature trails, you've done a solid 2-plus miles so far.

Turn right to pick up the **Crest Trail (170)** 0.5 mile ahead, then turn right and follow it another 0.25 mile. (A new trail segment splits left along the way but soon rejoins the same trail.) Mosca Peak comes into dramatic view before a meadow, where you might find grazing cattle, opens on the right. Incidentally, bovine encounters on this trail commonly end with panicky cows fleeing into the forest. To fully appreciate a heifer stampede in the upper-mountain forest, you must witness the spectacle yourself.

Thickets of Gambel oak start to squeeze in, narrowing the trail. Press through to the clearing on the other side, then take a moment to rest on the stone bench and enjoy the view. From nearly 8,700 feet, it appears that the closest major towns are mere specks in the vast Rio Grande Valley. It's more than tempting to gaze until the sun sinks behind Arizona, but there's still the matter of getting off this mountain. (For reference, Ojito Trail [171] drops into the canyon of the same name straight ahead, but it is no longer maintained. The Crest Trail goes less than 1 mile to the east side of Mosca Peak before officially ending at the southern boundary of the Isleta Reservation. From there, the 0.8-mile Mosca Trail [58] links to the Albuquerque Trail.)

To continue on this hike, backtrack to the junction of the Fourth of July and Cerro Blanco trails. From there, continue straight along **Cerro Blanco Trail.** The remaining 1.5-mile descent to FR 55 is a cakewalk. The trail is well established and navigable up to the last flicker of dusk. After a few switchbacks, it squeezes between rocky outcrops and looming cliffs as it drops down to a stream that's often flowing.

At the junction ahead, consider turning right for a detour to a grottolike bend in the canyon. The foliage on this 0.3-mile spur matches Fourth of July's, making it an attractive option for a romantic stroll on its own. (Starting from the Cerro Blanco trailhead on FR 55, this easy hike is about 0.8 mile out-and-back.) Otherwise, bear left at the junction, and you'll soon arrive at FR 55. Turn left, and follow this pleasant creekside road 1.4 miles downhill to the gate at the Fourth of July Campground.

NEARBY ACTIVITIES

Whether it's from the picnic-area barbecue grills or the high-altitude heifers, I always get a craving for steak after this hike. The **Ponderosa Eatery & Saloon** is just your typical local diner–biker bar, but its steak rellenos plate is an authentic feast. To find the restaurant, look for a log-cabin lodge on NM 337, about 7 miles north of Chilili or 12 miles south of Tijeras. (505) 281-8278 (call for hours); **ponderosaeateryandsaloon.com.**

16 BOX SPRING-RED CANYON

KEY AT-A-GLANCE INFORMATION

LENGTH: 8.6-mile loop

DIFFICULTY: Moderate

SCENERY: Quartzite cliffs, dense woodland, subalpine meadows, views over the Estancia and Rio Grande valleys

EXPOSURE: Mostly shaded

TRAIL TRAFFIC: Moderate

SHARED USE: Low (equestrians, camping)

TRAIL SURFACE: Dirt, rock

HIKING TIME: 4–5 hours

DRIVING DISTANCE: 62 miles

ACCESS: Year-round; free day use or $7 campsite fee

LAND STATUS: Cibola National Forest

MAPS: Mountainair Ranger District–Manzano Division; Manzano Mountain Wilderness–South Half; USGS Manzano Peak; Capilla Peak

FACILITIES: Restrooms (no water), picnic tables, grills, and corrals at Red Canyon Campground.

LAST-CHANCE FOOD/GAS: Convenience store in Manzano, 6 miles from the trailhead; convenience store–gas station in Tajique, 15 miles from the trailhead.

GPS TRAILHEAD COORDINATES

Latitude   N34° 37' 18"

Longitude   W106° 24' 42"

IN BRIEF

Most hikers come here for a 7.5-mile loop that incorporates Spruce Spring Trail and a short spur to Gallo Peak. This slightly longer route explores a wider diversity of landscapes along paths less traveled, namely Box Spring Trail, Ox Canyon Trail, and a lonely stretch of the Manzano Crest Trail. Either way you'll witness old-growth conifer, mountain meadows, and the main attraction—the towering quartzite outcrops of Red Canyon (aka Cañon Colorado).

DESCRIPTION

The best way to hike this route is open to debate. Photographers prefer to start with Red Canyon to take advantage of early daylight. Summer hikers start on Box Spring Trail to avoid the heat in Ox Canyon's exposed sections. The route described here opts for the latter in a strategy that simply saves the best for last.

Box Spring Trail (99)—or Box Canyon Trail, according to some maps—is an easy, well-shaded 1.4-mile path that climbs gently

----

Directions

From I-40 East, take Exit 175 to Tijeras. Drive south on NM 337 and NM 55 about 41 miles, passing through the villages of Escobosa, Chilili, Tajique, Torreon, and Manzano. On the south side of Manzano, veer right at the fork onto NM 131, following the signs toward Red Canyon. Go 2.4 miles, then turn right before the entrance to Manzano State Park. NM 131 soon becomes Forest Road 253. About 2.5 miles past the Manzano State Park entrance, turn right and continue 0.4 mile toward the Red Canyon Campground. Unless you plan to stay the night, park in the day-use area.

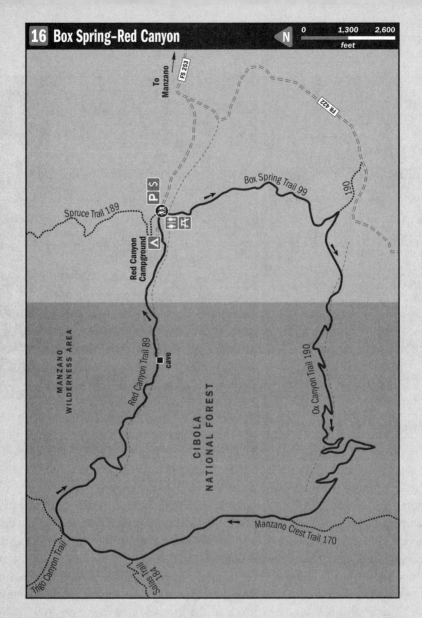

0   1,300   2,600

feet

N

To Manzano

FS 253

FR 422

Box Spring Trail 99

190

P S

Spruce Trail 189

Red Canyon Campground

Red Canyon Trail 89

cave

Ox Canyon Trail 190

MANZANO WILDERNESS AREA

CIBOLA NATIONAL FOREST

Trigo Canyon Trail

Salas Trail 184

Manzano Crest Trail 170

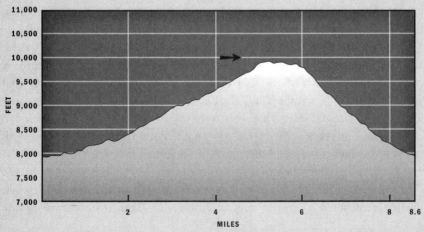

FEET

11,000
10,500
10,000
9,500
9,000
8,500
8,000
7,500
7,000

2   4   6   8   8.6

MILES

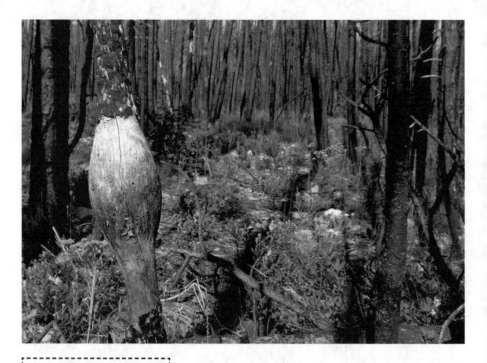

Burn zone on Box Spring Trail

around the bulging ridge between Red Canyon and Ox Canyon. A sign for its trailhead stands on the south side of the road in the day-use area, near the restrooms and picnic grounds. It starts by dropping south to cross an occasionally damp creek bed, then soon passes through an equestrian/pedestrian gate. From there it's a casual stroll on a narrow but obvious path that dips in and out of steep drainages. Aside from a few freakishly fat and contorted specimens of alligator juniper, some of the forest appears healthy and green, and dense enough to shield views of the plains down east. Some areas, however, are in dire need of thinning.

A natural forest fire burns close to the ground, clearing undergrowth while leaving the big trees intact. Excess timber in the form of scrawny trees often referred to as "doghair" can add fuel to the fire, often with disastrous results, as you'll soon see. A few blackened pines are the first hint of a major forest fire not too long ago. Then suddenly, about a mile into the hike, you turn a corner and hit the burn zone—remnants of the Ojo Peak fire, a 19-day blaze that consumed nearly 7,000 acres in November 2007. Box Spring Trail comes to an end at a junction in a field of charred stalks that were once tall trees.

Ox Canyon Trail (190) is the intersecting path. Four years after the Ojo Peak fire, the scorched terrain around this junction remained, in a word, otherworldly. A stony peak once hidden behind tall stands of pine now glares down from the west. (You won't visit it on this hike, but you'll come close.) A nearby signpost, presumably reinstalled after the fire, indicates that Trail 190 runs 0.5 mile

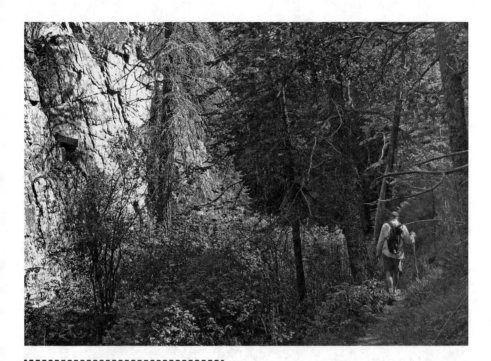

Heading downstream on Red Canyon Trail

southeast to FR 422 and 3.5 miles west to join the Crest Trail. Turn right here and start climbing west. The lower trail is as broad as a boulevard and as easy to follow. Trail workers installed numerous signs and laid down branches to keep you from straying onto discontinued routes, and mature pines emphasize the way with rectangular blazes scored many decades ago.

Though the fire spread deep into Ox Canyon, crossing over the near entirety of its trail, evidence of it soon fades as the singed landscape yields to lush woodland ripe with fern, moss, and mushrooms. The trail stays near the canyon floor, meandering near the intermittent stream that (sometimes) flows from the upper and lower Ox Springs. It switches back to traverse a rockslide and continues climbing to a point at 8,840 feet. By now you're in aspen territory, and just high enough to catch a glimpse of salt lakes in the Estancia Basin. They're sometimes hard to spot, but at the right time of day they seem to mirror the sky. The big one, Laguna del Perro, is about 12 miles long and 1 mile wide. Pueblo Indians harvested salt from these *salinas* to trade with Plains Indians. Early Spaniards valued salt for its use in extracting silver from its ores. Vying for dominion over the Salinas Province, they established Franciscan missions at three nearby pueblos. (See Nearby Activities.)

After a brief respite on relatively level terrain, the trail crosses to the south side of the stream and the switchbacks turn severe. Over the next 1.2 miles or so on this narrow and coiled trail, you'll travel a linear distance of

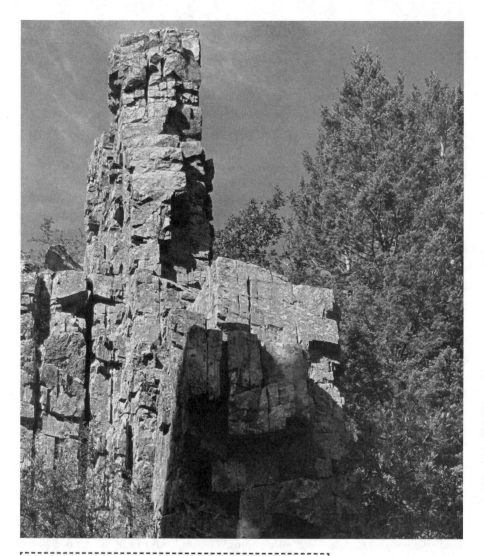

A quartzite outcrop resembles a cubist tower over Red Canyon Trail.

only 0.18 mile, half of which is in a gain in elevation. After the fifth switch-back, the trail eases over a hump to arrive at a perfect spot on the crest to break for lunch, and maybe a nap.

The **Manzano Crest Trail (170)** starts out deceptively easy. Monumental cairns stand along the stretch heading south, and a cluster of signs gives distances in all directions. The segment for this hike is 1.5 miles north to Red Canyon Trail. You soon enter a steep meadow where the trail fades out. Maintain your direction and you should be able to spot diminutive cairns in the tall grass. The trail regains its definition farther uphill. The saddle just ahead is the high point of this hike. Gallinas Peak is visible about 45 miles southeast. Climb the rocks on your left for better views west over the Rio Grande Valley and down into Monte Largo Canyon (Hike 49).

The Crest Trail then descends on the west side of the ridge. Rest assured it will soon return to the east side, where it enters dense woodland and fades out. Again, maintain your direction and you should soon spot the posted junction with Salas Trail (184). Continue on the Crest Trail into a meadow where it vanishes once again. You know the drill by now. The next posted junction is about 200 feet northeast.

Red Canyon Trail (89) is the steepest segment of this hike, but it's all downhill from here, and its entire 2.4 miles is easy to follow. A signpost here points the ways to trails running north, south, and east but says nothing of the one running west. (Take a quick jog in that direction to find its sign. TRIGO is the only word remaining on this bear-clawed sign. It refers to an old alignment of the discontinued Trigo Canyon Trail, which last met the Crest Trail 2 miles north of this point.)

Back at the junction, head east on Red Canyon Trail. It quickly drops into the shade of fir, spruce, and a smattering of massive ponderosa. The narrow path crosses a creek a few times. Crossings can get tricky with a good spring runoff, but that usually dies down to a trickle by summer. Stony walls rise to flank both sides of the stream. (Geologists, take note: In this area, where the Sais directly overlies the White Ridge Quartzite without the intervening Estadio Schist, the two quartzites look very much alike. It's also interesting to note that bedding, which was originally horizontal, is now subvertical due to folding and thrusting during the Precambrian.) Just past a waterfall is an alcove with the shelter cave. From there, the canyon widens and the trail continues about 0.7 mile to the campground.

The Red Canyon trailhead is marked with the standard map and info board. It's located at the top of the campground loop, so either way you go is less than 0.2 mile back to the day-use area.

NEARBY ACTIVITIES

Salinas Pueblo Missions National Monument: Like the plantations that would later come to plague the American South, these imposing missions fueled fierce discontent. Three far-flung units—Abó, Quarai, and Gran Quivira—now make up the National Monument. Quarai is the nearest and is open daily, Memorial Day–Labor Day, 9 a.m.–6 p.m. The rest of the year you can visit 9 a.m.–5 p.m. Entry is free. To get there from Manzano, drive 5 miles southeast on NM 55. Turn right at Punta de Agua and go west 1 mile. For more information, call (505) 847-2290 or visit **nps.gov/sapu**.

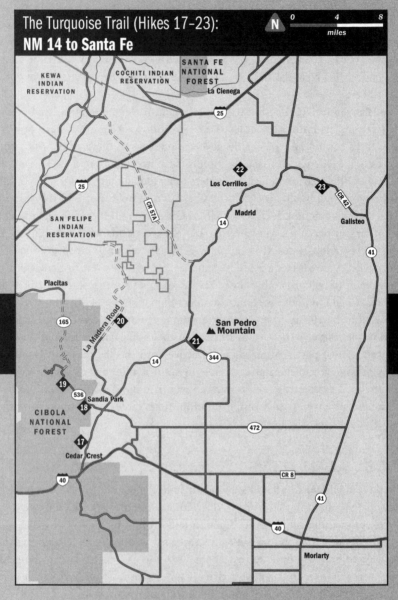

The Turquoise Trail (Hikes 17–23): NM 14 to Santa Fe

N

0   4   8
miles

KEWA INDIAN RESERVATION

COCHITI INDIAN RESERVATION

SANTA FE NATIONAL FOREST

La Cienega

25

22

Los Cerrillos

23

CR 42

25

CR 57A

Madrid

14

Galisteo

SAN FELIPE INDIAN RESERVATION

41

Placitas

La Madera Road

165

20

San Pedro Mountain

19

21

14

344

536   Sandia Park

18

472

CIBOLA NATIONAL FOREST

17

Cedar Crest

CR 8

40

41

40

Moriarty

THE TURQUOISE TRAIL
(NM 14 TO SANTA FE)

17 MUD SPRING-CAÑONCITO

KEY AT-A-GLANCE INFORMATION

LENGTH: 5.5-mile or 10-mile balloon options

DIFFICULTY: Easy or strenuous

SCENERY: Travertine falls, early-20th-century ruins, wooded canyons; crest views on 10-mile route

EXPOSURE: Mostly shaded

TRAIL TRAFFIC: Moderate

SHARED USE: Low (educational activities; no dogs on first 0.3 mile)

TRAIL SURFACE: Packed dirt, loose rock, pine bedding

HIKING TIME: 2–5 hours

DRIVING DISTANCE: 19 miles

ACCESS: Limited (see Special Comments)

LAND STATUS: City of Albuquerque; Cibola National Forest–Sandia Mountain Wilderness

MAPS: Sandia Ranger District; USGS Sandia Crest

FACILITIES: Restrooms, interpretive information

LAST-CHANCE FOOD/GAS: All services in Cedar Crest on NM 14

SPECIAL COMMENTS: The Sandia Mountain History Center is not open to the public during school hours. Their trails are accessible during some public events. For more information, visit nmnaturalhistory.org/smnhc.

GPS TRAILHEAD COORDINATES

Latitude   35° 07' 33"
Longitude   106° 22' 43"

IN BRIEF

Hikes on the trails at the Sandia Mountain Natural History Center can be extended into the Sandia Mountain Wilderness. The long route incorporates a mile of the Crest Trail. Overlooks from 9,200 feet alternate between eastern and western vistas. A shorter loop via Faulty Trail misses the views but visits waterfalls on the lower Cañoncito Trail.

DESCRIPTION

Most visitors who drive the Turquoise Trail National Scenic Byway don't realize that behind the contemporary facade of Cedar Crest lie small but culturally vibrant villages. Many of the families here are the descendants of those who came to settle the Spanish Crown's 90,000-acre Cañon de Carnué land grant.

Cañoncito is an exception. The initial attempt to establish El Cañoncito de Nuanes predates Mexican independence, but its would-be founder, Juan Nuanes, abandoned his efforts in the wake of an Apache attack. His family returned in the 1850s to finish the job, and eventually the modest agrarian community boasted a gypsum mine, a quarry, a church, and two dance halls. However, when a 1901 U.S. government survey excluded Cañoncito from the Cañon de Carnué land grant, the Nuanes family lost their entitlement to the land.

Directions

From I-40 East, take Exit 175 toward Cedar Crest on NM 14. About 2.6 miles north of the I-40 overpass, turn left on Columbine Lane (immediately after the coffee shop). Follow this gravel road 0.7 mile up to the visitor parking area at the Sandia Mountain Natural History Center.

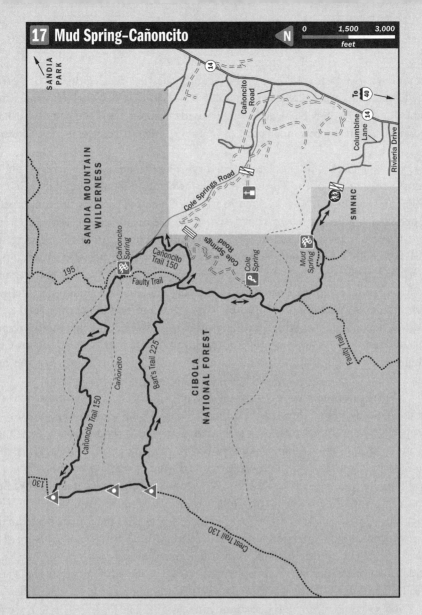

N

0	1,500	3,000

feet

SANDIA PARK

SANDIA MOUNTAIN WILDERNESS

Cañoncito Road

14

To 40

14

Columbine Lane

Riviera Drive

Cole Springs Road

SMNHC

Cañoncito Spring

Cole Springs Road

Cole Spring

Mud Spring

Cañoncito Trail 150

Faulty Trail

195

Cañoncito

Bart's Trail 225

Cañoncito Trail 150

Faulty Trail

CIBOLA NATIONAL FOREST

130

Crest Trail 130

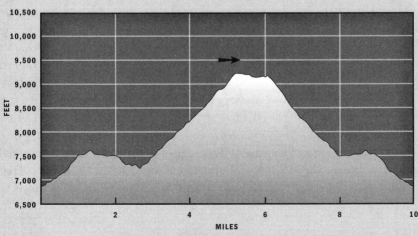

10,500					
10,000					
9,500					
9,000					
8,500					
8,000					
7,500					
7,000					
6,500					

FEET

MILES

2   4   6   8   10

Given the history, you might call into question the legitimacy of current landownership, especially when you arrive to find that today's landowners have shut down the access road traditionally used to access the Cañoncito and Bart's trailheads. But there's no point in arguing. Instead, consider this alternate approach:

The Sandia Mountain Natural History Center stands on 128 acres of piñon–juniper forest west of the Turquoise Trail. Owned by Albuquerque Public Schools (APS) and run by the New Mexico Museum of Natural History, the center offers more than 5 miles of hiking trails, two self-guided trails, interpretive programs, and numerous picnic areas. Access, however, is limited. As of this writing, the SMNHC and its trails are closed to the public, except for special events and public days. Further, the SMNHC does not encourage the use of its 0.3-mile segment of Mud Spring Loop to access trails in the adjacent Sandia Mountain Wilderness. Truth is, nobody along the Turquoise Trail wants to be the gateway to the east side of the mountains, which is why both the SMNHC and the Sandia Ranger District recommend approaching Cañoncito and Bart's trails from Sandia Crest Highway—an option that would add about 4 miles to this route. See the next hike, Armijo Trail–Cienega Spring, if you wish to explore that option.

Mud Spring Loop starts on the west side of the office. Go around the right side of the building to find the signed trailhead. The 0.3-mile segment that crosses APS property is a groomed path that meanders alongside a shaded arroyo, visiting a picnic area and an outdoor classroom before arriving at the Sandia Wilderness boundary. Continue uphill to the aptly named Mud Spring. Ruins of a stone cabin and a ponderosa tagged CUSTER'S LAST STAND TREE are located nearby. Both are marked with numbers that correlate to an interpretive map. Bear left at the fork ahead, right at the next one, and left at the one after that. Signs posted along the way indicate the direction to the Faulty Trail. Mud Spring Trail splits from the loop and becomes steep and rocky as it continues west. It soon bends northwest and becomes steeper yet before arriving at an unsigned T-junction the Faulty Trail, just under a mile into the hike. Before turning right here, remember this junction so you don't miss the turn on your way back.

Faulty Trail (195) is an easy north–south trail that spans the east side of the mountains from the Crest Trail near Canyon Estates (Hike 10) to Bill Spring Trail near the Doc Long Picnic Ground—8.7 miles end to end. This route uses a 1-mile segment to reach Bart's Trail, or 1.4 miles to Cañoncito Trail. You can make that decision later. For now enjoy the stroll north, dipping in and out of shallow drainages along the way and bypassing the spur on the right to the Cole Spring Picnic Area, which closed long ago when local property owners first gated Cole Springs Road.

At 2.0 miles into the hike, Bart's Trail crosses the Faulty Trail at a signed junction. Those here for the 5.5-mile route can continue on the Faulty Trail another 0.4 mile. Turn right on Cañoncito Trail and follow it 0.7 mile down to

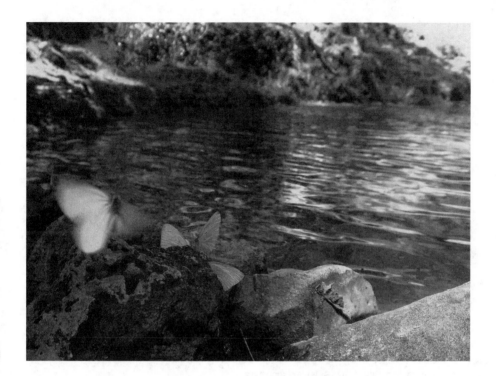

Bart's trailhead on Cole Springs Road. From there it's 0.3 mile back up Bart's Trail to return here at its junction with the Faulty Trail.

For the 10-mile route, turn right to commence on a strenuous counterclockwise loop, using the lower section of Bart's Trail to reach the Cañoncito trailhead. Other loop options should spring to mind, so choose wisely, grasshopper. But before making a decision, read on to learn more about the trails involved. Also, if you're parked in the SMNHC visitors lot, allow yourself ample time to return before they close for the day and lock the gate on Columbine Lane.

Cañoncito Trail (150) reaches the Crest Trail in 3 miles. It starts on a modest climb northeast from Cole Springs Road, traversing piñon-and-juniper-forested slopes. The path soon turns northwest to drop into its namesake "little canyon." After 0.4 mile on this trail, you might see the stone foundation of an old cabin on the right, though it's been increasingly difficult to spot in the midst of bark-beetle devastation. A marshy area just ahead indicates the lower reaches of Cañoncito Spring. You'll usually find it flowing stronger as you ascend closer to the source.

Unlike the sudden drop of the travertine falls near Canyon Estates, deposits here create a gradual, stepped decline. Water spills down a series of terraces, some of which form pools just deep enough to soak your feet. Farther upstream, water gushes down a 20-foot embankment. The trail splits here, with an informal path staying close to the stream while the proper trail turns wide to avoid eroding the embankment. Both soon pass by a streamside campsite.

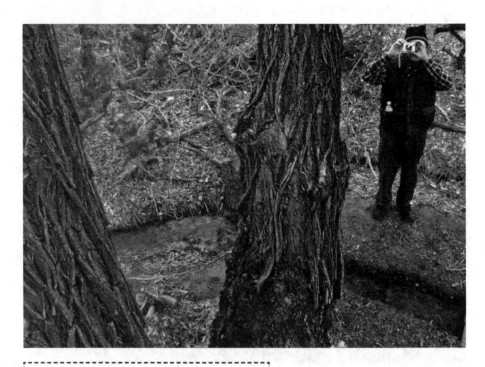

A few notable features close ahead: a small sign (easy to miss) marks Cañon-cito Spring; a limestone outcrop forms a cliff, which kids will find irresistibly climbable; and a junction signpost on the Faulty Trail gives directions and distances for multiple trails and destinations. From the junction, Cañoncito Trail soon becomes steeper and rockier. Limestone in this area is rich with marine fossils. About a mile past Faulty Trail junction, tree cover thins and the trail narrows. It can get lost in overgrowth along this stretch. Just when you think you're on the wrong path, square-and-rectangle blazes indicate you're still on course. Shade is still spotty, but now it's coming from spruce and fir, with a hint of aspen. A wooden post ahead marks the T-junction with the Crest Trail.

Crest Trail (130) is your connector to Bart's Trail. But before going south for the transfer, turn right for a quick detour. Just a few yards north, the Crest Trail jogs right. Turn left here for a fantastic overlook directly above Bear Canyon. For what it's worth, the canyon crosses the western forest boundary at an elevation of 6,200 feet. Your elevation at the overlook is slightly over 9,200 feet.

Now go south on the Crest Trail, keeping an eye out for numerous overlooks just off the trail. Good views to the east come up on the left about 0.4 mile ahead, and on the uppermost segment of Bart's Trail. If you find yourself walking through a tunnel of bowed oak on the Crest Trail, you've just missed the wooden post that marks the upper terminus of Bart's Trail.

Bart's Trail (225) climbs (or, in this direction, descends) 1,800 feet in elevation in just 2 miles. For comparison, the Cañoncito Trail segment from the cabin ruin (its lowest elevation point) to the crest gains 1,900 feet in 2.5 miles. Yet Bart's is notorious for being the hard way up to the crest—and worse, for wearing out downhill hikers' knees. Its overblown bad-boy reputation probably stems from its designed purpose. Constructed to provide quick access to the South Peak area, the trail intentionally lacked froufrou amenities like switchbacks. Credit for its brilliant design and construction goes to Fayette "Bart" Barton and the New Mexico Mountain Club. The trail was completed in 1979, and the Forest Service has since adopted it into their trail system with few modifications.

But what makes Bart's Trail less challenging is the absence of the vegetation that occasionally overwhelms the upper Cañoncito. Bart's holds its shape better, making it easier to follow. And though it lacks Cañoncito's splendid water and rock features, it does have its own *cañoncito*.

Coming from the crest, you cross the head of the little canyon about 1.4 miles down the trail. Stay close to the north rim for the next 0.25 mile or so. About 1.7 miles from the crest, it returns you to the junction with the Faulty Trail. Turn right here and backtrack 2 miles to the parking area.

NEARBY ACTIVITIES

The 88-acre **Ojito de San Antonio Open Space** features a meadow, an apple orchard, and piñon–juniper forest on the surrounding slopes. Spend a lazy afternoon in the shade of an ancient willow by the side of a historic acequia. Two natural springs have provided drinking water for wildlife and the nearby community for centuries. To get there from Cañoncito, return to NM 14 and go south 2.4 miles. Turn west on San Antonio Drive. A parking lot and access to the open space are hidden behind the San Antonio de Padua Church. For more information, call Bernalillo Open Space at (505) 314-0400 or visit **bernco.gov/openspace**.

18 | ARMIJO TRAIL-CIENEGA SPRING

KEY AT-A-GLANCE INFORMATION

LENGTH: 4.8-mile loop; (5.2-mile loop in winter)

DIFFICULTY: Moderate

SCENERY: Mountain pine forest, springs, tipi village

EXPOSURE: Mostly shaded

TRAIL TRAFFIC: Moderate; heavy on weekends

SHARED USE: Moderate (equestrians, limited vehicle access, popular with dog owners)

TRAIL SURFACE: Dirt, asphalt

HIKING TIME: 2–4 hours

DRIVING DISTANCE: 24 miles

ACCESS: Year-round (see Directions for seasonal access notes); day-use fee $3 per car; free with Sandia Mountain Annual Permit or National Parks and Federal Recreation Lands Annual Pass

LAND STATUS: Cibola National Forest

MAPS: Sandia Ranger District; USGS Sandia Crest; Sandia Park

FACILITIES: Picnic shelters, restrooms, drinking water, nature trail, wheelchair access

LAST-CHANCE FOOD/GAS: Convenience store–gas station at the junction of NM 14 and NM 536

GPS TRAILHEAD COORDINATES

Latitude   35° 09' 54"

Longitude   106° 22' 33"

IN BRIEF

Wooded trails on the lower slopes of the Sandias' east side are ideal for casual hikes in any season. This route has it all—travertine springs, an overlook, a trailside stream, and a few unnatural objects that aren't as easy to explain.

DESCRIPTION

Driving up Sandia Crest National Scenic Byway, your first opportunity to pull over for a hike is the turnoff for the Sulphur Canyon and Cienega Spring picnic areas. There the dilemma begins. Faced with numerous hiking options, I'm often drawn between two old favorites: the Cienega Canyon and Armijo trails. Cienega was always best for a long steady climb to a 9,200-foot junction on the Crest Trail. On Armijo, I rarely made it past 7,200 feet, opting instead to explore side trails of a curiosity sometimes referred to as the "tipi village." On one winter's day of exceptional indecisiveness, I opted for both, using Faulty Trail as the connecting link. It turned into an exhausting 8-mile slog through mud and snow and semifrozen springs. The route description that follows is an abbreviated version, a loop optimized for all seasons.

Directions ───────────────────→

From I-40 East, take Exit 175 toward Cedar Crest. From the I-40 overpass, go north 5.9 miles on NM 14. Turn left on NM 536 (Sandia Crest Scenic Byway) and drive 1.8 miles west. Turn left at the Sulphur Canyon/Cienega Spring picnic areas. Turn left again at the junction just ahead and drive another half-mile up to the Cienega Canyon site. From November to April, the road is gated, but you can park at the Cienega Horse Bypass trailhead area and hike a slightly different loop.

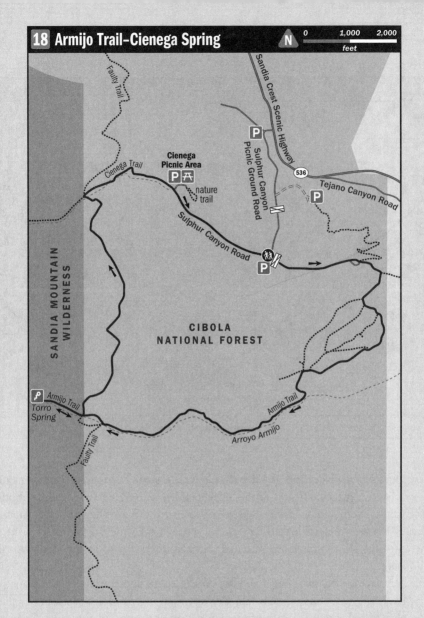

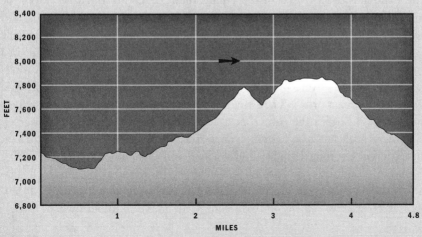

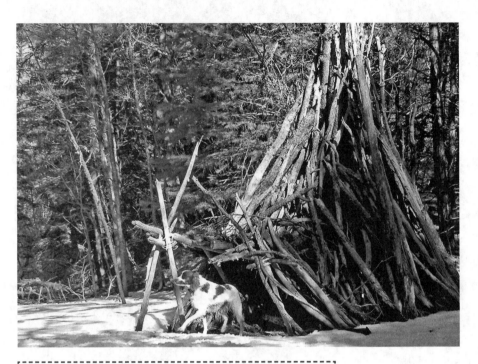

Cone-shaped stacks of deadwood are sometimes modified into shelters.

The hike begins at the upper parking area, Cienega Spring. In the event of a snow closure, the hike begins at the Sulpher Canyon parking area, adding about a mile to the overall route. From November to April, the hike begins at the Cienega Horse Bypass trailhead area. From there you can take the 0.75-mile Trail 98 to the east end of Sulphur Canyon Road and rejoin the route below at the Armijo trailhead.

Interesting structures turn up early en route. An anonymous pair of stone pillars, likely the remnants of a Civilian Conservation Corps project, lurk in the shadows near the northwest corner of the T-junction at the top of the drive. From the T-junction, turn left past the site attendant's trailer and head east past the barrier. The asphalt road continues downhill. More stoneworks, remnants of the old picnic area, crop up on your left about a quarter-mile past the barrier. The road ends in a small loop, and Armijo Trail begins. Continue east until you see a wagon-wheel fence (which marks private property). A post on your right indicates where you should turn to stay on Armijo Trail, which soon descends into a shallow ravine. Less than a quarter-mile past the Armijo post, an unmarked trail splits left. Detour up this unofficial trail and you'll soon spot a cone-shaped stand of deadwood that resembles a tipi. Continue uphill to find another, and yet another. Many hikers have wondered out loud over the purpose and meaning of this array of unusual formations. Is it an environmental art installation? A colony of mountain beavers? Primitive portals to another dimension that's completely identical to our own?

The explanation is simple, and a lot less fun than you might imagine. The "cones" are what's left of a Forest Service thinning project that began around 2001. Trunks and brush cut during thinning were stacked, piled, or spread in arroyos for erosion control. A bit higher up, deadfall was stacked into cone structures. This cleanup gives the area an open, parklike feel and improves the forage in the area.

The so-called "tipi village" or "cone zone" occupies a 200-foot ridge between Armijo Trail and Arroyo Armijo. You can explore it via a 2-mile network of informal trails that tend to hold up well year-round. In spots where pine straw or snow obscures the paths, the cones act as cairns to get you back on track, and private-property boundaries to the east prevent you from straying off too far. Near the top of the ridge, past a clearing with a supersized cone, the trail splits and forces a decision: continue following cones or begin following rock pyramids? (The latter also raises obvious questions: Who had time to stack so many rocks? And why?)

Either way you'll eventually end up back on Armijo Trail, where you can continue hiking southwest. The trail soon drops down to the arroyo streambed, then follows it west as it climbs a mile to the marked intersection with Faulty Trail. To visit Torro Spring, continue another 0.2 mile west on a diminishing trail. The spring is said to be one of the prettiest travertine formations in the Sandias. (I've only seen it buried in snow.)

You can revisit the cone zone by returning to the parking area the way you came, or complete the loop via Faulty and Cienega trails. At this point, the return distance is about the same either way.

To complete the loop, head north on Faulty Trail. It's a fairly flat mile to a splendid overlook above Cienega Canyon, immediately followed by a short, steep drop that can be treacherous with snow or rain. To follow my example, slip, slide, and tumble down to Cienega Trail, then turn right. The picnic area is less than a half-mile south. Bark-beetle outbreaks along this trail, especially the lower section, have been devastating. Restoration efforts are ongoing, and the trail is usually clear. A pleasant stream crosses the trail once or twice, occasionally transforming the picnic area below into a true *cienega* (marsh or wet meadow).

Note: Bears in the area are allegedly hostile. Review the protocol for ursine diplomacy (page 12) before hiking here.

NEARBY ACTIVITIES

Tinkertown Museum is on the south side of the Sandia Crest National Scenic Byway. No doubt you saw the sign en route to the Cienega Spring turnoff. Within the walls of this ramshackle compound lies the labyrinthine *Wunderkammer* of Ross J. Ward, a creator and curator of unusual things. Open daily, 9 a.m.–6 p.m., April–October. For more information, call (505) 281-5233 or visit **tinkertown.com**.

19 TREE SPRINGS-CREST TRAIL

KEY AT-A-GLANCE INFORMATION

LENGTH: 7.2-mile out-and-back

DIFFICULTY: Moderate

SCENERY: Marine fossils, aspen and fir, ski runs, world's longest aerial tramway

EXPOSURE: Mostly shaded

TRAIL TRAFFIC: Popular

SHARED USE: Low (skiing; limited mountain bike and equestrian access; no motor vehicles)

TRAIL SURFACE: Dirt, rock

HIKING TIME: 4 hours

DRIVING DISTANCE: 27 miles

ACCESS: Year-round; day-use fee $3 per car; free with Sandia Mountain Annual Pass or National Parks and Federal Recreation Lands Annual Pass

LAND STATUS: Cibola National Forest

MAPS: Sandia Ranger District; USGS Sandia Crest

FACILITIES: Restrooms (no water) at trailhead; visitor center, tramway terminus, restaurant, restrooms, and emergency phone at Sandia Peak

LAST-CHANCE FOOD/GAS: All services in San Antonito, 6 miles from the trailhead.

GPS TRAILHEAD COORDINATES

Latitude   35° 11' 38"

Longitude   106° 24' 17"

IN BRIEF

This classic hike combines the 2-mile Tree Springs Trail with a 1.6-mile segment of the Crest Trail to reach the upper terminal of the Sandia Peak Tramway. Aspen shades the upper trail to the subalpine mountaintop, where views encompass 11,000 square miles.

DESCRIPTION

In 1936 the U.S. Forest Service cleared the slopes and established a system of trails at Tree Spring to accommodate the fledgling Albuquerque Ski Club. These were the first runs in what would become La Madera Ski Area. By 1946 it expanded to the current location of Sandia Peak Ski Area and featured the nation's longest T-bar lift. A lift ticket cost $1. Diminutive by comparison, the original slopes at Tree Spring were soon considered a mere practice area.

You won't see a trace of ski runs at Tree Spring today, but the fee box standing at the trailhead is hard to miss. A large board displays the usual rules, safety info, and trail map. Nearby signs alternate between the singular and plural of spelling of the trail, but there's no mistaking the way.

Tree Spring(s) Trail (147) starts out as a paved sidewalk that leads straight to the latrines. This unfortunate decision in trailhead management is soon corrected with a right

----

Directions

From I-40 East, take Exit 175 toward Cedar Crest. From the I-40 overpass, go north 5.9 miles on NM 14. Turn left on NM 536 (Sandia Crest Scenic Byway) and follow it 5.7 miles up to the Tree Spring parking area on the left.

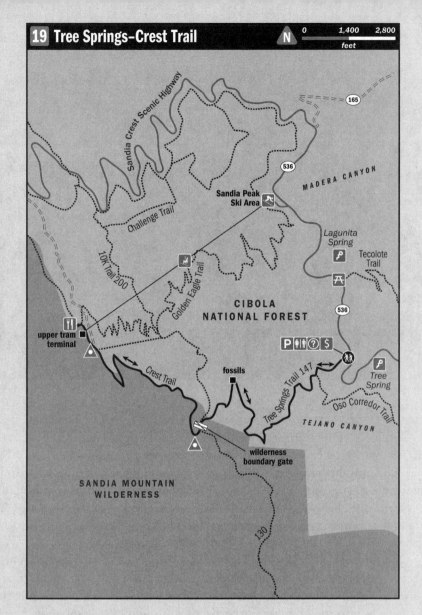

N

0   1,400   2,800
feet

165

Sandia Crest Scenic Highway

536

MADERA CANYON

Sandia Peak
Ski Area

Challenge Trail

Lagunita
Spring

Tecolote
Trail

10K Trail 200

Golden Eagle Trail

CIBOLA
NATIONAL FOREST

536

upper tram
terminal

Crest Trail

fossils

Tree Springs Trail 147

Tree
Spring

Oso Corredor Trail

wilderness
boundary gate

TEJANO CANYON

SANDIA MOUNTAIN
WILDERNESS

130

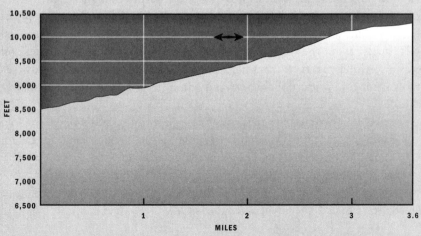

10,500
10,000
9,500
9,000
8,500
8,000
7,500
7,000
6,500

FEET

1   2   3   3.6

MILES

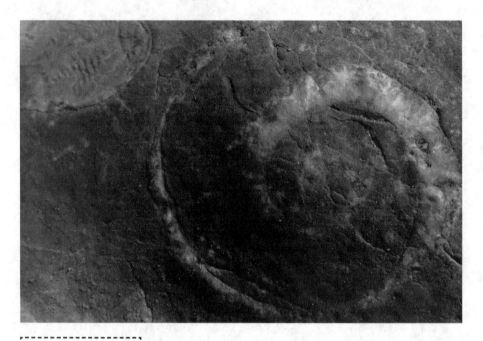

Trilobite and gastropod

turn that puts you back on the original broad path of hard-packed dirt. About 0.75 mile into the hike, it gets rocky and crooks to the left at a faded path that climbs straight up. Just ahead on the left is the marker for Oso Corredor (265), semi-Anglicized here as Oso Corridor. This easy, though occasionally soggy, 2.7-mile side trail was named for the numerous black-bear sightings in its inaugural season in 1989, a particularly dry summer in the Sandias.

Fine attention to grooming Tree Springs Trail shows on its steeper sections, where erosion might otherwise erase it. Credit the Adopt-a-Trail volunteers who cast aside large stones and terraced the grounds to facilitate your ascent. Just over a mile into the hike, the forest opens to meadows that thrive with wild-flowers in warmer seasons. After 1.5 miles, the Sandias' limestone cap pokes through the soil. Look closely at the smooth gray rock for marine fossils. Gastropods (snails) about the size of a quarter are the easiest to spot. Trilobites and crinoids also riddle the rock from here to the peak. Visitors often ask how sea creatures managed to cross the desert and climb these mountains. The answer lies ahead.

For now, a bigger mystery: the limestone is part of the 300-million-year-old Madera group. Beneath it is Precambrian granite that dates back some 1.4 billion years. It seems a few intermediary layers have gone missing. Landscapes often lose bits of their geologic records. Such absentmindedness is called an "unconformity." The Sandias, however, blacked out for more than a billion years in what geologists worldwide refer to as "The Great Unconformity."

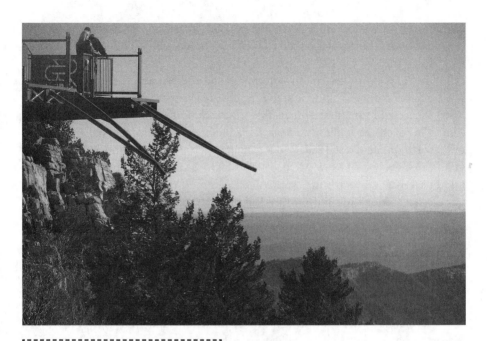

Upper terminus of Sandia Peak Tramway

Tree Springs Trail nears its end at the boundary of Sandia Mountain Wilderness, marked with a wooden post fence and signs reminding you to check your chainsaws, motorized vehicles, bicycles, and hang gliders at the gate.

Alternate routes: The 10K Trail extends to the right. If you prefer a loop in your route, follow its blue diamonds to the ski slopes. Turn left at the first ski run and climb about 0.5 mile uphill to the tram terminal. Beware of high-speed bikes when crossing Golden Eagle Trail. For the return segment, follow the Crest Trail back to the wilderness-boundary gate. Just be sure not to miss this turn back onto Tree Springs Trail or you'll end up following the Crest Trail down to Canyon Estates, 13 miles to the south—or farther. The Crest Trail is part of the Grand Enchantment Trail, a hiking route between Albuquerque and Phoenix, so you could extend your hike another 700 miles.

The **Crest Trail (130)** is just beyond the gate. To stay on the planned route, continue straight ahead about 600 yards to the edge of a precipitous drop-off. It's a good spot for a snack break as the next 2 miles are a little strenuous.

Refueled and ready to roll, backtrack halfway to the gate, and turn left to resume north on the Crest Trail. Pass through dense stands of mature fir, intermittent groves of aspen, and colonies of mushrooms and lichens. The green shaggy growths resembling Spanish moss are an unrelated plant known as "old man's beard."

After a couple of long switchbacks, the trail runs near the ridgeline. Opportunities abound for short detours to secluded overlooks. If the wind dies down for a moment, you'll hear the hum of the tram's pulley system. Follow that sound and you'll soon emerge from the woods at the top of the ski trails. The red benches and blue poles of the chairlifts are impossible to miss, as is the steep view down the slopes.

The stairs up to the tramway terminal and the restaurant are by the second lift. Once on the wooden deck above, you've reached an altitude nearing 10,400 feet—squarely in subalpine spruce–fir forest archaically known as the Hudsonian Zone. To reach the highest point in the Sandias, you'd have to hike another 1.8 miles north on the Crest Trail. Peaking at a mere 10,678 feet, Sandia Crest doesn't quite crack the list of New Mexico's 100 highest summits. But if you're a dedicated peak-bagger, go for it.

Three stations located on the deck identify peaks and landmarks in every direction. On an average day, the view overlooks 11,000 square miles—essentially everything within 60 miles of Albuquerque. They're also enjoyable from inside the adjacent restaurant. High Finance serves up hearty fare and magnificent microbrews. (*Warning:* Alcohol packs a stronger punch at this altitude.) On summer weekends and holidays, an outdoor grill lures hungry hikers from all over the mountain.

The Sandia Peak Tramway is the main attraction. At 2.7 miles, it's the world's longest aerial tramway. The longest span between towers is 7,720 feet, and a tramcar at midspan hangs 900 feet above the ground. "Flights" depart every 20–30 minutes, in all seasons, about 10,500 times per year, and have carried more than 9 million passengers since 1966.

At the upper tram terminal, the Four Seasons Visitor Center (open spring, summer, and fall) contains interpretive exhibits on natural history, including an explanation of how fossilized sea creatures ended up atop these mountains.

Note: If any hikers in your group balk at a trail with a 2,000-foot gain in elevation, consider dropping them off at the Sandia Peak chairlift and meeting them at the top. The chairlift runs scenic rides on summer weekends and holidays, and during Balloon Fiesta in October. Mountain bikers can also ride up with their bikes to take advantage of 8 miles of downhill singletrack. The chairlift starts from the Sandia Peak Ski Area base lodge, 1.3 miles up the road from the Tree Springs trailhead. Also note that the trails in the ski area tend to stay open when the Forest Service trails shut down for drought-mandated closures. For more info, call (505) 242-9052 or visit **sandiapeak.com**. Check with the Sandia Ranger District for local road and trail conditions in the winter and fire danger updates in the summer: (505) 281-3304 or **fs.usda.gov/cibola**.

NEARBY ACTIVITIES

At least a dozen official trails start near the Sandia Crest Scenic Byway. **Tecolote Trail (264)**, a nicely shaded ridgeline route that features a mineshaft, is a relatively flat 1.3-mile out-and-back with a turnaround loop at the end. The trailhead is at the back of the Dry Camp Picnic Ground, 0.5 mile up on the right from the Tree Spring parking area.

GOLDEN OPEN SPACE 20

IN BRIEF

"Best-kept secret" is the worst cliché, but the City of Albuquerque kept this one hidden in a neighboring county for more than 40 years. Established trails now allow you to walk the rim above San Pedro Creek and Arroyo Seco. Newer trails explore these deep-red drainages.

DESCRIPTION

The City of Albuquerque acquired this 1,200-acre parcel in Sandoval County in 1964 under the federal Recreation and Public Purposes Act, which required the city to develop it for recreational purposes or return it to the BLM. Early plans for the property had it slated as a campground, one of several that would form a camping ring around the city. The idea never reached fruition. In retrospect, it's probably best it didn't.

Set aside for the preservation of nature, the land has since remained relatively undisturbed. Viewing it from La Madera Road, you might guess it extends for miles as monotonous grazing lands, but a short hike beyond the fence reveals a fascinating corrugated landscape.

The Golden Open Space appears on maps not as public land but rather as an anonymous parcel 6 miles west of its namesake

Directions

From I-40 East, take Exit 175 toward Cedar Crest. From the I-40 overpass, go 6.9 miles north on NM 14. Turn left on La Madera Road and go 9.5 miles to the signed gate on the right. *Note:* The first 7.5 miles of La Madera Road are paved but narrow and twisty, and can be difficult in winter conditions. The remaining 2 miles are gravel and dirt but adequately maintained and fairly level.

KEY AT-A-GLANCE INFORMATION

LENGTH: 2.25-mile loop; 5.6 miles with spurs

DIFFICULTY: Easy (moderate with spurs)

SCENERY: Views of multiple mountain ranges; mesa-rim overlooks of the Arroyo Seco and San Pedro Creek

EXPOSURE: Little shade above; canyon shade below

TRAIL TRAFFIC: Moderate

SHARED USED: Moderate (mountain bikers, equestrians; pets must be leashed; no motor vehicles)

TRAIL SURFACE: Packed dirt, sand

HIKING TIME: 1-hour loop; 3 hours with spurs

DRIVING DISTANCE: 31 miles

ACCESS: Daylight hours

LAND STATUS: Albuquerque Open Space

MAPS: USGS Hagan

FACILITIES: None

LAST-CHANCE FOOD/GAS: All services in San Antonito on NM 14, about 16 miles from the trailhead.

SPECIAL COMMENTS: The trail system at the Golden Open Space is an ongoing project. For updates, contact the Albuquerque Open Space Division at (505) 542-5200 or visit cabq.gov/openspace.

GPS TRAILHEAD COORDINATES

Latitude	35° 16' 18"
Longitude	106° 19' 42"

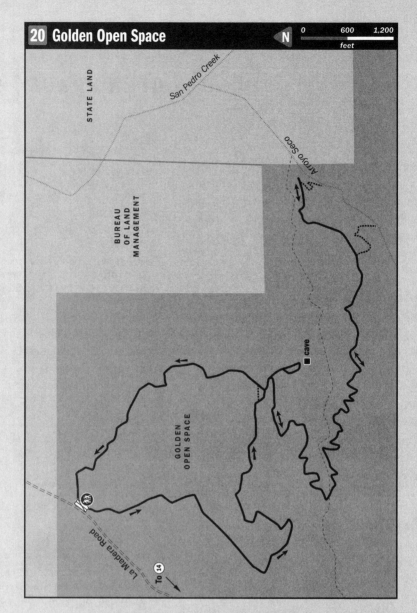

N

| 0 | 600 | 1,200 |

feet

STATE LAND

San Pedro Creek

Arroyo Seco

BUREAU OF LAND MANAGEMENT

GOLDEN OPEN SPACE

■ cave

La Madera Road

To 14

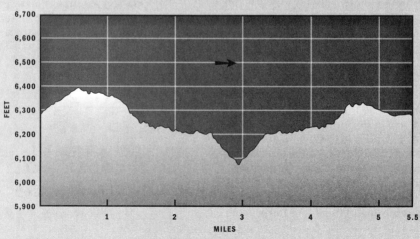

FEET

6,700
6,600
6,500
6,400
6,300
6,200
6,100
6,000
5,900

1   2   3   4   5   5.5

MILES

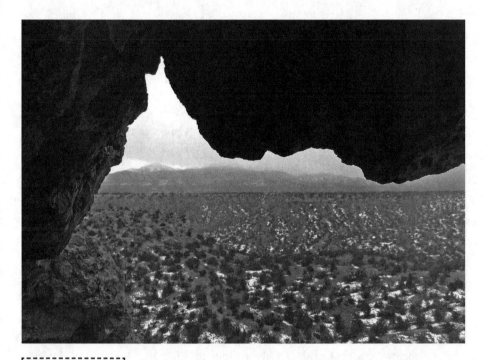

A cave with a view

ghost town. I had driven along its barbwire fences perhaps a half-dozen times in as many years, assuming it was private ranchland. But then small OPEN SPACE signs mysteriously appeared on the posts of its padlocked gates. Later, pink survey flags sprouted from the gritty earth, forming a dotted line that wended through juniper savanna. Weeks passed, and the flags were replaced with a freshly scraped path marked with cairns. Unable to locate anyone to take credit for the trail work, I reached the only logical conclusion: the land was beset with *los duendes.*

Some people describe them as industrious elves, others as evil dwarfs. In his 1910 paper "New-Mexican Spanish Folk-Lore," Aurelio Macedonio Espinosa identified *los duendes* as "individuals of small stature who frighten the lazy, the wicked and in particular the filthy." Their origins and motives remain a mystery.

In August 2007, I led a reconnaissance expedition to inspect their progress. Our extensive fieldwork unearthed several pertinent details, the most important of which is this: August really isn't the best time for extensive fieldwork in the Golden Open Space. It's insanely hot. Quite frankly, I don't know how the evil dwarfs can stand it.

The hike begins at a GOLDEN OPEN SPACE sign behind an equestrian access gate. Rules for the Open Space are posted nearby.

A groomed trail runs south up a gently sloping plain. After 0.6 mile of ordinary juniper scenery, the trail arrives at an overlook on the cusp of Arroyo Seco. The main channel of the arroyo heads from the eastern side of Capulin Peak, about 5 miles southwest of the overlook. Once it crosses La Madera Road, numerous tributary washes emerge and converge, creating the vast drainage network before you. At the point due south of the overlook, it's more than 1 mile wide and nearly 200 feet deep, and it is divided into four or five major channels. At an elevation of 6,400 feet, this overlook is the highest point in the hike.

If you plan to explore the drainages, this overlook will make a useful reference point for navigation. To help you recognize it later, take a moment to study nearby details and try to visualize them as viewed from below.

Continuing with the hike, follow the trail along the mesa rim. At 1.2 miles, the trail splits. The left fork is your option for an easy 2.25-mile loop. The right fork leads to a better hike. About 100 yards later, the trail splits again. This time the left fork starts on a narrow quarter-mile loop out to a cave just beneath the rim. It's a little tricky to reach. Follow the rim to the southernmost tip of the overlook, then turn east and look for an easy way to reach the shelf below. Within a few yards, you should find a point where the descent won't require a scramble. Once on the shelf, turn right. If you don't spot it in less than a minute, you probably descended too far. If you still can't find it, no worries. It's easy to spot from the trail below. It's no Carlsbad Caverns, but it is big and airy enough for five sweaty hikers to kick back in shaded comfort. (I've also taken refuge here from sudden storms, both summer and winter.) Though the ceiling is smudged from past campfires, both camping and fires are prohibited at the Golden.

Loop back around to the last fork and consider this 1.7-mile spur carefully. It's not easy, but it leads to the best part of the Golden. It begins with a steep drop west toward the Arroyo Seco. The earth darkens to rust red as the trail rounds the first headcut and stays above the drainages. It's the perfect singletrack for beginner to moderate-level mountain bikers. Toward the end of the spur are two short trails that dip down to the Arroyo Seco. You can use these, along with the streambed itself, to add a loop to the end of the spur, and about a quarter-mile to the overall hike.

Pedestrians might be more impressed with a hike down the streambeds. I've explored them countless times without once repeating the same route. They trench deeper and steeper as they cut east toward San Pedro Creek. The colors and contours make it worth revisiting again and again. One caveat: transfer between drainages and trail only where they intersect. Shortcuts between the two are the quickest way to get disoriented. Also, backtracking is your best option to save both time and the land itself. High-desert vegetation—the kind you'll encounter on most hikes in this book—looks tough, but it's extremely fragile. It doesn't take much foot traffic to create competing paths. Also, cryptobiotic soil is particularly sensitive. This crusty black layer is a balanced community of mosses, algae, microfungi, and bacteria. It binds sandy soil, keeping it from eroding, and it helps seedlings gain footholds in the ground. Watch your step when hiking off-trail in arid lands— a single misstep can wipe out centuries of growth.

Losing yourself in the tributaries of the Arroyo Seco is half the fun. Just be sure to hang on to enough of your bearings to find your way back to the trail that brought you down here, and leave yourself extra time to follow it back to the loop above the rim. The Open Space trail crew, aka "Los Duendes," promises many more miles of great trails like these over the next few years. They also insist that they are *not* evil dwarfs, but rather industrious gnomes who summon their superpowers from Pulaskis, Mattocks, and McLeods.

NEARBY ACTIVITIES

La Madera Road (also appearing on maps as Madera Road, Hagan Road, Indian Route 844, and County Highway 53) deteriorates quickly with a little rain or snow. But if conditions are good, reset your odometer at the Golden Open Space gate and continue north. The sites listed below are on private land but can be viewed from the road.

1.8 miles: A few rock walls are all that remain of a forgotten settlement on the right.

4.2 miles: The ruins of Hagan appear on the east bank of the Arroyo Tuerto. In the mid-1920s, the town boasted a grand hotel, a train station, and a mercantile store, but by 1950 Hagan was officially a ghost town.

5.1 miles: Petroglyphs can be found in the facing cliff almost within reach from the road. Look for the shapes of deer or antelope. One of the more curious works features a head with a pair of lollipop-shaped extensions. Is it an Indian with a feathered headband? An insectlike character stemming from Anasazi mythology? Evidence of a prehistoric visitation from antennaed aliens? Interpretation is open to debate.

7.5 miles: The little town of Coyote emerged in anticipation of the Hagan Spur of the Rio Grande Eastern Railroad. The train finally arrived in 1924—three years after citizens of Coyote had given up waiting for it. A few rock foundations remain on the right, along with pieces of off-white bricks stamped TONQUE.

8.8 miles: The ruins of Tonque Brick Factory are on the left, near the site of a precolonial pueblo of the same name. The road soon crosses onto the San Felipe Reservation and continues 5 miles to the Casino Hollywood on I-25, about 20 miles north of Albuquerque.

21 CERRO COLUMBO

GPS TRAILHEAD COORDINATES

Latitude   35° 14' 27"

Longitude   106° 12' 33"

IN BRIEF

A web of old roads and a little bushwhacking make up this route through the western hills of the San Pedro Mountains. Riddled with holes and scraped to the bone, this stout, rugged range bore the brunt of gold fever.

DESCRIPTION

The San Pedro (formerly Tuerto) Mountains stand near the south end of a mining belt that has endured at least 10,000 years of continuous human occupation. Evidence of early mining activity includes remnants of an ancient Native American copper-smelting industry found in the Canon del Agua, near to the west of Cerro Columbo.

In 1839 the Mexican government awarded the San Pedro Land Grant to families in the area, hoping that development here would deter Plains Indians from raiding the main settlements farther west. That same year, gold was discovered in the mountain streambeds. Two history books published in the late 19th century mention a nugget weighing 11 pounds, 9 ounces, found by a Pueblo Indian, who traded it for "a little whisky, a blind pony, and a crownless hat."

Mining settlements sprang up overnight and quickly developed into formal town sites with hotels, mercantile stores, and saloons.

Directions ⟶

From I-40 East, take Exit 175 toward Cedar Crest. From the I-40 overpass, go 16 miles north on NM 14 and turn right on NM 344. Drive 0.9 mile southeast and turn left at the double gate. Drive about 0.2 mile northeast on this dirt road. Park in a clearing near the five-way intersection.

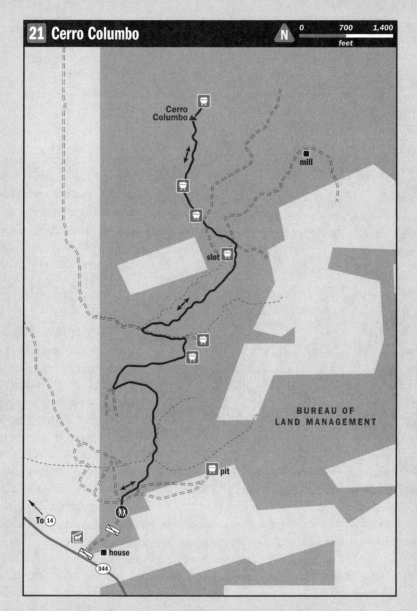

N

0   700   1,400
feet

Cerro
Columbo

mill

slot

BUREAU OF
LAND MANAGEMENT

pit

To 14

house

344

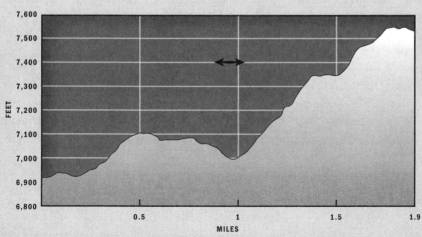

7,600
7,500
7,400
7,300
7,200
7,100
7,000
6,900
6,800

FEET

0.5   1   1.5   1.9

MILES

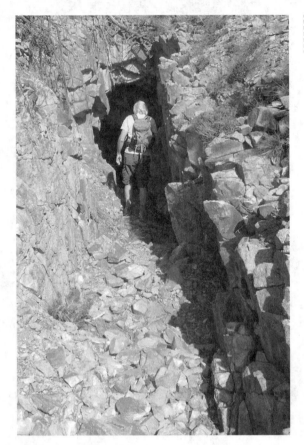

Slot mine

Within a decade, miners scalped the peaks of their natural surface terrain and essentially transformed the slopes into giant prairie-dog colonies. An 1849 report estimated the annual output of gold at $500,000, or $13 million in today's dollars.

In July 1880, President Ulysses S. Grant, on leave from politics and fast approaching bankruptcy, came to examine prospects in the San Pedros. He left discouraged. In a letter to a leading stockholder in the San Pedro Mining Company, he cautioned: "Every valuable claim in New Mexico, particularly those held under Spanish Grants, will be embarrassed by lawsuits of some sort." Indeed, litigation over property ownership and mineral rights was rampant, but the biggest challenge to working the ground was the scarcity of water. Shortly after World War I, large-scale operations ceased and town sites were razed.

In recent years most residents of the San Pedro community have consistently opposed attempts to revive mining operations, but they have no jurisdiction over 2,200 acres of BLM land in the San Pedro Mountains. Yet for decades this chunk of public land was available for recreation in theory only. A ring of private holdings kept it strictly off-limits, making the San Pedro Mountains the missing link in Santa Fe County's master trail plan.

The private stranglehold on public land did not escape the notice of the BLM–Taos office. Their plan for securing a public-access corridor was more than 20 years in the making, but on November 19, 2010, they succeeded in obtaining a 30-foot-wide ribbon of land totaling 2.96 acres—the piece that connects Highway 344 with the mountain interior.

The hike begins at a multiple junction about a quarter-mile northeast of Highway 344. Two gravel roads are on your right. Start northeast on the second one. Within 100 yards or so, turn left, then bear left at the fork just ahead. Stay on the main road as it crosses a couple of dry washes and passes numerous mines. It soon climbs north, then hooks west onto a ridgetop. About 0.5 mile into the hike, you arrive at a junction. Take a sharp right to stay on the ridgetop road. Also take a look back at the junction so you'll recognize it on your return.

The ridgetop road ends at a mine surrounded by tree debris. It's time to trailblaze. Turn left and bushwhack north about 250 feet downhill until you reach the road below. The road runs on the near side of a streambed. You'll find several mines in the area, along with signs of prospecting that seems both recent and unorthodox. Among the repurposed items I encountered were folding chairs, a wooden yoke, and a bathtub. Whatever oddities you find here should certainly help you recognize the way back.

Turn left and follow the road downstream to a Y-junction, where you'll take a sharp right and start a steep climb northeast. Stick to the right at a Y-junction near the top. As the road levels out, look down to your left for a slot. It leads to a horizontal shaft that extends through rock directly beneath your feet.

Turn left at the junction just ahead. Take a good look around and memorize the turn, because it's the easiest one to miss on the way back. Proceed about a quarter-mile northwest. Just before the road bends right and heads downhill, look for a campfire ring in the clearing on the left. Continue straight past it, going off road to climb the hill. About a quarter-mile up, cairns mark the 7,572-foot summit of Cerro Columbo. A stamp mill stands out among the abandoned structures in the valley to the immediate east. The view also includes San Pedro Mountain peaking at 8,242 feet, less than a mile southeast. Placer Mountain, the high point of the Ortiz, stands at 8,897 feet, 6 miles north-northeast.

The plan at Santa Fe County Open Space shows the San Pedro Mountains as the hub of a multiuse nonmotorized system with trails radiating south to Edgewood, north to the Pecos Wilderness, and west to the Sandia Mountains. With the access corridor finally secure, the Open Space program's vision is positioned to become a reality for future generations to enjoy. For now, you can visualize the glory of it all here on the peak of Cerro Columbo. First look for South Mountain, which tops out at 8,650 feet, about 5 miles south. Edgewood is another 8 miles south. Now look for Sandia Crest. It's the one rising to 10,678 feet, 14 miles west. And finally, look to the Santa Fe Mountains, the massive cluster on the horizon 35 miles northeast. That's the near side of the Pecos.

22 CERRILLOS HILLS STATE PARK

KEY AT-A-GLANCE INFORMATION

LENGTH: 4.6-mile loop with spurs

DIFFICULTY: Moderate

SCENERY: Rolling hills, canyons, abandoned mines, various reptiles

EXPOSURE: Some canyon shade

TRAIL TRAFFIC: Moderate

SHARED USE: Moderate (popular with equestrians; upper trails are suitable for mountain biking, but the canyon segments are too sandy; no motorized vehicles)

TRAIL SURFACE: Sandy streambeds, dirt trails

HIKING TIME: 3 hours

DRIVING DISTANCE: 55 miles

ACCESS: Sunrise–9 p.m. daily; $5 per vehicle or NMSP pass

LAND STATUS: State park; BLM–Taos Field Office

MAPS: USGS Madrid

FACILITIES: Restrooms (no water) at main parking area; Visitor Center in Cerrillos

LAST-CHANCE FOOD/GAS: Convenience store—gas stations on NM 14, about 26 miles south and 7 miles north of Cerrillos. Cafe and bar in Cerrillos.

SPECIAL COMMENTS: For special events and other park info, contact the CHSP office: (505) 474-0196 or www.emnrd.state.nm.us/SPD/cerrilloshillsstatepark.html.

GPS TRAILHEAD COORDINATES

Latitude   35° 26' 57"

Longitude   106° 08' 27"

IN BRIEF

Cerrillos Hills State Park is divided into two distinct areas. In the northwest corner, an unmarked network of canyons, closed dirt roads, and horse trails create several possibilities for extensive wandering between Waldo Canyon Road and Grand Central Mountain. The map and **Exploratory routes** section that follow focus on navigating that area. In the heart of it, trails are well marked and stocked with enough interpretive signage for a dissertation on local history and geology. The **Interpretive trails** section outlines a recommended loop there.

DESCRIPTION

To fully appreciate the appeal of Cerrillos Hill State Park, you need to go back, oh, let's say 30 million years. That's about when the Rio

----

Directions ———————————→

From I-40 East, take Exit 175 toward Cedar Crest. From the I-40 overpass, go 32 miles north on NM 14 and turn left onto Main Street toward Cerrillos. Once in the village, turn right at the first stop sign onto First Street. Cross the railroad tracks, take an immediate left onto CR 57 (Waldo Canyon Road), and go 1.3 miles northwest. (If you cross a cattle guard after the horseshoe curve, you've gone about 0.15 mile too far.) Turn right onto an unmarked dirt road, drive about 500 feet north to a state-park boundary sign, and park by the gravel pit on the left.

Alternate route (50 miles): From I-25 North, take Exit 267 and turn right on CR 57. Drive 6.5 miles south-southeast, then look for the unmarked dirt road on the left about 0.15 mile past the cattle guard. Note that most of Waldo Canyon Road is unpaved and can get tricky in wet weather.

N

0   1,000   2,000

feet

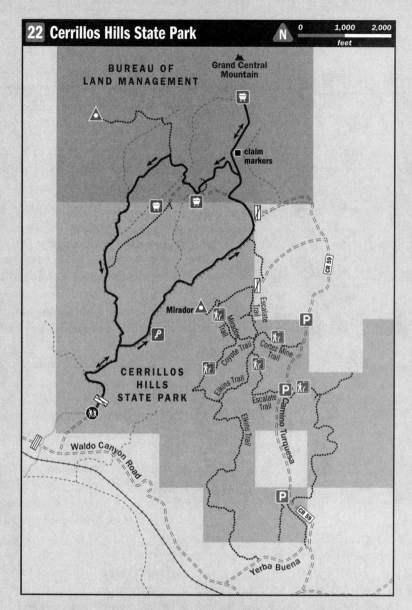

BUREAU OF
LAND MANAGEMENT

Grand Central
Mountain

claim
markers

CR 59

Escalate
Trail

Mirador

Mirador
Trail

Cortez Mine
Trail

Coyote Trail

Elkins Trail

CERRILLOS
HILLS
STATE PARK

Escalate
Trail

P

Camino Turquesa

Elkins Trail

P

CR 59

Waldo Canyon Road

Yerba Buena

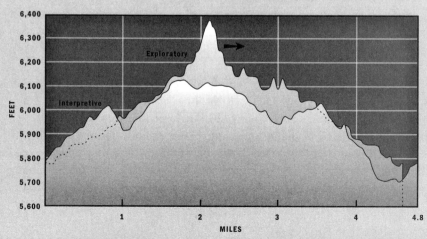

6,400
6,300
6,200
6,100
6,000
5,900
5,800
5,700
5,600

FEET

Exploratory

Interpretive

1   2   3   4   4.8

MILES

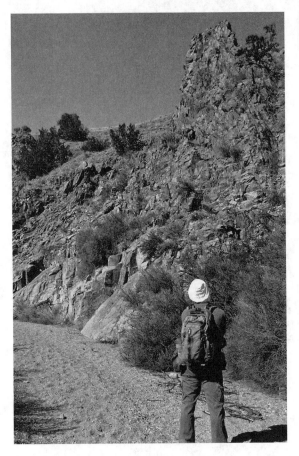

The main canyon provides access to exploratory routes.

Grande Rift yawned, stretched, and ultimately stirred up several deeply embedded laccoliths in what would become Cerrillos Hills. These massive igneous bodies never broke through as volcanoes, but they did fracture the overlying rocks as they rumpled the crust into mountains. Over the ensuing eons, weathering eroded the range down to a chain of cone-shaped hills, while pressured mineral springs flowed into the cracks to form ore veins.

Starting around AD 900, Puebloans began mining veins of blue-green stones. Believed to be an effective evil-repellent, worked turquoise was strong currency in the Rio Grande Valley, particularly at the commerce center now known as Chaco Canyon, about 100 miles northwest. Galena (lead sulfide) further boosted the mining economy when lead-glazed pottery suddenly became a hot commodity.

Credit for this technological breakthrough in ceramics goes to early-14th-century potters at what is now known as San Marcos Pueblo, about 2 miles east of Cerrillos Hills. With a stronghold on the turquoise and pottery markets, San Marcos grew, and pueblo developments filled the surrounding Galisteo Basin over the next few centuries.

The mining activity in Cerrillos Hills did not escape the notice of early Spaniards. Priorities in order, they launched the first silver operation in 1581 and established a mission at San Marcos in 1620. Anglo prospectors began moving in on the digs in 1846 and would assume control over the hills in time for the Cerrillos Mining Boom of 1879–1884. The promise of an industrial future earned Cerrillos the nickname "Little Pittsburgh," but by 1898 a millennium of mining had exhausted the hills. In the wake of the bust, they abandoned numerous towns and camps, and well over 5,000 holes in the ground.

Few commercial operations survived into the 20th century, with all but a gravel mine having closed by the 1960s. In the 1990s, the New Mexico Abandoned Mine Land Program sealed the last of the hazardous shafts.

The 1,100-acre Cerrillos Hills Historic Park opened in 2003. Since then, its developed trail system has grown to exceed 8 miles. In 2009 the State Parks and Recreation Division assumed management and officially reintroduced it as Cerrillos Hills State Park. Aside from the new $5 parking fee at the main trailhead, little has changed as of 2011. The CHSP Visitor Center was completed in 2012.

Exploratory routes begin at the gravel pit. The unmarked road runs up the east side of an alluvial fan that empties into Galisteo Creek, about 0.2 mile south of the gravel pit. About the same distance northeast, the main channel emerges from the mouth of a canyon. A cable gate has been installed here to prevent unauthorized vehicles from entering. Numerous waterways, old roads, and horse trails multiply the possibilities for navigating the rolling terrain beyond the gate.

The scenery changes dramatically once you step inside the craw of the canyon. Rock shelves and overhangs on the walls are inviting for a shaded respite on hotter days. Deep pockets of sand on the canyon floor can slow the pace, so take advantage of rest stops where you can. After a 0.6-mile walk north from the gate, note a prominent sandy wash fanning out from a canyon on the left—that's the branch you'll use to close the loop. For now, bear right to stay in the main canyon. You'll soon encounter a series of low rock dams designed to rehabilitate a small spring. Less than 0.25 mile past the spring, an outcrop resembling a stone wall points downstream. The narrow canyon on the left is worth a quick look. (It's also a shortcut to the capped mine mentioned later in the hike.) To continue on this route, stay right in the main canyon. About 0.4 mile ahead, or 1.5 miles from the cable gate, you'll see a second cable gate on the right and a road rising on the left. Exit the wash and follow the road northwest. Nearby signage indicates the state-park boundary. BLM (public) land lies to the north.

The landscape soon opens to a tangle of interwoven and overlapping old dirt roads and active horse trails. Head uphill about 0.1 mile along the road and go right at the Y-junction. About the same distance ahead, a horse trail starts on the left. To cut a steep spur from this hike, veer left. Otherwise, continue along the road another 0.1 mile. Three wooden posts propped up in rock piles are claim markers. The road from here fades fast as it climbs the mountain. Less than 0.25 mile past the claim markers, down in the arroyo on the left, is a boarded mine that's losing its battle against the elements. A nearby clearing is a good spot to enjoy the views to the south and contemplate your next move.

If you intend to climb Grand Central Mountain, formerly known as Cerro del Oso ("hill of the bear"), the route from here is clear: it's all uphill—a quarter-mile scramble for and elevation gain of about 600 feet. Loose rock and maybe an ornery rattler or two can complicate this last leg of the trip to its 6,976-foot peak. Climb if you must, but give it at least 30 minutes, and be careful not to trample vegetation. The view from the top includes Cerro Bonanza (7,088 feet), about 2 miles north.

The escarpment of La Bajada (Hike 28) starts about 3.5 miles to the northwest and stretches another 4 miles from there. If you've already done that hike, you might find greater appreciation for it here. No other vantage point reveals the enormity of that obstacle quite like the view from Grand Central Mountain.

Go back down the road and return to the junction with the horse trail mentioned earlier. (The route from here gets a little more complicated. If you get off course, just remember that all drainages funnel back down into the main canyon.) Turn right on the horse trail. In about 0.25 mile, it splits three ways. Keep going straight down the middle until you pick up the dirt road again, where you'll see a capped mine and a couple of stern warnings about entering abandoned mines. Turn right on the road. It soon splits, with the left fork climbing a steep hill. Maintain a straight course and cross the wash ahead. From here a well-worn singletrack starts on a 0.8-mile course northwest. For the next half-mile, all drainages on your left feed back into the main canyon, so take your pick whenever you're ready to start closing the loop. If you follow the singletrack to its end, you'll arrive at a spectacular overlook. However, you'll need to backtrack at least 0.2 mile before heading downstream. Otherwise you'll end up in the wrong watershed.

When you return to the main canyon, turn right and follow it 0.5 mile downstream to the cable gate.

Interpretive trails begin at the main trailhead. To get there from Cerrillos, cross the railroad tracks and drive another 0.25 mile to the Y. Bear left onto CR 59 (Camino Turquesa) and go 0.5 mile north, following the signs for Cerrillos Hills State Park.

We need more parks like this, with hikes to exercise both body and brain. Interpretive trails here amount to a seminar in New Mexico culture and natural history. Only instead of a sleep-inducing lecture hall, the classroom is rolling terrain with scenic vistas, high-desert wildlife, and historic mines. A recommended 4.8-mile loop starts at the trailhead across the road from the main parking area. Begin on the steep, wide Jane Calvin Sanchez Trail. Within 1 mile, you'll pass three fenced mine shafts then descend to the springs on Camino Turquesa. A sign here details the mineral and organic contents of the small but vibrant springs. (In summary: don't drink the water.)

Turn left and head down the road about 60 yards to pick up Escalante Trail on the right. After a steep 0.5-mile climb past Cortez Mine Trail, look left for a 60-yard spur to Escalante View, the highest point on this route.

Return to the main trail and continue 0.1 mile north to a fence that crosses the road. Take a sharp left before the gate and follow signs to the Mirador. A sign there identifies the many mountain peaks and ranges in view.

From the Mirador, return to the main trail and turn right. Within the 0.5-mile descent ahead, four mines dot the trailside. Protective mesh allows you to gape into each one without the risk of falling in. When the trail starts uphill again, you have slightly more than a 0.5-mile climb before the sharp drop into Elkins Canyon.

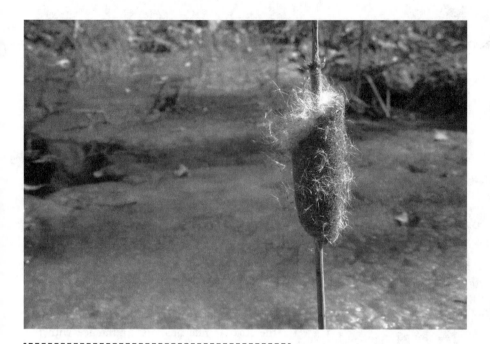

Cattails grow from algae-rich springs on Camino Turquesa.

At the canyon floor, turn right and follow the streambed trail as it squeezes through a rocky chute. When you emerge from the south end, take the first path on the left and follow a 300-yard easement to Yerba Buena (CR 59A). Turn left on this dirt road and go 0.25 mile to Camino Turquesa. Turn left again to go north past the cemetery and return to the parking area.

NEARBY ACTIVITIES

Waldo, a coal-mining town on the Santa Fe Railroad, was named for Henry L. Waldo, Grand Master of the New Mexico Masons (1878) and Chief Justice of the New Mexico Territory Supreme Court (1881). The Colorado Fuel and Iron Company built 15 coke ovens in Waldo in the 1890s but closed the mines in 1906. The town persevered by supplying Madrid with well water, hauling up to 150,000 gallons in rail tank cars per day. As Madrid's mining economy began to falter, so did Waldo. A salvage company purchased the town in 1937 and stripped it down by the end of the 1940s. A couple of structural foundations and ruins of the coke ovens can be spotted from Waldo Canyon Road northwest of the cattle guard.

For more local lore, visit the Casa Grande Trading Post & Mining Museum, at the west end of Waldo Street in Cerrillos. Call (505) 438-3008 or visit **casa grandetradingpost.com.**

23 CAÑADA DE LA CUEVA

KEY AT-A-GLANCE INFORMATION

LENGTH: 7.4-mile out-and-back

DIFFICULTY: Moderate

SCENERY: Sinuous arroyos, piñon–juniper hills, views of the Sangre de Cristo and Jemez mountain ranges

EXPOSURE: Some canyon shade

TRAIL TRAFFIC: Low

SHARED USE: Low

TRAIL SURFACE: Sand

HIKING TIME: 3–4 hours

DRIVING DISTANCE: 55 miles

ACCESS: Year-round

LAND STATUS: BLM–Taos Field Office

MAPS: USGS Picture Rock

FACILITIES: None

LAST-CHANCE FOOD/GAS: Restaurants in Madrid, 10 miles from the trailhead; convenience store–gas station in Cedar Crest, 33 miles from the trailhead

SPECIAL COMMENTS: This route follows an intermittent stream that can be hazardous with heavy rainfall.

GPS TRAILHEAD COORDINATES

Latitude   35° 26' 19"

Longitude   106° 01' 07"

IN BRIEF

An unofficial, yet intuitive route follows a dry wash across seldom-visited terrain in the hill country of the Galisteo Basin. Steep rock walls punctuate 20 twists and turns in this fascinating segment of the Cañada de la Cueva.

DESCRIPTION

The Galisteo Basin, as defined by the Galisteo Creek watershed, encompasses approximately 470,000 acres spanning northeast to the Sangre de Cristo Mountains, southwest to San Pedro Mountain, and reaching as far west as the Rio Grande near its confluence with the Santa Fe River.

This vast lowland is a sag in the earth's crust formed where rock layers are depressed and thickened. Runoff from surrounding mountains flows into the basin and carves numerous arroyos, creeks, and cañadas. Throughout New Mexico's fractured landscape, many places use the Spanish word *cañada* to describe a gulch or shallow ravine made by erosion or by volcanic activity.

A 3.3-mile segment of the Cañada de la Cueva snakes diagonally across 2,000 acres of land that's still (tentatively) open to the public.

Stream corridors like this support willow, tamarisk, and cottonwood trees. They also function as convenient avenues for animal life. Local species include frogs, salamanders, antelope, bear, chipmunk, coyote, deer, fox, prairie dog, and rabbit. These avenues are part of

Directions ⟶

From I-40 West, take Exit 175 (Tijeras) and go 36 miles north on NM 14. Turn right on CR 42 and go 3.8 miles east to the San Marcos Station. Park in the dirt pulloff by the gate.

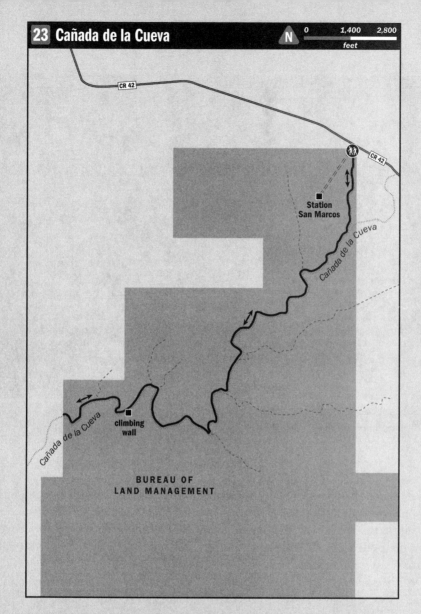

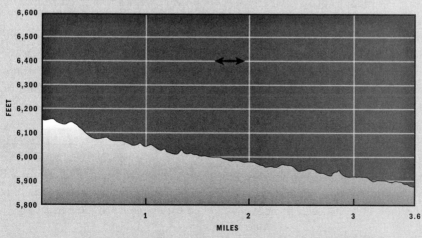

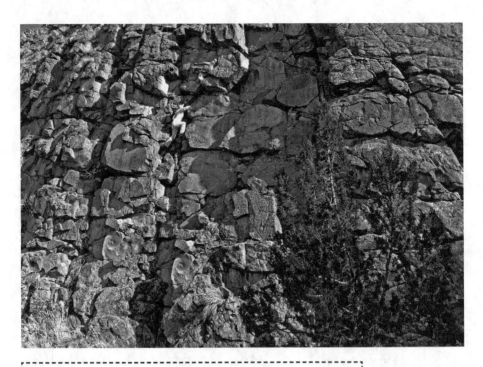

Climbing this so-called climbing wall could be more dangerous than it looks.

a larger migration corridor for wildlife, a kind of mass-transit system that animals use to commute between the surrounding rivers and ranges. Species that prefer aerial routes depend on the flora and fauna below for rest and refueling layovers. The bird checklist includes hawks, eagles, falcons, owls, hummingbirds, and a virtual choir of songbird species.

The popularity of this wildlife corridor owes largely to the relative scarcity of humans. Though it's poised to become Santa Fe's next major subdivision, great efforts are in place to protect what lives here now, as well as things left behind by those who lived here long ago.

Archaeological surveys conducted between 2002 and 2006 turned up more than 180 sites in the vicinity. Innocent strollers would be hard-pressed to distinguish any one of these pueblo mounds from a hole in the ground. The route described below sticks to the streambed to avoid the inadvertent trampling of fragile ruins. If you must wander off-course, please tread lightly. And remember: whatever you find there stays there.

The hike begins at the gate to Station San Marcos, a solid-waste and recycling facility. No, it's not an ideal way to kick off a backcountry trek, but rest assured the scenery soon improves. And don't worry about the fortified gate and reinforced chainlink fence. They're just there to secure the waste station. You need only step over a strand of barbed wire to access land filled with sensitive archeological sites.

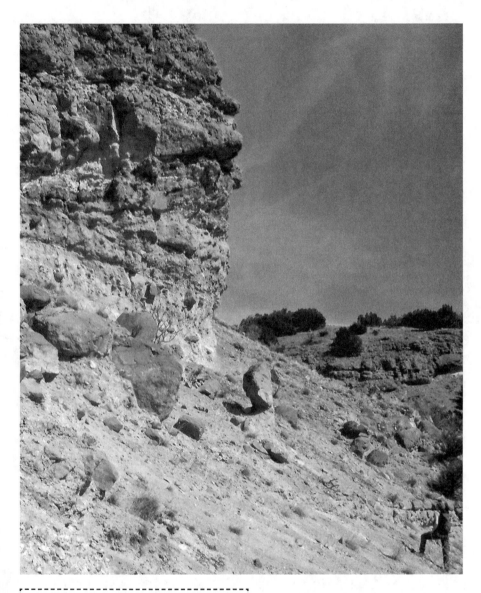

Erosion leaves softer cliffs with a certain character.

A BLM sign reading NO MOTOR VEHICLES marks the trailhead on the left side of the station gate. Start by heading due south on a faint doubletrack. You'll intersect the Cañada de la Cueva in less than half a mile. At this point the streambed is shallow and nearly 200 feet wide. Turn right and follow it downstream. Within minutes you'll pass bulging walls of rock as the arroyo narrows to 20 feet across. It soon widens again, and rock features grow more impressive at every turn. Though the route is simple to follow, what awaits around the next bend is often unpredictable.

About 3 miles into the hike, the arroyo bows northeast, then U-turns south-west. There a solitary hoodoo stands on the right near the base of the steep, white bank. A quarter-mile farther downstream, a dark formation resembling stacked blocks seems perfect for an impromptu climb. A similar wall crops up less than a half-mile downstream. Beyond that, the channel spreads out more than 200 feet across and fills up with chamisa. This is about where you run out of public land, according to the maps. Nothing on the ground indicates the transition to private holdings; however, if you were to keep going another 0.2 mile, you would hit a locked gate with a sign indicating that you're trespassing. And if you made it that far, it's past time to turn back anyway. You've got nearly 4 miles to backtrack to the trailhead, and the slight upward grade on soft sand makes the return notice-ably more difficult than the way down.

On the other hand, if you still have the energy, you'll find many opportuni-ties to exit the arroyo for short scrambles to higher ground. Cliff tops along the embankment are ideal for views over hilly terrain that extend to the Sangre de Cristo and Jemez mountain ranges. Additionally, several tributaries radiate from the main cañada. These tighter drainages also feature rock walls, some with caves that you might enjoy from a safe distance. (If nearby bear scat and mountain lion tracks don't deter you from entering caves, take into consideration that these rocky niches are also ideal for rattlesnakes.)

NEARBY ACTIVITIES

Garden of the Gods is a mini-preview of the park of the same name in Colorado Springs, Colorado. Both feature ancient sedimentary beds tilted vertically by immense mountain-building forces during the Laramide Orogeny, the upthrust that gave rise to the Rocky Mountains. Until recently, visits to New Mexico's version of the garden were confined to a roadside pulloff. Now, the Turquoise Trail Sculpture Garden and Studio is on a mission to make this convoluted landscape accessible to the community through an educational sculpture garden. It's just off NM 14 at Ambush Rock, about 3 miles north of Cerrillos. Tours are available by appoint-ment. Call (505) 471-4688 or visit **www.sculpturegarden.com**.

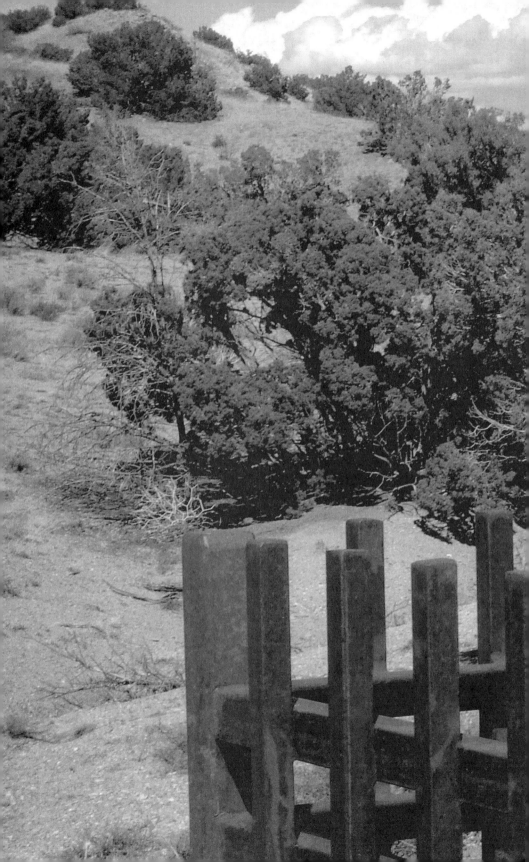

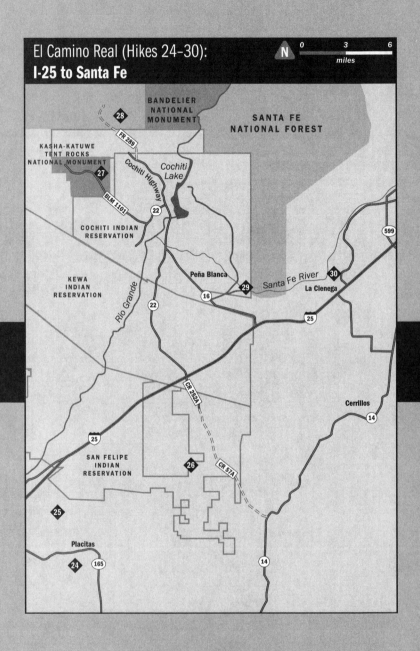

El Camino Real (Hikes 24–30): I-25 to Santa Fe

N

0   3   6
miles

BANDELIER
NATIONAL
MONUMENT

SANTA FE
NATIONAL FOREST

28

FR 289

KASHA-KATUWE
TENT ROCKS
NATIONAL MONUMENT

27

Cochiti Highway

Cochiti
Lake

BLM 1101

22

COCHITI INDIAN
RESERVATION

Rio Grande

KEWA
INDIAN
RESERVATION

Peña Blanca

Santa Fe River

599

30

La Cienega

29

16

22

25

25

CR 252A

Cerrillos

14

SAN FELIPE
INDIAN
RESERVATION

26

CR 57A

25

Placitas

24 **165**

14

EL CAMINO REAL
(I-25 TO SANTA FE)

24 TUNNEL SPRING-AGUA SARCA

KEY AT-A-GLANCE INFORMATION

LENGTH: 9.5-, 7.2-, or 4.5-mile loop options

DIFFICULTY: Strenuous

SCENERY: Canyon and valley overlooks, mixed-conifer forest, seasonal wildflowers, riparian habitat, marine fossils

EXPOSURE: Some forest and canyon shade

TRAIL TRAFFIC: Moderate

SHARED USE: Low (equestrians; closed to all mechanized vehicles)

TRAIL SURFACE: Gravel, packed dirt, loose rock

HIKING TIME: 5–7 hours

DRIVING DISTANCE: 21 miles

ACCESS: Year-round

LAND STATUS: Cibola National Forest–Sandia Mountain Wilderness

MAPS: Sandia Ranger District; USGS Placitas

FACILITIES: Restrooms (no water)

LAST-CHANCE FOOD/GAS: All services available in Bernalillo and Placitas

GPS TRAILHEAD COORDINATES

Latitude 35° 17' 30"

Longitude 106° 26' 22"

IN BRIEF

Three trails of varying designations add up to adventurous loop options on the northern end of the Sandia Mountains. Dizzying overlooks and mountain vistas punctuate this scenic journey.

DESCRIPTION

The route described here links two designated trails to form one big loop. Throw in a third trail—an unofficial shortcut known as Ojo del Orno Route—and your loop options multiply. Consider all possibilities to plan a hike that best serves your interests. For example: to minimize downhill impact on bad knees, follow the hike description in reverse; that is, go up the steep Agua Sarca Trail and return on the gentler Crest Trail.

The Crest Trail (130) begins on the south side of the Tunnel Spring parking area. Start from the gate on the left side of the map and information board. A nearby sign reports the distances to destinations along this majestic trail: Agua Sarca Overlook, 5 miles; Del Agua Overlook, 8 miles; Sandia Crest, 11 miles. In fact, it extends 26 miles to the Canyon Estates trailhead, visited in Hike 11 at Hondo Canyon.

Directions ⟶

From I-25 North, take Exit 242 toward Placitas. Follow NM 165 for about 5 miles east, then turn right on Forest Road 231. (Look for a bank of mailboxes and a green street sign for Tunnel Spring Road on the right. The 5-mile marker is about 50 yards too far.) Follow this steep and rugged dirt road 1.4 miles to its end at the Tunnel Spring trailhead.

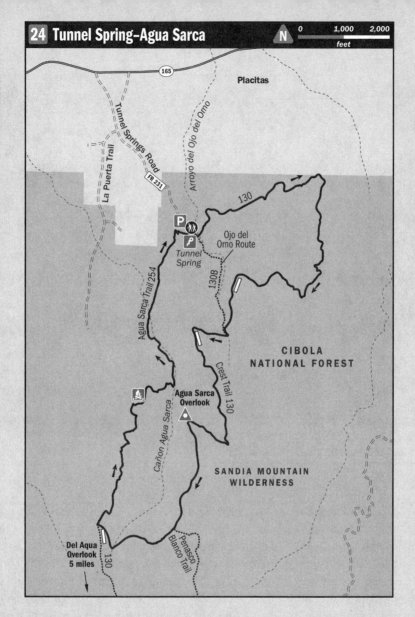

N

0   1,000   2,000
feet

165

Placitas

Tunnel Springs Road

La Puerta Trail

FR 231

Arroyo del Ojo del Orno

P

Ojo del Orno Route

Tunnel Spring

130

130B

Agua Sarca Trail 254

CIBOLA NATIONAL FOREST

Crest Trail 130

Agua Sarca Overlook

Cañon Agua Sarca

SANDIA MOUNTAIN WILDERNESS

Del Aqua Overlook 5 miles

130

Peñasco Blanco Trail

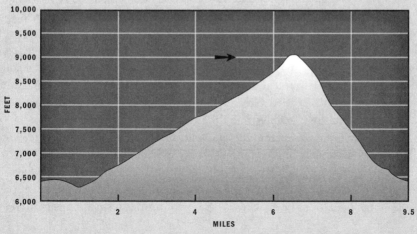

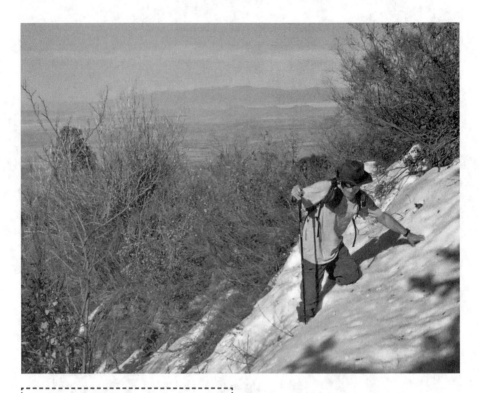

Snow in April is not unusual on the Crest Trail.

A sign indicating the wilderness boundary stands about 100 yards down the trail. Just past the sign, the Arroyo Ojo del Orno crosses the trail. A right turn immediately after the sign puts you on the following shortcut.

The shortcut: If you prefer to cut straight to the action, the 1.1-mile Ojo del Orno route will get your heart (and lungs) pounding in the first 5 minutes. It'll cut 2.6 miles from the big loop, but it's brutally steep. It starts and stays mainly on the right side of the streambed. You'll find a fork about 0.4 mile up. The right branch ends at a nearby mine. As an unofficial route, Ojo del Orno receives no maintenance. It appears as an unidentified line of thin red dashes on the map at the Tunnel Spring trailhead but has been omitted from later forest maps. Although it gets enough use to keep the way fairly clear, you may encounter drainage debris and overgrown vegetation. If you take the shortcut, turn left near the top to climb out of the drainage, and then turn right on the trail above. Resume following the directions from **Crest Trail (continued),** on the next page.

The long way: Some hikers find the first few miles of the Crest Trail somewhat dull, but if you enjoy slow-building drama, this is definitely the way to go.

To resume on the Crest Trail, cross the arroyo and continue past a few more posted signs. The trail roughly follows the wilderness boundary. Look for remnants of mining operations in this area. Ovens used for metal smelting were called *hornos,* for their resemblance to beehives. The name of the aforementioned arroyo, Ojo del Orno, refers to these furnace ovens. Sealed mineshafts and scattered rubble also serve as vague reminders of the mining era.

About 1.3 miles into the hike, the trail rounds the point of a ridge and climbs south. You'll notice a few old jeep roads running near and crossing the trail ahead. Pay attention to cairns and tree-branch edgings to stay on track. A potentially confusing junction sits 2.4 miles into the hike (about 200 yards past a major bend to the northeast). Continue climbing for another 0.5 mile until you reach the east rim of Ojo del Orno, now decidedly a canyon. A stone retaining wall just around the corner makes a convenient bench. Another 0.3 mile south, or 3.4 miles into the hike, the Crest Trail takes sharp right to cross the head of the canyon.

Crest Trail (continued): Just 0.3 mile east of the upper Ojo del Orno, a second stone bench overlooks Agua Sarca Canyon. Though this is not the official overlook, the view is breathtaking. Nearing 7,600 feet, you may notice a drop in temperature, particularly if strong winds greet you at the canyon rim. Say goodbye to the piñon–juniper zone as you prepare to wade through a waist-high canopy of scrub oak. Long pants are a wise choice on this hike, especially in the summer.

The trail angles south-southeast, veering away from the ridgeline for just under a mile, then switchbacks sharply to your right (northwest) to return to the rim at the Agua Sarca Overlook. It's a good 500 feet higher than the last one. Marine fossils are abundant in nearby limestone outcrops. The trail continues roughly south for about 0.8 mile before reaching the northern end of Peñasco Blanco Trail, which dives through thickets of oak on your left. The namesake "white bluff" (more of a gray limestone formation) is visible to the east.

From here the trees thin out, allowing for profusions of wildflowers in the spring and summer. Orange and red versions of the Western wallflower stand out against white blooms of fendlerbush. Near the head of Agua Sarca Canyon, a distinctive boulder is a good place to sit and enjoy the view. About 100 yards or so later, cross the shallow Agua Sarca streambed. Older maps show a path following the west side of the drainage almost all the way back to the Agua Sarca trailhead. If such a route still exists, it would be easier to navigate than the designated trail ahead, but then it probably wouldn't be quite as scenic. Go another 0.2 mile northwest to the next switchback. Those who went the long way are now 6.5 miles into the hike.

Agua Sarca Trail (254): This 3-mile route meets the Crest Trail at the bend in the switchback. There's no marker here, but the low end of a long retaining wall points directly at the trailhead. Turn right and prepare to follow a sporadic path. Give yourself a minimum of 2 hours to complete this section.

Study four different maps of Sandia Mountain trails and you will find as many incarnations of Agua Sarca Trail. Adding to the confusion are scores of small cairns placed by well-intentioned hikers who thought they knew the best way but then gave up at obvious points of uncertainty. On the plus side, all this really means is there's more than one way to get through the canyon.

For the upper portion of the Agua Sarca route, your best bet is to stick to paths closest to the ridgeline. The drop on the other side is a sheer 300 feet or more, and views to the west are spectacular. The path often ducks down to the right (east) to avoid outcrops and dense vegetation, only to vanish momentarily in scrub, exposed limestone, and scree. You should find several opportunities to return to the edge for more views over the Rio Grande Valley. The parting glance comes about 0.8 mile down the line, where a more clearly defined but particularly steep section of trail angles northeastward, deeper into the canyon.

The grade lessens slightly on a brief stretch heading north. (According to a 2006 forest map, Trail 254 crosses through here, with a right turn leading down to the canyon floor. I didn't notice it and so stayed north on the old trail.) A fork soon gives you a choice between a steep path (left) and a steeper one (straight ahead). Both lead to a prominent landmark that's either an elaborate fire pit or a crude stone hearth. A lean-to and other Boy Scout projects are nearby. Exit the east side of the site, and turn left to begin the descent toward the stream below. On this 0.5-mile final approach to the canyon floor, dense vegetation occasionally simulates jungle conditions, and musky aromas heighten your awareness of local wildlife.

Once you spot the stream, you're in the clear. Just turn left (north) and follow it down for the next 0.7 mile, crossing it a few times along the way as the path widens into an old jeep road. (Intersecting roads and trails are easy to ignore on the way down but can be confusing on the way up. Likewise, old mines along this stretch are easy to miss on the way down, but obvious on the way up.) After the third crossing, the road leaves the sandy streambed to climb over a saddle to the northeast. From there it's all downhill to FR 231, where you'll turn right to return to the parking area.

LAS HUERTAS DE PLACITAS 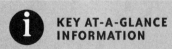 25

IN BRIEF

Near the village of Placitas, this hike relies on natural waterways cut through low rolling foothills in the Las Huertas Basin. The 560-acre Placitas Open Space and 4,000 acres of adjacent BLM land add up to a roomy place to roam in the footsteps of ancient Puebloans, conquistadors, homesteaders, miners, and others.

DESCRIPTION

The village of Placitas has a certain charm that belies its turbulent past. Troubles in the area escalated in the early 1820s with a series of Apache raids on Las Huertas. The walled town was evacuated in 1823, and most families retreated to Algodones, 6 miles northwest. Many returned 17 years later to start over. Struggling to reestablish their community, they called their scattered collection of small farms Las Placitas ("the villages"). But the problems didn't end there.

The 1850s brought a rush of Anglo miners. By the 19th century's end, a violent grudge had developed between Catholics and Presbyterians. But perhaps the most unsettling period started in the 1960s with the arrival of the counterculture movement. What began as experiments in communal

KEY AT-A-GLANCE INFORMATION

LENGTH: 4-mile loop

DIFFICULTY: Easy

SCENERY: Juniper grassland, mountain and mesa views, lizards, rabbits, and maybe wild horses

EXPOSURE: Little shade

TRAIL TRAFFIC: Moderate

SHARED USE: Low (off-road vehicles on BLM segments)

TRAIL SURFACE: Sand, river rock

HIKING TIME: 2 hours

DRIVING DISTANCE: 27 miles

ACCESS: Daylight hours

LAND STATUS: Albuquerque Open Space; BLM–Rio Puerco Field Office

MAPS: USGS Placitas

FACILITIES: None

LAST-CHANCE FOOD/GAS: All services on NM 165 in Placitas

SPECIAL COMMENTS: For information on events involving Placitas Open Space and Las Huertas Creek Watershed Project, contact Las Placitas Association at (505) 867-5477 or lasplacitas.org. You can download the Placitas Open Space Bird Checklist and the List of Flowering Plants from the website.

Directions

From I-25 North, take Exit 242 toward Placitas. Turn right (east) on NM 165 and go 6.9 miles. Turn left on Camino de Las Huertas and go 2.8 miles. Turn left on Palomino Road. Follow this paved road 0.7 mile to a dirt road (Llano del Norte). Turn left and go 0.3 mile to two gates. Go through the first gateway (but not the second one) and turn left. Drive 0.2 mile and park near the green gate at the end of the road.

GPS TRAILHEAD COORDINATES

Latitude 35° 20' 23"

Longitude 106° 27' 38"

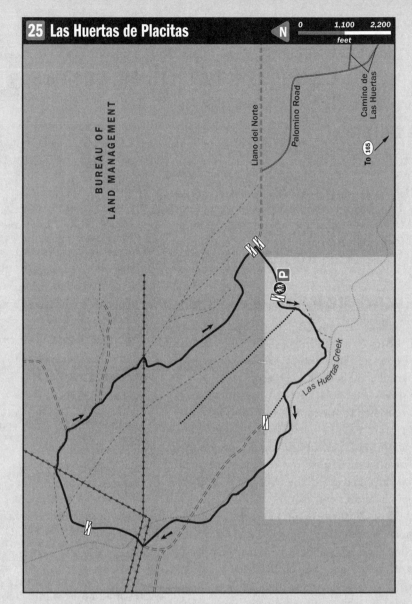

N

| 0 | 1,100 | 2,200 |
feet

BUREAU OF
LAND MANAGEMENT

Llano del Norte

Palomino Road

Camino de
Las Huertas

To 165

Las Huertas Creek

P

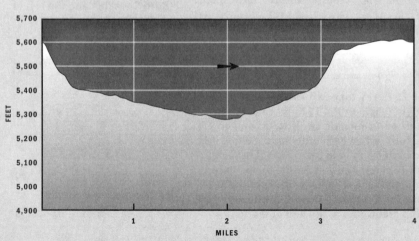

living ultimately devolved into enough drug-addled mayhem to rival that of the Manson Family.

Today the seemingly endless construction of millionaire homes suggests that the curse of Placitas has finally lifted, though some longtime residents would argue that this marks only the beginning of another one. Either way, the ruins of the old and ancient settlements hidden throughout the hills have not been forgotten. Recent area surveys recorded at least 72 archeological sites, not counting hippie ruins. So far, 16 are eligible for the National Register of Historic Places, some dating back 11,000 years. Site locations are not made public, but here's a hint: you'll pass within a whisper of at least three of them and probably won't notice anything more than grass and rock.

The City of Albuquerque acquired these 560 acres near Placitas in 1966 under the federal Recreation and Public Purposes Act, which required the city to develop them for recreational purposes or return them to the BLM. Lacking a hard deadline, they left the property undisturbed for 29 years. In 1995 an Albuquerque resident proposed a shooting range for Placitas Open Space. The proposal was denied, and local community organizations have since assumed a more proactive approach to minding the open space and other public lands along the lower Las Huertas watershed.

Las Placitas Association completed its Open Space Master Plan in 2002, proposing a designated trail system, interpretive signage, picnic shelters, restroom facilities, native revegetation projects, fence removals, and gates affording easier access. As of 2011, little has changed, indicating that priorities strongly favor conservation.

The land north of Placitas Open Space is one of the most desired properties in the BLM's Rio Puerco inventory. At least three Indian pueblos have aboriginal land claims relating to this land. The Wild Horse Association wants to turn it into a horse preserve. Ranchers want to use it for cattle grazing. Oil companies want to drill it. Mining companies want to dig gravel quarries. The Placitas Board of Realtors has asked the BLM to dispose of lands for real-estate development. Hikers, enjoy it while you can.

At the trailhead, views are wide open in all directions. Forty miles northwest, Cabezon resembles a cork in an anthill. Five miles south, the dramatic tilt of the Sandia range is revealed in profile. Las Huertas Creek starts just below Capulin Peak, about 8,600 feet up in the Sandias. The creek runs 15 miles as though aiming toward Cabezon but empties into the Rio Grande near Algodones.

In past centuries, it was a reliable stream that supported populations of elk, pronghorn antelope, gray wolf, and bighorn sheep. Human activity since the mid-1800s has devastated the habitat. In 1906 just 5 miles south of Placitas, local rancher Augie Ellis shot the Sandias' last grizzly bear. The last trout was fished from the pools of Las Huertas Creek sometime in the 1930s. (One of only two perennial streams in the Sandias, the upper creek in Las Huertas Canyon receives an occasional restocking.)

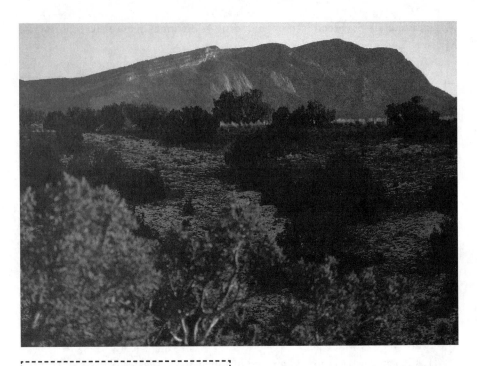

The Sandia Mountains, as seen from Placitas

At least 20 horses have been known to frequent the Placitas environs in the early-morning hours. Their origins are unclear. Some local residents believe them to be descendants of Spanish mustangs. Others regard them as feral nuisances and hope to have them removed.

Animal life today still includes coyote and gray fox. Bald eagle, peregrine falcon, and the rare willow flycatcher have been spotted along the creek. Jackrabbit and cottontail are far more common, and several lizard species run riot in warm months.

The segment of the creek on this hike is about 80 yards wide, on average. While you probably won't find much evidence of water in its sand and cobblestone streambed, it can overrun its banks after a heavy downpour.

The hike begins on the other side of the green gate. A pedestrian-access gate on the right leads to a marked trailhead pointing north. A distinct path heads downhill and soon curves around to a fork. The right branch extends northwest along a ridge (or drumlin, as some folks here see it). It's a pleasant option for a short, easy stroll. This route, however, continues to descend along the left branch and soon braids with a wash. Stick to the right side of the wash until you reach a fading doubletrack. You can turn right here for a slightly shorter hike with even footing, or continue straight to the creek and turn right to explore its wide, cobbled streambed. Both aim for the power lines about a mile downstream, crossing each other and three fencelines along the way.

If you follow the road over to the west side of the creek, be sure to bear right at the Y ahead and follow it back down to the streambed. Directly beneath the power lines, it crosses back over the creek and splits off to the right. Follow it up to a gate 0.25 mile northeast. Stay on the road as it curves around the northwest end of the ridge. Continue east, past a wide draw opening on your right. Go around the end of the next ridge. Directly beneath the utility lines, turn right onto a doubletrack heading into the second draw.

Walk up the wide sand-and-gravel streambed/road southeast 0.7 mile. Once again, directly beneath the power lines, you'll find a doubletrack splitting off to the right. Exit the wash and follow the road straight up the ridge. You'll soon climb high enough to look down into both draws. Take a moment to look behind you for a view of mesa country on the Santa Ana and San Felipe reservations.

After 0.25 mile of steady climbing, the road levels out. Soon you should be able to spot your car through the juniper ahead on your right. Stay on the main road as it bends left. Once past the head of the second draw, the road bends right and leads you straight back to the two gates. Go through the first one (but not the second one), and turn right. Return to the parking area the same way you drove in.

NEARBY ACTIVITIES

Built in the old hacienda style and surrounded by spring-fed orchards, **Anasazi Fields Winery** provides a relaxing oasis for wine tasting and tours. The winery is open Wednesday–Sunday, 12–5 p.m. Special events are held seasonally. To get there from Placitas Open Space, return to NM 165 and go 0.8 mile west to Camino de los Pueblitos. Turn right and go northeast 0.2 mile to the winery. For more information, call (505) 867-3062 or visit **anasazifieldswinery.com**.

26 BALL RANCH

KEY AT-A-GLANCE INFORMATION

LENGTH: 4.6-mile loop, 9.2-mile balloon without gate key

DIFFICULTY: Moderate

SCENERY: Winding canyon, petrified wood, red mesas, hilltop overlook

EXPOSURE: Some canyon shade

TRAIL TRAFFIC: Low

SHARED USE: Low (equestrians, mountain bikers; livestock; limited motor-vehicle access)

TRAIL SURFACE: Sand, dirt

HIKING TIME: 2 hours, 4.5 hours without gate key

DRIVING DISTANCE: 41 miles (one-way) from the I-40/I-25 exchange

ACCESS: Year-round (but see Special Comments)

LAND STATUS: BLM–Rio Puerco Field Office (ACEC)

MAPS: Map available from BLM office; USGS San Felipe Pueblo NE

FACILITIES: None

LAST-CHANCE FOOD/GAS: Convenience store, food, gas at Exit 259

SPECIAL COMMENTS: For roads beyond the gate, a high-clearance vehicle or mountain bike is helpful. Four-wheel drive recommended after wet weather. Pick up a gate key from the BLM office at 435 Montano Road NE in Albuquerque: (505) 761-8700.

GPS TRAILHEAD COORDINATES

Latitude   35° 23' 10"

Longitude   106° 18' 08"

IN BRIEF

Surrounded by tribal lands and accessed by rough easement roads behind locked gates, the trailhead can be a challenge to reach—but it's worth the extra effort. This hike follows arroyos and old ranch roads from the lowest canyon to the highest ridge to give you the full flavor of this seldom-visited public land.

DESCRIPTION

If you use the BLM map to navigate the BLM easement road, you may soon realize the lines don't fully articulate the twisted reality of the roads. Fortunately, signs installed in 2006 effectively spell out where you can and cannot go. Unfortunately, signs in remote areas often disappear or get shot beyond recognition.

If that happens to be the case, use these road directions to get from the locked gate to the drop gate: About 0.8 mile past the locked gate, the road bends south and then arrives at a fork. Bear left and cross the arroyo. Take a sharp right at the junction ahead and go about

----

Directions ———————————→

From I-25 North, take Exit 259 and turn right on County Road 252A (formerly NM 22). Measuring from the top of the northbound exit ramp, go south 5.9 miles to the second gate on the right, marked BALL RANCH. (GPS coordinates for the gate are N 35° 23' 30", W 106° 16' 12".) If you have the key, unlock the gate. *Inspect the gateway area for objects that could puncture tires.* Drive through and lock the gate behind you. Follow the BLM signs 2.2 miles to the drop gate. (See Description for more details.) Unlatch the gate, drive through, and close it behind you. Continue straight (west) 0.1 mile and turn left (south) at the first junction. Go 0.3 mile and park near the windmill.

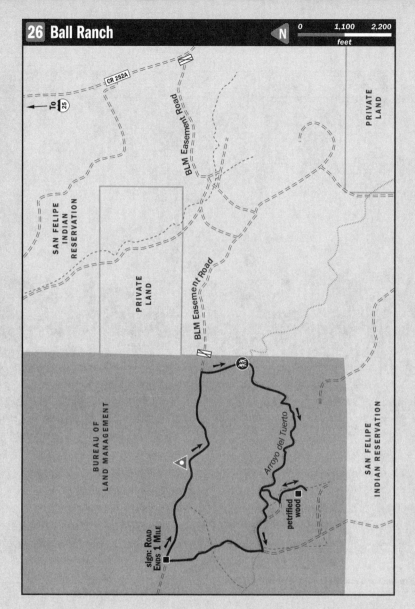

N

0   1,100   2,200
feet

CR 252A

To 25

BLM Easement Road

SAN FELIPE INDIAN RESERVATION

PRIVATE LAND

PRIVATE LAND

BLM Easement Road

BUREAU OF LAND MANAGEMENT

Arroyo del Tuerto

SAN FELIPE INDIAN RESERVATION

petrified wood

sign: ROAD ENDS 1 MILE

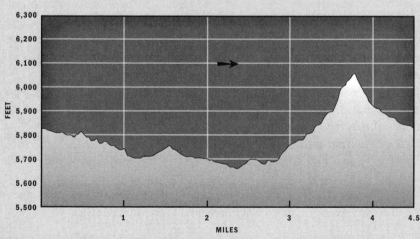

6,300
6,200
6,100
6,000
5,900
5,800
5,700
5,600
5,500

FEET

1   2   3   4   4.5

MILES

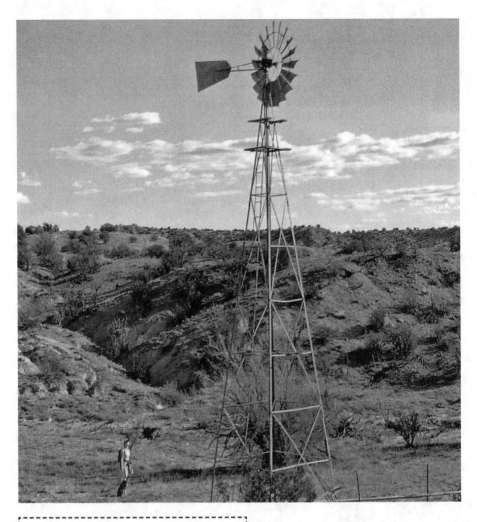

The windmill watches over the Arroyo del Tuerto.

80 yards west to cross another arroyo. Turn left at the junction ahead and go southwest 0.3 mile to the next junction. Take a sharp right, and go 1 mile west-northwest (0.6 mile northwest and 0.4 mile west) to the drop gate. Once through the gate, turn left and go downhill about 0.25 mile to the windmill.

When you reach the parking area, take a moment to get oriented. Check your tires for flats—I've had three in as many visits to Ball Ranch. Note that the last stretch of road you drove down is part of the return loop, as is the road that extends west from the junction and climbs over the hill.

There are a hundred different ways to explore this little BLM venue known as Ball Ranch, and twice as many ways to get lost or inadvertently trespass on tribal land. To keep things simple, this hike is confined to one of three small tracts in the Ball Ranch Area of Critical Environmental Concern (ACEC).

The ACEC status was set in part to protect five rare plants found here, including the Santa Fe milk vetch, a purplish perennial that went missing for a full century (from the 1840s to the 1940s), and the paper-spined cactus, which turned out to be not so much rare as difficult to spot for the way it mimics clumps of grama grass.

The ACEC also protects Stearns' Quarry, a deposit of fossilized wood and bone discovered in the late 1940s. Most of the bones belonged to titanotheres, an extinct group of mammals related to horses. They resembled rhinos with exaggerated horns but grew to the size of Indian elephants. Big as they were, you won't likely find any of their remains on this hike. Pay attention, though, and you'll find loads of petrified wood.

Begin the hike by heading past the windmill, straight into the Arroyo del Tuerto, which runs along the south side of the parking area. Like so many routes in this book, this one depends on both roads and waterways—rarely, however, is it more difficult to distinguish between the two. Despite a nearby sign forbidding vehicles beyond this point, you'll find tire tracks running up and down the wide, sandy wash. Turn to the right and follow them into the canyon ahead, keeping in mind the usual precaution about traveling in arroyos: beware of flash flooding.

The canyon soon narrows, running deep and sinuous as it squeezes between two hills. Look for birds' nests in the pocked walls. Keep an eye on the ground as well. On my first hike through here, I encountered a tarantula the size of a fried egg. It was recently deceased, regrettably, but still quite a surprise on a chilly December afternoon. I returned nine days later, a full week after a good snow, and found only the tracks of rabbits and bobcats.

After walking about 1 mile down the streambed, you'll notice that the canyon shallows and the arroyo straightens. At the top of the last sharp bend, the wall on the right reveals tan, pink, and green striations. Meanwhile, on the left, the wall shrinks down to a low bank. Exit the arroyo there, and pick up a doubletrack running south.

About 0.2 mile from the arroyo shorty after crossing a wash, the road splits. Take a sharp left and follow the road as it crooks southward. The road and wash soon merge and diverge. It's a mess, really, but just continue south, keeping the wash on your right.

About 0.2 mile from the sharp left, the wash shallows down to a sandy bed. You'll see it in a distinct clearing through the juniper on your right. This is where you'll exit the path for a short detour.

Cross straight over the wash and continue west about 200 feet until you see a hillside littered with strange dark rocks, some with a brilliant patchwork of lichen. Closer inspection reveals a woody grain in the stone surface. It doesn't take an expert eye to see they were once trees, albeit several million years ago. (The GPS coordinates for the petrified-wood area are N 35° 22' 52", W 106° 18' 58".)

Return to the Arroyo del Tuerto and continue downstream about a half-mile to an intersecting road. Turn right and follow the main road north 0.6 mile to the

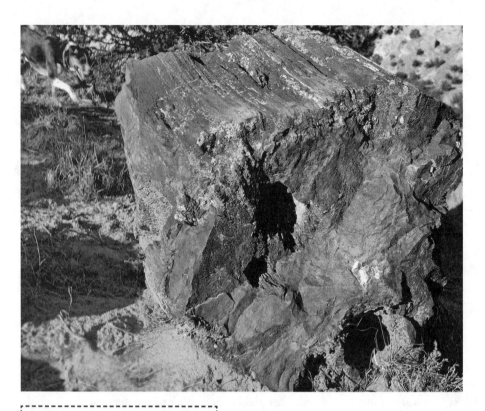

Petrified wood with a patchwork of lichen

BLM easement road. When you arrive at this T-junction, you'll see the backside of a sign that states ROAD ENDS 1 MILE (referring, of course, to the road you just traveled). Turn right and follow the easement road about 0.8 mile to the top of the hill. The views are gorgeous in all directions. It's even better at night, when Santa Fe glimmers to the northeast while the Sandias shield the glow of Albuquerque in the southwest.

To finish the loop, go straight down the east side of the hill and turn right at the bottom to get back to the windmill. (Or, if you parked outside the locked gate, continue straight ahead.)

As you drive out of Ball Ranch, secure both gates behind you. Also check your tires again before getting back on the interstate.

Trivia: Ball Ranch shares its namesake with the Indiana-based Ball Corporation (manufacturers of Ball canning jars) and Ball State University.

KASHA-KATUWE TENT ROCKS NATIONAL MONUMENT

IN BRIEF

Tapering hoodoos up to 90 feet tall are the primary attractions at Tent Rocks. Enter a sinuous slot canyon to admire them from below, then climb high upon a ridge to gaze down upon them. In warm seasons, wildlife comes in furred, feathered, and spiked varieties, and wildflower identification can turn into a full-day affair.

DESCRIPTION

Since it was designated a national monument in 2001, Tent Rocks has seen crowds in the lower Peralta Canyon increase steadily. Although you could arrive to find it virtually deserted, particularly in winter or on a midweek morning, you're almost as likely to find a camera safari or a busload of schoolchildren around every corner.

For now, hiking in the 4,148-acre monument is restricted to a total of 3.2 miles of developed trails. The BLM, in partnership with the Pueblo de Cochiti, is currently working on opportunities for visitors to enjoy other areas of the monument. Recent proposals indicate that an old pumice-mine road and nearby laterals will be converted into foot trails.

An invitational preview of the anticipated routes revealed a typical Pajarito

---

KEY AT-A-GLANCE INFORMATION

LENGTH: 3.3-mile loop and spur

DIFFICULTY: Moderate

SCENERY: Birds and wildlife, seasonal wildflowers, premium hoodoos

EXPOSURE: Some canyon shade

TRAIL TRAFFIC: Popular

SHARED USE: None

TRAIL SURFACE: Packed sand and gravel, bedrock

HIKING TIME: 2 hours

DRIVING DISTANCE: 55 miles

ACCESS: November 1–March 10: 8 a.m.–5 p.m.; March 11–October 31: 7 a.m.–7 p.m. Visitors must be out by closing time. On-site fee is $5 per noncommercial vehicle. Federal Land Recreation Passes are accepted.

LAND STATUS: BLM–Rio Puerco; Cochiti Pueblo

MAPS: Brochure map available at park entrance station; USGS Canada

FACILITIES: Picnic area, restrooms, Cave Loop Trail, and Veterans' Memorial Overlook are wheelchair-accessible.

(See additional information at end of Description.)

Directions

From I-25 North, take Exit 259 toward Peña Blanca. Turn left on NM 22 and go 12.2 miles north to the junction with Cochiti Highway. Turn left to stay on NM 22 another 1.8 miles. Turn right on Tribal Road 92, which connects to Forest Road 266 and BLM Road 1011. Go 0.5 mile west to the fee station. Continue 4.7 miles to the designated parking area on the right.

GPS TRAILHEAD COORDINATES

Latitude   35° 39' 27"

Longitude   106° 24' 41"

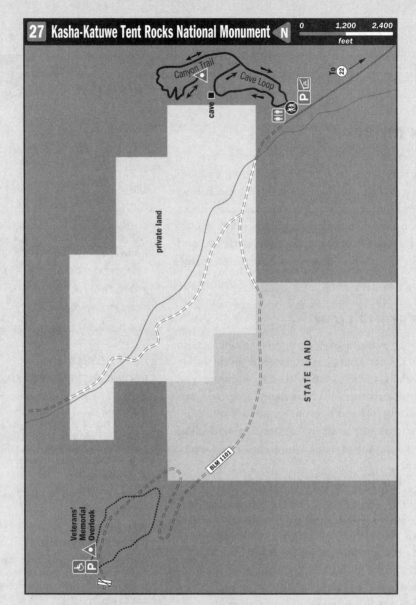

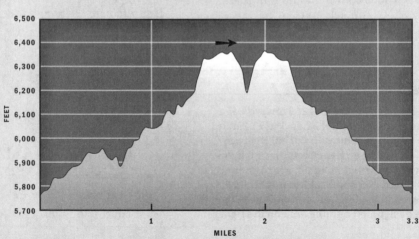

Plateau landscape of juniper and ponderosa. Those who have hiked the main area a dozen times already might appreciate the upper canyon trails when they open. Or if nothing else, the extra space should help disperse the crowds. But if you haven't yet seen the jaw-dropping spectacle in the lower canyon, make it your top priority.

The National Recreation Trail is composed of two segments: Cave Loop Trail and its spur, Canyon Trail. Both segments are well groomed and clearly marked. An information kiosk at the trailhead will further help keep you on the right track.

The big attraction here is Kasha-Katuwe, but there's more to it than the words imply. Meaning "white cliffs" in the traditional language of the Cochiti people, Kasha-Katuwe is packed with fascinating formations. To summarize the complex geologic processes at work: When the Jemez volcanic field erupted 6–7 million years ago, it piled 1,000 feet of pumice, ash, and tuff upon the Pajarito Plateau. Over the ensuing millennia, wind and rain cut into the soft rock layers, eventually carving deep canyons. But in places where durable caprock withstood erosion, it protected the soft rock directly beneath it. The result: hundreds of towering conical spires known as tent rocks, each donning a boulder for a hat. Their shapes resemble tipis and castle towers. When covered in snow, they evoke the soft-serve creations of Tastee Freez. It's a bizarre landscape, to say the least. To see another one like it, you'd need to travel to Cappadocia in central Turkey.

Cave Loop Trail begins at the kiosk north of the parking area and soon splits in two. Take the left path for the long way to Canyon Trail—it leads you through a small party of tent rocks, with the tallest among them standing no higher than a streetlight. These hoodoos have lost their caps and are gradually melting.

As the lesser-traveled of the two trails, Cave Loop is where you're more likely to spot animal life. Ground squirrels, chipmunks, coyotes, and rabbits are prevalent. Also keep an eye out for horned lizards, or "horny toads," in the traditional language of Texans. A member of the iguana family, the short-horned lizard is common throughout much of New Mexico, from desert grasslands to mixed conifer forests and mountain meadows. Colored and patterned to match their environment, these spiked reptiles are difficult to spot unless they're moving, and they often stay perfectly still until they're a step away from getting trampled. In addition to using camouflage and their spiny heads, they can defend themselves by squirting a noxious dose of blood into a predator's eyes and mouth. You'll sometimes find these charming creatures plunging their sticky tongues into anthills.

Located at the top of the loop, the cave is a scooped-out hole in the wall. Its ceiling is charred from ancient woodfires. The trail follows the wall down to a drainage. After 0.7 mile on the loop, you arrive at a T-junction. Turn left into the canyon.

Canyon Trail is easily one of the best short hikes in New Mexico. This 1.1-mile spur features tent rocks up to 90 feet tall, and a slot canyon more than 1,000 feet long. Mind your step in winter—a little snow and ice can turn the narrow,

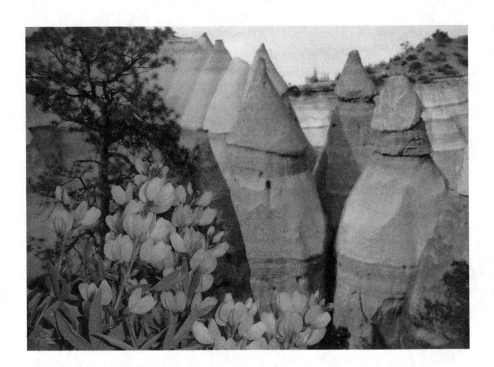

winding segments into a bobsled run. In wide sections, scan the base of the wall for petroglyphs and handprints. It takes a sharp eye to find them. (*Hint:* Pay special attention to the left wall near a stray tent rock paired with a ponderosa.)

In spring and summer, white-throated swifts spend their days careening through the canyon. Unlike swallows, they won't stop to rest until the sun goes down. At night they roost in cantaloupe-sized niches high in the rock walls.

At the head of the canyon, the trail turns steep, climbing 200 feet in 0.3 mile. A couple of steps require some upper-body effort, but if you can climb up on a kitchen counter, you'll manage. When you reach the top, the trail splits. The short spur on the left leads to an overlook. The right branch runs 0.3 mile. Refrain from exploring informal paths along the way. They enter private property to the immediate west. The designated trail descends southeast, culminating with a brief vertigo-inducing ridge traverse to the overlook. There are gorgeous views in every direction. You can also spot the trailhead about 0.5 mile southwest and 500 feet lower than the vista point. To get there, however, you need to backtrack a mile to the mouth of the canyon. From there, continue straight on Cave Loop Trail 0.4 mile to the parking lot.

The Veterans' Memorial Scenic Overlook was dedicated in 2004 to American veterans, with special recognition to those from the Pueblo de Cochiti. This stately terrace perched on the ridge overlooks Cañada Camada ("similar canyon") near its confluence with Peralta Canyon. Views include the Dome Wilderness and Jemez Mountains, and tent rock assemblies in the upper canyon. These ghostly regiments of ashen spires stand on the far side of an unseen river below.

Dead piñon trees surround the overlook. As elsewhere on the plateau, pine-bark beetles (genus *Ips*) have proved themselves merciless throughout the monument. But the manzanita still thrives on cliffs and ridges. This evergreen shrub can be identified from its emerald leaves, red-orange bark, and pinkish-white flowers in warm seasons. Banana yucca, golden pea, and redwhisker clammyweed provide additional color. You can explore this landscape on the Veterans' Memorial Trail. This 1-mile loop, installed in 2010, is broad, relatively flat, and hard-packed, making it suitable for wheelchairs.

Relatively few visitors go to the Veterans' Memorial Scenic Overlook. The road is probably the primary deterrent, though most cars should be fine in dry conditions. From the National Recreation Trail parking area, turn right and drive 3.8 miles up the washboarded road. En route, you'll ford a shallow stream (or dry streambed), then bear left at a fork. About 0.6 mile past the second hairpin turn, pull over into the parking area on the right. Note that a gate along the road is locked an hour earlier than closing time.

NEARBY ACTIVITIES

No doubt you saw Cochiti Dam on the east side of NM 22. It's the world's 11th-largest earth-filled dam. Behind it lies **Cochiti Lake,** a popular area for camping, bird-watching, fishing, swimming, and no-wake boating. Basic food and gas services are available in the nearby town of Cochiti Lake. To get there, return to the junction of NM 22 and Cochiti Highway, where you'll turn left. Access to the lake is 1 mile north on the right. A plaza with a convenience store–gas station is 0.4 mile farther north. For more information, visit **pueblodecochiti.org.**

MORE KEY AT-A-GLANCE INFORMATION

LAST-CHANCE FOOD/GAS: Convenience store–gas station in the town of Cochiti Lake (see Nearby Activities above).

SPECIAL COMMENTS: No dogs allowed at Kasha-Katuwe Tent Rocks National Monument. The monument is subject to closures due to inclement weather and by order of the Pueblo de Cochiti Governor. Check with the Pueblo main office for current conditions or closures: (505) 465-2244. For other information, contact the BLM office in Albuquerque at (505) 761-8768 or nm.blm.gov/recreation/albuquerque/kasha_katuwe.htm.

28 DOME WILDERNESS– BANDELIER BACKCOUNTRY

KEY AT-A-GLANCE INFORMATION

LENGTH: 8.4-mile out-and-back

DIFFICULTY: Moderate–difficult

SCENERY: Rocky canyons, volcanic cliff formations, scorced landspace

EXPOSURE: No shade

TRAIL TRAFFIC: Low–moderate

SHARED USE: Low (equestrians; closed to all mechanized vehicles)

TRAIL SURFACE: Fine gravel, dirt, sand

HIKING TIME: 4–5 hours

DRIVING DISTANCE: 53 miles

ACCESS: Year-round, but note Special Comments on possible gate closures. Permits required for backpacking in Bandelier National Monument.

LAND STATUS: Jemez Ranger District; Bandelier National Monument

MAPS: Santa Fe National Forest– West Half; USGS Canada, Cochiti Dam

FACILITIES: None

LAST-CHANCE FOOD/GAS: Convenience store–gas station on Cochiti Highway, 2.8 miles south of the turnoff for FR 289

SPECIAL COMMENTS: FR 289 is rough, rocky, treacherous when wet, poorly maintained, and subject to weather-related closures.

GPS TRAILHEAD COORDINATES

Latitude   35° 42' 42"

Longitude   106° 23' 03"

IN BRIEF

This rugged wilderness trail from FR 289 to Turkey Springs crosses three canyons and drops into a fourth, visiting massive volcanic formations along the way. You can hit this route's scenic highlights with a 6-mile out-and-back. But if your goal is to sneak through the back door of Bandelier National Monument, be prepared for 8 miles minimum on roller-coaster terrain.

DESCRIPTION

Both the Dome Wilderness and Bandelier backcountry suffered in the 2011 Las Conchas Fire and subsequent flooding, but trails reopened in 2012—much sooner than expected. Trail reports in 2014 started out "good." But then with a robust monsoon season, soon became "poor" with waist- to head-high weeds and extreme erosion in places, making it difficult see at times. The first section from the trailhead down to the canyon floor was in the worst shape; and though it improved from there, a few little scrub oak were the only living trees to be seen in the area. To complicate matters more, FR 289 was washed out about 2.5 miles shy of the trailhead. In spite of that, a visit to the Dome Wilderness is still worth the extra effort. And besides, it's no stranger to catastrophe.

Directions _____→

From I-25 North, take Exit 259. Turn left and go north 12.2 miles on NM 22 to the junction at Cochiti Dam. Continue straight 4.5 miles on Cochiti Highway, or 0.9 mile past Cochiti Lake Golf Course. Turn right on FR 289. (Note Special Comments.) Follow the dirt road about 3.5 miles to a hairpin turn. Park on the right side of the road just before the turn.

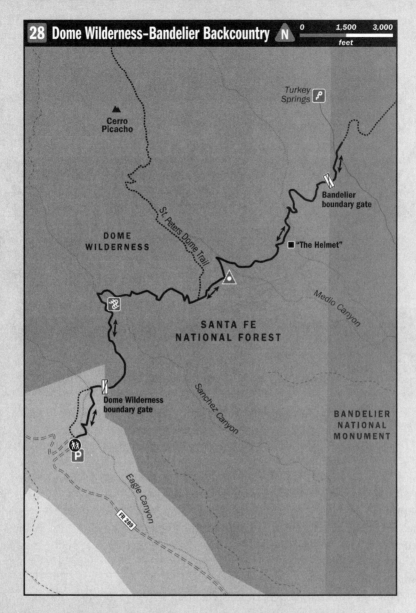

N

0   1,500   3,000

feet

Turkey
Springs

Cerro
Picacho

Bandelier
boundary gate

DOME
WILDERNESS

St. Peters Dome Trail

"The Helmet"

Medio Canyon

SANTA FE
NATIONAL FOREST

Dome Wilderness
boundary gate

Sanchez Canyon

BANDELIER
NATIONAL
MONUMENT

P

Eagle Canyon

FR 289

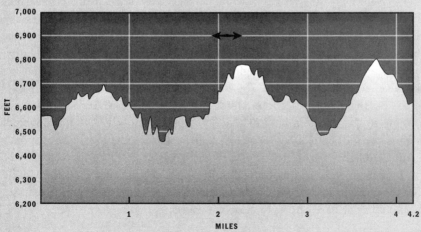

7,000

6,900

6,800

6,700

6,600

6,500

6,400

6,300

6,200

FEET

1   2   3   4 4.2

MILES

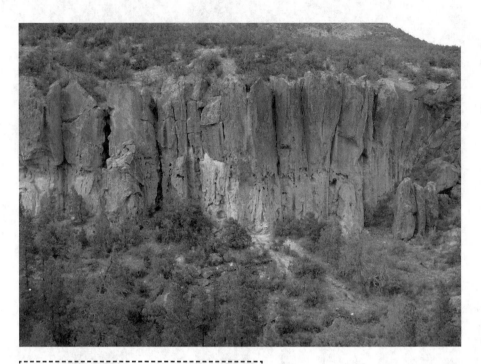

View at the southern rim of a branch of Medio Canyon

On April 26, 1996, a fire raged 25 miles west of Santa Fe, blackening the skies and casting an eerie Halloween glow over The City Different. The culprit: a camper who had failed to heed New Mexico's most celebrated native son, Smokey Bear. The damage: more than 16,500 acres burned, including most of Dome Wilderness and the neighboring wilderness area in Bandelier National Monument. More than a decade later, charred and desolate slopes on St. Peter's Dome still remind us of the notorious Dome Fire.

The 8,464-foot St. Peter's Dome, which supposedly resembles the dome on its namesake basilica in Rome, stands near the northern end of the smallest wilderness area in the Southwest. At 5,200 acres, the Dome Wilderness is a complex landscape where the Sanchez and Medio canyons reach up into the San Miguel Mountains. Combined, these features amount to challenging hiking terrain. Each canyon crossing on the route described below might not seem like much on fresh legs, but the cumulative effect approximates a 1,700-foot gain and loss in elevation.

To ease the hike, this route avoids the area's steepest trails by roughly conforming to the southern base of the San Miguels. However, piñon downfall poses a unique set of small but frequent challenges. As if the Dome Fire weren't devastating enough, bark beetles have been particularly vicious in this backcountry region. Trail maintenance is occasionally left to volunteer units, such as the Middle Rio Grande chapter of the Back Country Horsemen of America. Natural processes often outpace their hard efforts to clear the trails.

Where the trail gets sketchy, keep a sharp eye out for ducks (small versions of cairns, often assembled from two or three rocks). Watch for arrangements of rocks or branches laid across side paths. These are subtle but important signs meant to deter you from straying off in the wrong direction. Also, take a moment to look back every so often so that the return route will seem familiar.

The hike starts out on the right side of the road, heading north from the outer bend of a hairpin turn on FR 289. DOME WILDERNESS appears on a Forest Service sign. Just beyond that is a sign for Dome Trail (118). (Incidentally, maps and signage rarely agree on the names and numbers of trails in the Dome Wilderness.)

The fine gravel trail leads into the conifer shade of Eagle Canyon, so named for Joseph Eagle, a key developer of the Cochiti Gold Mining District in the late 19th and early 20th centuries. A wooden marker posted at the canyon floor directs you out via a natural staircase in the rock wall. Less than 0.5 mile into the hike, an arrow on a post points you right. A gateway just ahead marks the southwestern boundary of the Dome Wilderness.

The trail soon curves north to gradually descend into Sanchez Canyon. About 1.4 miles into the hike, you arrive at a stream that has been described elsewhere as "reliable" and "permanent." You'll likely find it better described as "slightly moist." If, however, you do find it flowing steadily, check it carefully before crossing. A short distance downstream, it plunges 80 feet deeper into Sanchez Canyon.

From the stream crossing, the trail climbs east 0.8 mile. You'll find an overlook of the falls within the first 100 yards or so. Farther up on your left are good views of cliff formations that compose a south-facing wall of Sanchez Canyon. Details in this volcanic mass evoke ancient temples, castle towers, and cathedral facades with lancet windows. After a couple of switchbacks to the ridge, the trail fades as it crosses bedrock. Turn to your right for a view of Cochiti Lake, about 7 miles to the southeast. Resume your east-northeastward trajectory and, after about 100 feet, you'll reach a T-junction. Here, at 2.2 miles into the hike, a sign *should* indicate that the Dome Trail (118) climbs north, while Turkey Springs Trail (119) commences to run northeast to Bandelier National Monument. Continue straight toward Turkey Springs.

About 0.3 mile past the junction, you arrive at the southern rim of a branch of Medio Canyon. Before turning left for the descent, go straight to reach the prominent outcrop ahead for a preview of the cliffs on the other side. Unlike the formal architectural details found in Sanchez Canyon, the gas-bubbled and wind-sculpted tuff formations here evoke quirkier moods. (The caricatured expressions of tiki masks come to mind.)

For a closer look, follow the trail across the pine-shaded canyon. Amusing hoodoos stand near the base of the cliff. Cholla cacti crowd the narrow path, so watch your step. The trail continues southeast and squeezes between a pair of natural shelters, then gradually curves northeast to aim directly toward a formation that a fellow hiker likened to a helmet, (specifically, a *Pickelhaube*). This freestanding tower of tuff is in a shaded area next to a deep streambed at the top

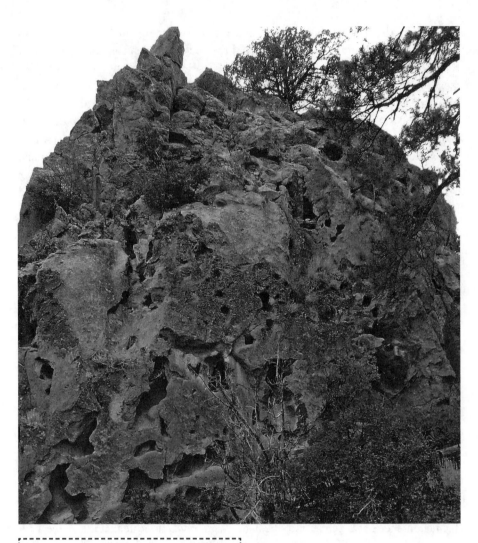

The area around "the helmet" is worth exploring.

of a (usually) dry waterfall. Marking the 3-mile notch on this hike, it's an ideal place to take a break, explore, and reconsider your hiking objectives. The trail ahead is the most strenuous, with diminishing returns in terms of scenic value. Maintenance also seems to taper off, making it increasingly difficult to follow. In short, novice hikers, (particularly those experiencing visions of tiki masks and *Pickelhauben*) might be better off turning back here.

Those determined to visit Bandelier backcountry can continue onward. West of "the helmet," the trail hooks to cross a shallow channel, then crosses a deeper one about 0.25 mile north. A rock slide comes into view on your left. The trail does *not* continue north past the rock slide. Instead, it hooks south in the first of a 0.4-mile series of switchbacks to climb out of Medio Canyon.

From the ridgetop, the boundary gate is a mere 300 yards away, but a disaster area of downfall swallows the trail. For those with GPS units, these are the coordinates for the boundary gate: N 35° 44' 05", W 106° 21' 25".

Aim downhill to the north-northeast until you intercept a shallow gully. (If you walk by a stout pair of old alligator junipers with whitish trunks, you're on the right track.) Follow it as it curves east to the boundary gate. Prominent signage here clearly identifies the monument boundary and its rules. Read the fine print for an interesting footnote about this backcountry wilderness: ELECTRONIC SENSORS AND REMOTE VIDEO SURVEILLANCE SYSTEMS MAY BE IN USE.

The trail improves as it curves north down a red slope to an outflow of Turkey Springs. It's little more than a trickle, barely audible from more than 50 feet away, but you should find more than enough running water to cool your feet for the return hike. (As with any wilderness stream, it must be treated before drinking.)

A nearby sign indicates that Capulin Canyon is 4 miles to the north and Cañada Ranch is 6.5 miles back the way you came. Retrace your steps 4.2 miles to return to the trailhead.

29 LA BAJADA

KEY AT-A-GLANCE INFORMATION

LENGTH: 6.8-mile loop

DIFFICULTY: Moderate, with one difficult descent

SCENERY: Views from atop 500-foot cliffs; petroglyphs and pueblo ruins; river canyon

EXPOSURE: Minimal shade

TRAIL TRAFFIC: Low–moderate

SHARED USE: Moderate (mountain bikers, equestrians, camping; livestock; limited motor-vehicle access)

TRAIL SURFACE: Dirt, rock

HIKING TIME: 4 hours

DRIVING DISTANCE: 45 miles

ACCESS: Year-round

LAND STATUS: Cochiti Indian Reservation; Española Ranger District

MAPS: Santa Fe National Forest (West Half); USGS Tetilla Peak

FACILITIES: None

LAST-CHANCE FOOD/GAS: Convenience store, food services, gas station at Exit 259, about 12 miles from the trailhead

SPECIAL COMMENTS: This hike begins and ends on Cochiti land. Respect the privacy of local residents and the authority of pueblo officials, who have been gracious in allowing access to the river and the mesa.

GPS TRAILHEAD COORDINATES

Latitude   35° 33' 05"

Longitude   106° 14' 13"

IN BRIEF

A hike in the nearest corner of the Santa Fe National Forest takes a legendary route to a mesa top, skirts the rim of an expansive canyon, then drops down to follow the Santa Fe River back to the start.

DESCRIPTION

A bit of local history will help you prepare for a few obstacles you'll face on this hike. In the Spanish colonial era, New Mexico was divided into two major governmental and economic regions: the Rio Arriba and the Rio Abajo, the upper river and lower river, respectively. The physical boundary between them was a steep slope on the edge of La Bajada Mesa.

From 1598 to the mid-19th century, La Bajada, or "the descent," was a traffic nightmare for oxcart travelers along the Camino Real. An ostensibly gentler route ran through the Santa Fe River Canyon, but it was vulnerable to rain and snowmelt. Accordingly, the community at the eastern end of the canyon is La Cienega, which translates from Extremaduran as "marsh" or "swampy land." Indeed, with snowmelt or summer monsoons, the canyon floor is *muy cienegoso*. To complicate matters more, the river insists on a curvaceous route, bouncing side-to-side between canyon

- -

Directions ⟶

From I-25 North, take Exit 264 and drive 3.8 miles north-northwest on NM 16. Turn right for La Bajada and the Tetilla Peak Recreation Area, and go 1 mile east. Turn right again and follow the road 1.5 miles. (As you cross the bridge, note river conditions.) Immediately after crossing the bridge, park in the dirt clearing on the right.

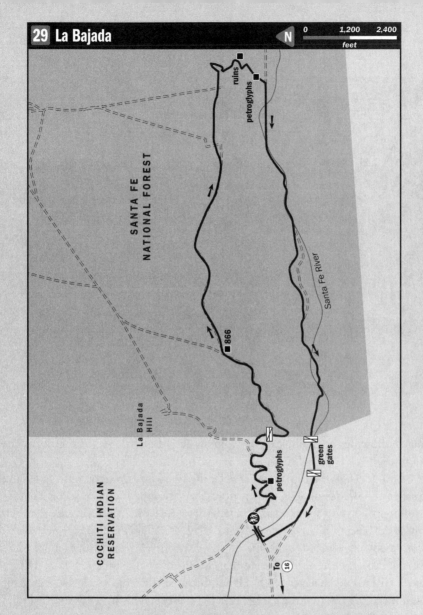

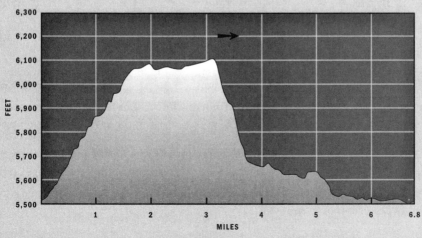

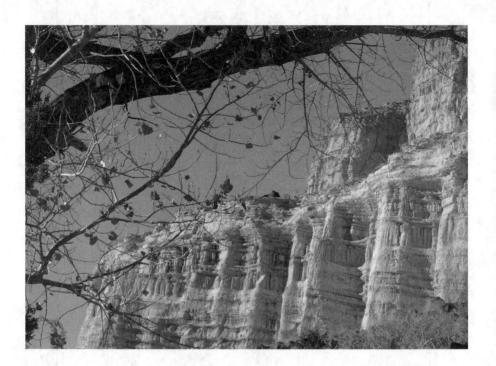

walls. Following the 2-mile canyon segment described below, you'll cross the river five times.

Around 1860 the U.S. Army opened the first known wagon road to climb the mesa. In the winter of 1923–24, prison labor equipped with pickaxes and dynamite modified the wagon road, reducing its grade by 2 percent and eliminating 7 of its 23 hairpin turns. From 1926 to 1932, La Bajada Hill was regarded as the most harrowing segment of Route 66. In 1932 the alignment that would become Interstate 25 was laid out 5 miles to the east. From then on, the redundantly named Bajada Hill would be neglected by all but the most adventurous travelers. No doubt you noticed the twisted trail carved into the escarpment as you approached the village of La Bajada.

The hike begins at the junction about 100 feet past the parking area. Turn right and follow the main road uphill, avoiding shortcuts on footpaths between switchbacks.

As you ascend La Bajada, scan the basalt boulders for petroglyphs. Ancient designs appear alongside more-recent scribbles, initials, and dates. A gallery of these pecked rocks is located on the right side of the bend in the third switchback. The terrain is ideal for rattlesnakes, so watch out for those as you're poking around the rocks.

After rounding the sixth switchback, you'll hit a Y-junction. Unless you want to add a couple of miles to the hike via an older alignment, keep right. (See **Optional routes** on page 168.) At this point, you're nearly halfway up the 1.8-mile segment to the top of the 500-foot escarpment.

After two more switchbacks, or 1 mile into the hike, you'll pass through an open gate. It should be closed, but at last check, it looked as though a truck had run over it. The north–south fence approximates the boundary between Cochiti land and the national forest. (For the remainder of the hike, you may wonder how this treeless land ever came to be regarded as any kind of forest.) After one more switchback and another 200-foot elevation gain, the road tops out at the rim of the mesa. Congratulations, you've just conquered La Bajada Hill.

Actually, it's not so much a hill as a volcanic escarpment. Note the volcano, Tetilla ("breast" or "nipple") Peak, rising 3.5 miles to the north. Its pointed appearance on the Caja del Rio Plateau makes it easy to identify. Now that you've got your bearings, the next stop on this route is 1.4 miles due east. Continue another 200 yards up the road to locate a solitary post inexplicably numbered 866. A line of whitish rocks extends about 100 yards north of the post. Turn right at the break in the rocks, and follow the road northeast. About 0.25 mile ahead, it'll bend slightly southeastward.

After crossing under two sets of power lines, the road turns sharply northeast, parallel to the lines.

At this point, leave the road and continue 0.3 mile straight east. Near the halfway point (about 0.15 mile from where you left the road), you'll walk up an embankment that rises slightly to the south. You might drift slightly to your left to avoid the steeper end. Once past it, be sure to continue straight east to the rim of an alcove. (If you don't find it within a minute after crossing a faded doubletrack, you probably drifted too far north.) Standing on the west rim of the alcove, you'll note the Santa Fe River winding along the canyon floor, about 450 feet below to the right. Straight ahead, the descent to a shelf in the alcove is only about 150 feet. Giant mounds of basalt boulders in the alcove resemble crumbled castles. Look carefully and you may be able to distinguish natural rock piles from the ruins of an ancient pueblo. Rock-lined paths between the mounds hint at where the more popular structures once stood.

Options for a safe descent are limited. Two notches in the west rim are about 100 yards apart. Locate the north one, which contains the rusted remains of a barbed wire fence. A well-worn path begins immediately below. Follow the rock-lined trail about a quarter mile down to a flat clearing. Ruins of the Tsinat Pueblo, last occupied between AD 1100 and 1300, include several room blocks and fieldhouses. Those easiest to identify are near the southern edge of the clearing.

Don't get discouraged if you can't find these low rock walls, there are plenty of petroglyphs to enjoy below. Most are facing south, so the easiest way to find them is to continue down to the canyon floor, then start working your way back up. Note that a thorough hunt for petroglyphs can easily add a mile to the overall hike.

When you're ready to continue on the hike, return to the canyon floor, locate the dirt road on the near side of the river, and turn right to follow it west. From here on out, the terrain remains relatively flat but is not necessarily any easier. Under normal conditions, you simply stroll downstream 2.8 miles until you're out of the canyon, and you might wonder how anyone could regard the trickle of water as a river.

However, as mentioned earlier, recent snowmelt or summer monsoons can cause problems. Some observations made on previous hikes may prove helpful: First, washed-out footbridges usually turn up on the opposite bank. Second, dead tree limbs make unreliable vaulting poles. Finally, wet feet aren't such a bad thing after all.

If you follow the main road diligently for about 2.3 miles, you'll pass through (or climb over) two green gates. Try not to spook the cows along the way. From the second green gate, it's 0.5 mile to the road you drove in on. Turn right and walk 0.1 mile to cross the bridge and return to the parking area.

Optional routes: In wet seasons, you may want to avoid the canyon floor. For a shorter, simpler hike, try the Bajada loop. Start by following the hike as described to the mesa top, but instead of turning right after post 866, continue straight toward Tetilla Peak just over 0.5 mile. Take a sharp left at the junction, then walk the road southwest about 0.5 mile to the western rim of the mesa. The road turns north for a tight M-shaped series of switchbacks. Once through those, stay on the main track south for about 0.75 mile back to the Y. Or, to extend this route, explore the various road alignments above and below the rim; some appear as linear depressions through the mesa-top grasslands, whereas others are hardscrabble tracks in the escarpment below.

LA CIENEGA AND LA CIENEGUILLA **30**

IN BRIEF

An improvised route at La Cienega climbs up one side of a 500-foot hill and down the other, then drops nearly 200 feet into the Santa Fe River Canyon for a streamside stroll. An easier alternate hike sticks to a designated trail for a close look at the petroglyphs of La Cieneguilla.

DESCRIPTION

Just a mile off the interstate, the southern Santa Fe suburb of La Cienega is oddly reminiscent of New Mexico's northern villas. Milagro, the fictional hamlet of John Nichols's *Beanfield* trilogy, comes to mind. And at times the narrow winding streets of La Cienega have the feel of an older, quieter country. Yet there's so much to see and do that you might not know where to begin. Then again, with its main attractions closed for most of the year, your best bet is to start on open land.

La Cienega Area of Critical Environmental Concern, designated in 1992, refers to 4,500 acres along the Santa Fe River Canyon. It contains riparian wildlife such as garter snakes, tree lizards, weasels, and several species of bats.

It also abounds in cultural resources associated with the Galisteo Basin. Evidence of prehistoric and early historic pueblos is scattered along the Santa Fe River. Determining

KEY AT-A-GLANCE INFORMATION

LENGTH: 3.5-mile figure-8 with spurs

DIFFICULTY: Moderate–difficult figure-8

SCENERY: Volcanic hills, broad mesas, river canyon, petroglyphs

EXPOSURE: Some canyon shade

TRAIL TRAFFIC: Light

SHARED USE: Low (limited mountain bike and equestrian access; motorized vehicles prohibited)

TRAIL SURFACE: Dirt, rock

HIKING TIME: 2 hours

DRIVING DISTANCE: 51 miles

ACCESS: Year-round

LAND STATUS: BLM–Taos Field Office

MAPS: USGS Tetilla Peak

FACILITIES: None

LAST-CHANCE FOOD/GAS: Convenience store, food services, gas station at Exit 259, 14 miles from the trailhead.

SPECIAL COMMENTS: Two hikes originating from different trailheads appear on the map and in the Description, but the elevation profile refers only to the tougher hike at La Cienega.

Directions ⟶

From I-25 North, take Exit 271. Turn left on NM 587 (Entrada La Cienega) and go north 1 mile. Turn left on County Road 54 (Camino Capilla Vieja) and go 0.4 mile. Pull over and park in a clearing on the right, across the street from a small sign for the Rael Ranch.

GPS TRAILHEAD COORDINATES

Latitude   35° 33' 46"

Longitude   106° 07' 56"

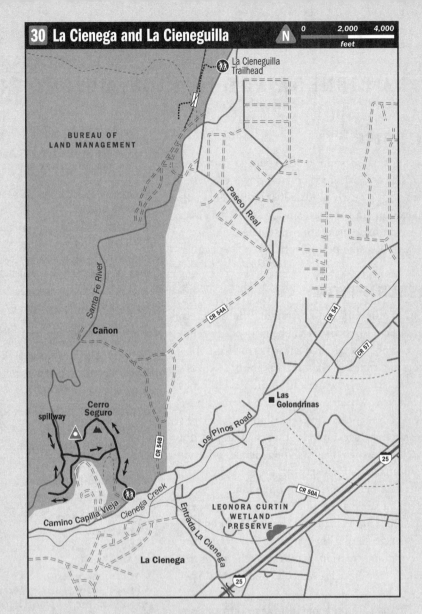

30 La Cienega and La Cieneguilla

N

0   2,000   4,000
feet

La Cieneguilla
Trailhead

BUREAU OF
LAND MANAGEMENT

Santa Fe River

Paseo Real

CR 54A

CR 54

CR 57

Cañon

Las
Golondrinas

Cerro
Seguro

spillway

Los Pinos Road

CR 54B

25

CR 50A

Camino Capilla Vieja

Cienega Creek

Entrada La Cienega

LEONORA CURTIN
WETLAND
PRESERVE

La Cienega

25

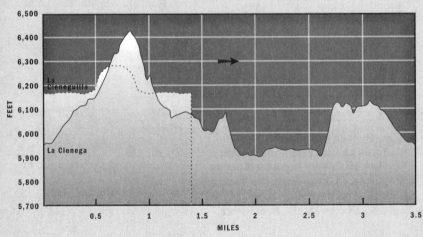

which ones constitute the pueblos of Cienega and Cieneguilla has been a matter of debate for centuries. The self-trained anthropologist Adolph Bandelier remarked on the considerable size of a pueblo he'd referenced earlier as "Cienega or Cieneguilla." However, later surveys failed to locate any major ruins in the area, suggesting that whatever he observed in 1892 had mostly vanished by 1915. Still, visitors today can easily spot pueblo mounds and petroglyphs in the area.. Whatever you happen to stumble upon, leave it the way you found it.

The hike at La Cienega begins on the dirt road directly across the street from mailbox 42. Start north and bear left at the Y close ahead. After a short, steep climb, note the road merging behind you; you'll want to avoid it on your return. Continue north toward the east side of Cerro Seguro. As you approach the hill, watch for a faint doubletrack that meets your road on the left. That's your return route. For now, continue uphill to a ridge on the northeastern flank of Cerro Seguro. Here you'll catch the first glimpse of the Santa Fe River Canyon. About 0.75 mile to the north, white stones form a cross on the sloping western wall of the canyon. Hidden beneath it on the canyon floor is the tiny community of Cañon.

Turn left on the ridge and follow a steep, rocky footpath to the summit. By this point you've gained 500 feet in elevation in 0.8 mile. What you find up here depends on the mood of local pilgrims. White picket crosses once stood here, later to be replaced with a curious assortment of offerings: a gold-lamé flag, river cobbles soaked in scented oils, and sprinklings of corn and salt.

Take a moment to get oriented. The Santa Fe River begins about 25 miles to the northeast, near Santa Fe Baldy in the Santa Fe Mountains and the Santa Fe National Forest. It crosses the Santa Fe Trail in the town of Santa Fe, passes north of the Santa Fe Municipal Airport, and then traverses the Santa Fe River Canyon directly in front of you. The river exits the canyon before crossing the western boundary of Santa Fe County and then bends north to join the Rio Grande near Cochiti Pueblo, about 12 miles to the northwest.

Visible landmarks from Cerro Seguro include Las Tetillas, hills of slightly lesser stature rising a mile to the west, and the somewhat larger Cerro Bonanza, 4.5 miles due south. At the same distance, to the east, is the former New Mexico State Penitentiary, the site of the bloodiest prison riot in American history (1980) and the filming location for the 2005 remake of the farcical prison romp *The Longest Yard.*

Continue walking south, heading downhill along the ridge. There's no obvious trail, so choose your steps carefully along the path of least impact; that is, try not to trample the vegetation. About halfway down, angle right toward a rocky bulge on the hillside that overlooks the canyon. The view from here gives you a better idea about what lies ahead on the lower portion of the route. This slight detour will also ease your descent on the slippery hillside. Proceed downhill, aiming for a bend in the road that runs near the canyon rim. Once on flat ground, note a rocky point protruding from the sloping canyon wall. It splits a drainage into two gullies. The one on its southern side is the way out of the canyon on the return part of this route. It's not as long of a climb as the hill, but it is steeper and just as slippery.

For now, follow the canyon rim about 0.25 mile south, until you come to a downed barbwire fence. Another 60 feet ahead, a cleft in the rim forms a natural staircase through the basalt caprock. Before stepping down, consider strolling along the rim another 0.25 mile or so to enjoy the views and look for petroglyphs in the caprock below. Collared lizards also lurk nearby in warm weather, but they're shier than their Albuquerque brethren.

Return to the cleft and head down toward the river. Once on the canyon floor, turn right at the acequia (irrigation canal), and follow it north. The wreckage of a Subaru is about 0.25 mile upstream. Another 60 yards ahead is the low end of the gully mentioned earlier. The absence of vegetation and caprock at the rim make this channel one of the few viable passages out of the canyon.

Continue upstream for now. How far you go may depend on the river. You'll have to cross it at least once to get to the spillway 0.3 mile ahead. At uncertain times of the year, a broad jump or stepping-stones will suffice. At other times, your best strategy is to just resign yourself to wet boots. The canyon floor is the highlight of the hike, particularly when the river actually flows like a river, or at least a decent creek.

The spillway is the turnaround point on this route. (An impressive pair of horseshoe canyons starts another 0.5 mile upstream, but I've never slogged up that far.) Return to the gully and climb up to the rim.

Once back on the mesa, head downhill. Do *not* take the obvious dirt road—it becomes a private drive. Instead, locate a faint path to the left of the dirt road; it runs between a drainage and the base of the hill and joins a doubletrack before turning north. If you can't pick it out, just hook around the base of the hill for a little more than 0.25 mile, until you cross an arroyo. (Head downhill too soon and you'll cross it twice in deeper sections.) The road you came up on is about 50 yards past the arroyo. Turn right and follow it 0.5 mile downhill to the car.

The hike at La Cieneguilla is an easy 1.4-mile round-trip out-and-back featuring a high concentration of fantastic petroglyphs. It's also much drier. To get there from the Cienega trailhead, drive back to the junction of Camino Capilla Vieja and Entrada La Cienega. Go 1 mile straight northeast on Los Pinos Road, where it bears north to become CR 56 (Paseo Real). Continue north another 2.8 miles. Turn left and park in a fenced parking area.

From the parking lot, walk 0.1 mile west, following arrows along the well-defined trail to a wire fence. Turn left and follow the trail south about 0.4 mile along the fence. Shortly after crossing a shallow arroyo, veer right on a path that stays closer to the fence. Go through the first gateway on the right and take the path straight up the escarpment. Look for petroglyphs as you approach the rim. A few panels have gone missing in recent years, but several dozen works remain. Turn left and stay on the path below the rim. Images you will see in the next 0.25 mile include stars, spirals, hands, elks, mustangs, a snake-headed eagle, and numerous versions of Kokopelli, the hunchback flutist.

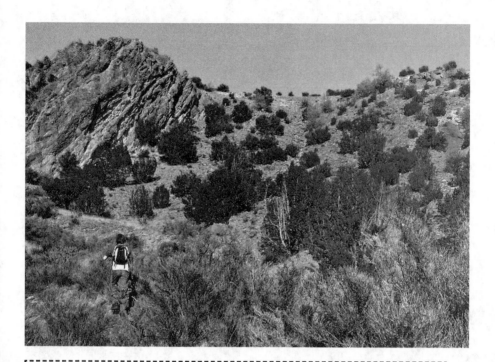

There's more than one way out of the canyon. Look for thin vegetation and breaks in the caprock.

NEARBY ACTIVITIES

El Rancho de las Golondrinas is a living-history museum in a 200-acre farming valley. Villagers in period clothing inhabit the original buildings, which date from the early 18th century. (Imagine a northern New Mexico version of Colonial Williamsburg, and you'll get the idea.) Admission fees range from $1 to $12. Open for self-guided walking tours June–September, Wednesday–Sunday, 10 a.m.–4 p.m. There are special events throughout the year. Call (505) 471-2261 or visit **golondrinas.org**. The entrance is on Los Pinos Road, 1 mile northeast of Entrada La Cienega.

Leonora Curtin Wetland Preserve is a 35-acre preserve featuring a nature trail that winds through an open meadow to a natural *ciénega,* or marsh. A second trail covers an arid upland area. Open May–October, 9 a.m.–noon Saturdays and 1–4 p.m. Sundays. For more information, call Santa Fe Botanical Gardens at (505) 471-9103 or visit **santafebotanicalgarden.org**. To get there, head back to I-25 and turn left onto West Frontage Road immediately before the exit ramps. The entrance to the preserve is 1.4 miles ahead on the left.

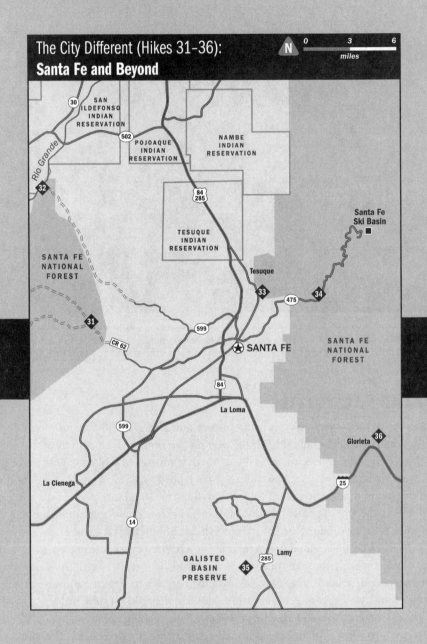

The City Different (Hikes 31–36):
Santa Fe and Beyond

N | 0 | 3 | 6
miles

30 SAN ILDEFONSO INDIAN RESERVATION

502 POJOAQUE INDIAN RESERVATION

NAMBE INDIAN RESERVATION

Rio Grande

32

84 285

Santa Fe Ski Basin

TESUQUE INDIAN RESERVATION

SANTA FE NATIONAL FOREST

Tesuque

33

475

34

31

CR 62

599

★ SANTA FE

SANTA FE NATIONAL FOREST

84

La Loma

599

Glorieta **36**

25

La Cienega

14

GALISTEO BASIN PRESERVE

285

Lamy

35

THE CITY DIFFERENT
(SANTA FE AND BEYOND)

31 TWIN HILLS

KEY AT-A-GLANCE INFORMATION

LENGTH: 6.9 miles

DIFFICULTY: Easy–moderate

SCENERY: Volcanic formations, hilly terrain, mountain vistas

EXPOSURE: Little shade

TRAIL TRAFFIC: Low

SHARED USE: Moderate (equestrians, mountain bikers, motorized vehicles; hunting, target shooting, primitive camping)

TRAIL SURFACE: Packed dirt, loose rock

HIKING TIME: 3 hours

DRIVING DISTANCE: 63 miles

ACCESS: Year-round, though subject to road closures

LAND STATUS: Española Ranger District

MAPS: Santa Fe National Forest (West Half); USGS Agua Fria, Montoso Peak

FACILITIES: None

SPECIAL COMMENTS: Rough roads provide the only access to hills on the plateau. This area is best enjoyed with a bike-and-hike.

LAST-CHANCE FOOD/GAS: Convenience store gas–station on Airport Road, 0.25 mile east of NM 599 (10 miles from trailhead)

GPS TRAILHEAD COORDINATES

Latitude　35° 42' 18"

Longitude　106° 06' 35"

IN BRIEF

Key advice for hiking on the plateau: head for the hills. Lightly forested volcanic formations provide a haven for unique geological sculptures and a flurry of wildlife.

DESCRIPTION

The Caja del Rio ("Box of the River") is a dissected volcanic plateau that stands between Santa Fe and the Rio Grande. Stretching about 20 miles north from La Bajada (Hike 28) to Buckman (Hike 31), it's mostly grassy plains with several clusters of moderate hills, few of which rise more than 500 feet. The plateau makes up the bulk of the exposed part of the Cerros del Rio volcanic field, which consists of about a dozen volcanoes and more than 70 vents of cinder cones, plugs, and tuff rings. Volcanic activity here peaked between 2.3 and 2.5 million years ago, leaving the basalts and intermediate-composition lavas that dominate the landscape today.

The plateau is also home to the Northern goshawk and Peregrine falcon. Bald eagles occasionally forage over the plateau in the winter. Other migratory bird species include the black-throated gray warbler and the gray

Directions　⟶

From I-25 North, take Exit 276 and turn left on Veterans Memorial Highway (NM 599). Go north 6 miles and turn left on CR 62, followed by a quick left on Frontage Road. Go southwest 1.4 miles and turn right on Caja del Rio Road. Go north 2.9 miles and turn left on CR 62. After 1.2 miles, CR 62 crosses the first cattle guard and becomes FR 24. Continue northwest another 1.6 miles, crossing two more cattle guards along the way. Turn left and park in a clearing at the T-junction.

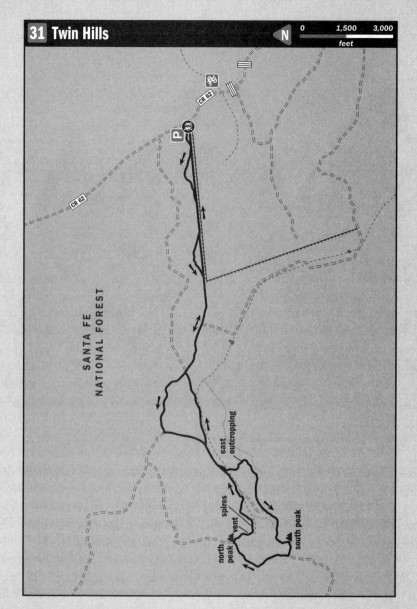

N

| 0 | 1,500 | 3,000 |

feet

SANTA FE
NATIONAL FOREST

CR 62

CR 62

P

east
outcropping

spires

vent

north
peak

south peak

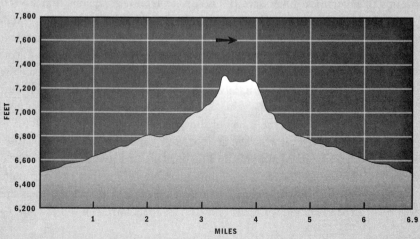

FEET

7,800
7,600
7,400
7,200
7,000
6,800
6,600
6,400
6,200

1   2   3   4   5   6   6.9

MILES

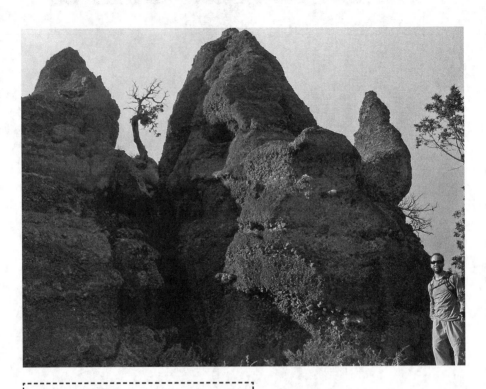

Spires between the north peak and main drainage

vireo. Kangaroo mice and a variety of lizards are common, as are coyotes, which are more frequently heard than seen.

Aside from stock ponds, you won't likely find much water on the plateau. Average rainfall amounts to less than an inch per month. Intermittent stream channels and ephemeral swales tend to stay dry outside of monsoon season.

The Caja del Rio Allotment of the Española Ranger District covers nearly 67,000 acres with well over 100 rugged roads and mapped trails. The area is popular with jeep tourists, target shooters, equestrians, and mountain bikers. What tends to deter most hikers are the relatively featureless plains that stretch (and yawn) between questionable roads and scenic hills. As a result, few hikers know what they're missing. These hills are packed with fascinating geologic features, abundant wildlife, and a smattering of remnants from ancient pueblos. You could wander for days out here and you'd still miss half of it. This hike just scratches the surface. The point is merely to get you into nearby hills quickly and effortlessly, without damaging your vehicle, and to acquaint you with endless possibilities for exploration upon the Caja del Rio Plateau.

The hike begins wherever you decide that your car has taken enough abuse. Under ideal conditions, the road holds up fine until you get past the second cattle guard, less than a mile up FR 24. A few bumpy patches follow over the next half-mile or so, but most cars with normal clearance can crawl over it to reach the T-junction. The road heading west from here is less forgiving. You can attempt to drive it to shave a few miles off the hike. For those eager to get their boots on the ground, it's probably best to get out here and start walking.

Navigating this route is simple, thanks to a prominent pair of stark, volcanic plugs (sometimes mistaken for Twin Hills, which stand less than a mile farther northwest). For the first mile, braided doubletracks follow a fenceline and aim directly at the plug on the north peak. Stay on the road another mile as it bends north. After it dips south, and just before turning north again, look for a lesser road veering south.

At this junction, you're 2 miles into the hike, and so far the immediate scenery has been a dusty display of overgrazed grasslands with a colorful potpourri of spent shotgun shells. Trust me, it gets better.

Turn left on the side road heading south. It soon curves right to pass between the points of two low ridges. Both ridges ramp up to peak at a pair of conjoined volcanic hills, roughly forming one continuous horseshoe-shaped ridgeline. The idea of the hike from here is simple: Follow the ridge on your left up to the south plug, cross over to visit the one to the north, then follow the other ridge back down to the road. (That's the basic idea, anyway, but be prepared for curiosities along the way that may cause you to deviate from this simple course.)

Start by looking for a rocky outcrop on the near end of the ridge on your left. It's not as prominent as either peak, but easy enough to spot from the road. Leave the road for a quick climb to that point. Views from here include an unobstructed panorama of the Sangre de Cristo range rising on the far side of Santa Fe. Also take a close look at the rock beneath your feet and you may find a metate, or grinding stone.

Climb southwest, toward the south peak. As the ridge bends west, a hogback begins to emerge on your right. Hiking on the upper side of an 0.3-mile-long wall is easier, due to thinner vegetation, though you'll better appreciate its immensity from below. If you stick to the high road, a good spot for a quick look below comes at a gap in the middle. A road once passed through here, though only a trace of it remains. Also keep an eye out for interesting rock formations on the far side of the drainage.

The hogback leads you to a short but steep ascent to the south plug. A red-dirt road parallels the ridge between the peaks. You can follow it to the north peak or stay on the ridge for better views. From the north peak, a short jeep road splits off to visit a volcanic vent. It's steep and deep, so watch your step. A local custom involves rolling old vehicles into the shaft, perhaps as a sacrifice to the volcano.

About 300 feet south of the vent are spires that you probably spotted from the hogback. They rise near the steep, vegetated head of the main drainage. You may spot a few more curiosities in this area. Feel free to wander off course to explore whatever catches your attention. You can return to the ridge above to finish the intended route, or just follow the drainage downstream for a shortcut to the road that brought you in. (The map shows the latter option.)

32 BUCKMAN-SODA SPRINGS

KEY AT-A-GLANCE INFORMATION

LENGTH: 6-mile out-and-back, 8-mile loop, or 10-mile loop and spur

DIFFICULTY: Moderate out-and-back, difficult loop

SCENERY: High desert chaparral, seasonal wildflowers, river gorge, volcanic mesas

EXPOSURE: Mostly sunny

TRAIL TRAFFIC: Moderate

SHARED USE: Moderate; heavy on weekends (mountain bikers, equestrians, rock climbing, limited motor-vehicle access)

TRAIL SURFACE: Dirt, sand, rock

HIKING TIME: 4–6 hours

DRIVING DISTANCE: 76 miles

ACCESS: Year-round

LAND STATUS: Santa Fe National Forest–Española District

MAPS: Santa Fe National Forest–West Half; USGS White Rock

FACILITIES: None

LAST-CHANCE FOOD/GAS: Convenience store–gas station on Airport Road, 0.25 mile east of NM 599 (20 miles from trailhead)

GPS TRAILHEAD COORDINATES

Latitude   35° 50' 00"

Longitude   106° 09' 52"

IN BRIEF

The first leg is a 3.2-mile hike down White Rock Canyon from the lost town of Buckman to a secluded meadow on the bank of the Rio Grande. From there you can embark on a challenging route over the northernmost tip of the Caja del Rio Plateau to the mouth of Diablo Canyon or just stroll back the way you came.

DESCRIPTION

The area around the northern tip of the Caja del Rio Plateau contains too many sights to see in one day. Make a sincere effort to run by as much as you can, because despite recent improvements the road to Buckman is not one you'll want to drive again soon. This loop covers a lot of ground, both high and low, so it helps to break it down into several segments.

To Soda Springs: Trail 306 from the parking area to Soda Springs is 3 miles of old double-track over gently rolling terrain above the east bank of the Rio Grande. The gate indicates how far motorized vehicles are permitted to drive in this part of the national forest, though lately no one seems to mind leaving it open to motorized traffic. The bunker just past the

----

Directions

From I-25 North, take Exit 276 and go 9.8 miles northeast on Veterans Memorial Highway (NM 599). Exit at Camino La Tierra, turn left, and go 4.8 miles northwest. Turn right off pavement onto Old Buckman Road and continue 10 miles northwest to the water-lift station. (It resembles a small prison in a sinkhole. You'll know it when you see it.) Bear left and follow the road 0.25 mile to a wide sandy wash. Park on either side of the wash and continue following the road uphill on foot. The hike begins at the gate about 100 feet south of the wash.

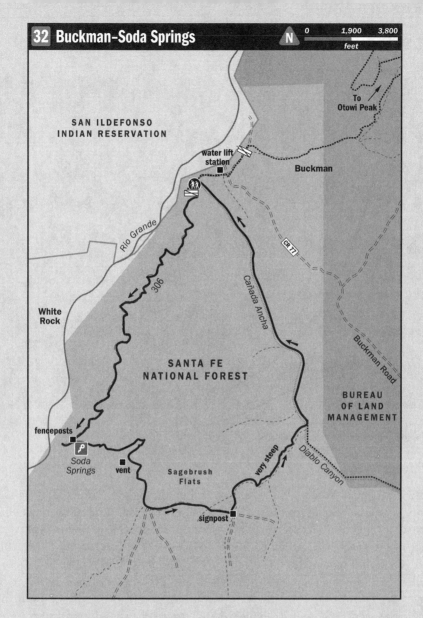

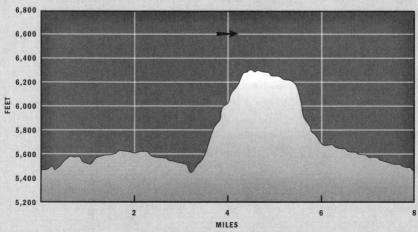

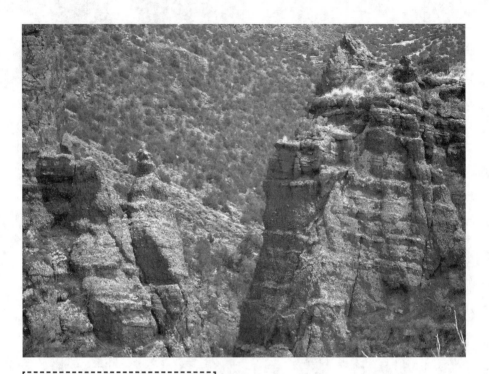

Spires along Trail 306 to Sagebrush Flats

gate is Buckman Well #8. Go around it, uphill to the right. Admittedly, the scenery can be unappealing for the first 0.5 mile, but once you get past the power lines ahead, it returns to relatively natural splendor (unless ATV yee-haws take advantage of the open gate). About 0.25 mile past the power lines, the trail splits. Bear left (the right branch goes down to the river). About 0.1 mile past that, the trail forks again; this time turn right (the left branch drops into an arroyo). From this point on, the way is clear. Just stick to the main road, put the book away, and enjoy the scenery. About 2.3 miles ahead, the road dies out as it drops into a wooded arroyo. Turn right before the arroyo, and follow a path down to a quiet, shaded spot on the edge of the Rio Grande.

Soda Springs to Sagebrush Flats: You can return to the parking area the way you came or take a challenging loop over the mesa. The segment to the rim of Sagebrush Flats gains more than 800 feet in elevation in 1.2 miles, most of it along a narrow, winding path best described as *jackassable* (fit for mules but not horses). Keep in mind that the climb up is easy compared with the climb down the other side. Read ahead so you know what you're in for before going up there.

As you're leaving the river, about 100 yards up the road, old metal and wooden fence posts stand at the roadside. The path beginning there on the right is the segment of Trail 306 to Sagebrush Flats. This end of it can nearly disappear under tall grass in a good monsoon season, but head straight east for 200 yards or so, and you'll pick up a trail of red lava rock winding up the steep cliffs. The trail is unmarked but shows signs of occasional use and light maintenance, so it's easy enough to follow. Any forks you encounter on the lower part are just shortcuts across switchbacks.

Rockslides occasionally erase crucial bits of the trail—proceed with caution. At 0.9 mile into the climb, the trail bends left and a volcanic vent opens on the right. Take a quick detour down the path west to check out red-lava formations and gaze into the dizzying depths of the vent.

Return to the trail and continue southeast another 500 feet to the confluence of two gullies. From here the trail begins to disintegrate. Aim south, heading uphill between the gullies, and pick up the road on the hilltop. Continue south on the road. You'll see two junctions within a quarter mile. Stay left at both, following the road as it bends east.

Sagebrush Flats to Cañada Ancha: The stretch across the aptly named Sagebrush Flats is 0.9 mile, rim-to-rim. From the second junction, follow the road about a half-mile east. Peaks just 20-odd miles due east may still be covered in snow, even when the flats are toasty hot. Cross two washes and turn left in the third. No worries if you turn too soon. All three flow to the same point. However, if you encounter a wooden signpost stripped of its sign, you just missed the third wash. Head north and follow the wash downstream.

The descent to Cañada Ancha drops nearly 600 feet in 0.8 mile, starting with a deceptively simple stroll down the wash. The first drop curves down like a grand staircase, but the second one plummets like an elevator shaft. Locate footholds beneath the edge. Once you find those, it's as easy as climbing down a kiva ladder. Just use care and common sense. Do not try it in wet or icy conditions.

None of the remaining drops is quite so drastic. However, they add up to a strenuous descent. And if the flats were hot, the rocks ahead are broiling. Summer afternoons you may need gloves to protect your hands from scalding. Give this segment at least an hour, during which time you might wonder if there are easier ways off this mesa. I'm sure there must be a few, probably another half-mile or so on the road east, but it seems unlikely that any could be more interesting than this one.

The drainage cuts through several distinct layers of basalt, ash, and cinders from multiple eruptions of both the local volcanic field and the Valles Caldera, which is about 20 miles west. At the low end of the drainage, an oasis of shade trees and maybe a few lingering pools offer cool respite. Take advantage of it before continuing out to Cañada Ancha at the mouth of the Caja del Rio Canyon. Assess your energy level, water supply, and remaining hours of daylight. If any of the preceding is almost out, turn left and follow the wash downstream for a flat 2 miles to close the loop.

Diablo Canyon spur: If, on the other hand, you're reinvigorated, turn right for a detour through the Caja del Rio Canyon, known locally as Diablo Canyon. An outstanding hike in its own right, this mile-long passage boasts an assortment of columns, slots, caves, cracks, crags, and cliffs. And with more than 100 routes to

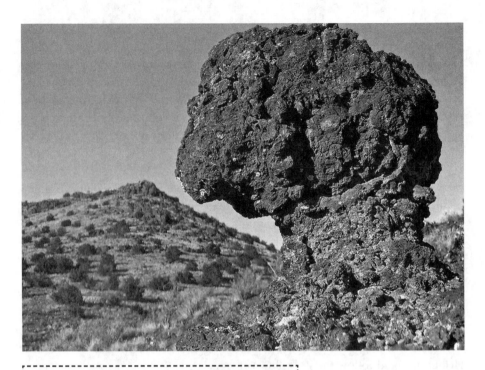

Encounter lava formations on the trail to nearby Otowi Peak.

conquer, it's a popular spot with rock climbers. The area was also the scene of a stagecoach ambush in the 2007 film *3:10 to Yuma.*

The canyon detour is 1.7 miles out-and-back, pushing the overall hike into the 10-mile range. Alternatively, you can drive around to the west end and hike in from there. Look for a turnoff on the right about 3 miles up Buckman Road from the parking area. Do not drive into the wash unless your vehicle is reliable in deep sand. Also be aware that flash flooding in the canyon has been known to carry away a vehicle or two.

NEARBY ACTIVITIES

Otowi Peak sits on the San Ildefonso reservation boundary, 1,100 feet above the Rio Grande. A rough, unmarked trail up the south side of La Mesita (aka Buckman Mesa) is the best approach. The hike is a moderate 4.6-mile out-and-back that starts on a road heading northeast from the lift station. Cross a cattle guard and turn right in the wash ahead. About 0.6 mile upstream, the wash turns southeast. Just past the uppermost bend, look for a rock cairn and an eroded path on your left. Exit the wash here to begin a hard 0.6-mile push to the rim. There you'll see the volcanic cone about a half-mile north, rising 300 feet from the mesa top to peak at 6,547 feet. It's a fairly straight shot out, but the most elaborate formations are along paths that run closest to the mesa's bowed west rim.

BISHOP'S LODGE– BIG TESUQUE CREEK

IN BRIEF

The Bishop's Lodge stands on the near corner of 1,500 contiguous square miles of national forest. Link its marked trails over hilly terrain with gentler designated trails in the Santa Fe National Forest for a hike that culminates with the cottonwood-shaded promenade along Big Tesuque Creek.

DESCRIPTION

Long before it became a premium resort, the Bishop's Lodge was the site of a small ranch, a private chapel, and splendid gardens. The bishop who first lodged here in the 1850s was Jean Baptiste Lamy, perhaps better known as Father Latour from Willa Cather's biographical novel, *Death Comes for the Archbishop.*

Christened the Villa Pintoresca, the bishop's ranch stood in the Little Tesuque Valley, about 4 miles north of St. Francis Cathedral. In reverence to the sanctity of a good long stroll, he often made the journey on foot and required his visitors to do the same.

Visitors today can put in a sufficient walk on the trails at the 450-acre resort. With a policy that no doubt appeals to the bishop's generous spirit, all are welcome to hike here. You might expect little more than sissified pathways for wine-and-cheese picnickers at

KEY AT-A-GLANCE INFORMATION

LENGTH: 4.3-mile loop

DIFFICULTY: Moderate

SCENERY: Piñon–juniper foothills in the Sangre de Cristo Mountains, riparian woodland, historic buildings, and gardens

EXPOSURE: Sunny on lodge trails, shaded on Forest Service trails

TRAIL TRAFFIC: High

SHARED USE: High (Forest Service trails popular with dog owners and mountain bikers; all trails popular with equestrians until the first snow; closed to all motorized vehicles)

TRAIL SURFACE: Dirt, sand, loose rock

HIKING TIME: 3 hours

DRIVING DISTANCE: 65 miles

ACCESS: Year-round, daylight hours. Some trails may be impassable in the winter.

LAND STATUS: Private; Santa Fe National Forest–Española Ranger District

MAPS: Santa Fe National Forest–East Half; USGS Santa Fe

FACILITIES: Resort and spa (See Nearby Activities)

LAST-CHANCE FOOD/GAS: All services in Santa Fe

Directions

From I-25 North, take Exit 282 and follow Saint Francis Drive (US 84) north 3.6 miles. Turn right on the *second* Paseo de Peralta. (It's a loop.) Head east 1 mile, then turn left on Bishop's Lodge Road. Go north 3 miles, following the signs to the Bishop's Lodge Resort. Turn right and follow the driveway to the parking area.

GPS TRAILHEAD COORDINATES

Latitude   35° 43' 56"

Longitude   105° 54' 38"

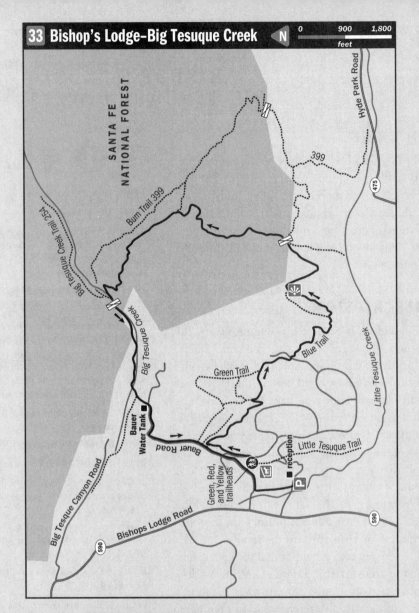

0   900   1,800
feet

SANTA FE
NATIONAL FOREST

Big Tesuque Creek Trail 254

Burn Trail 399

399

Hyde Park Road

475

Big Tesuque Creek

Blue Trail

Little Tesuque Creek

Green Trail

Bauer
Water Tank

Bauer Road

Little Tesuque Trail

reception

Green, Red,
and Yellow
trailheads

P

Big Tesuque Canyon Road

Bishops Lodge Road

590

590

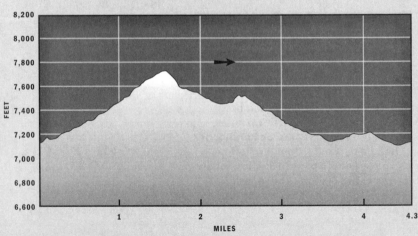

FEET

8,200
8,000
7,800
7,600
7,400
7,200
7,000
6,800
6,600

1   2   3   4   4.3

MILES

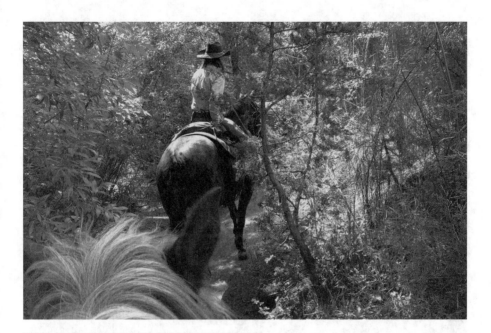

Big Tesuque Creek Trail is twice the fun on four legs.

such a swanky establishment, but you would be sorely mistaken. A few segments are tough enough to count as penance. Factor in connections with the Forest Service system, and you get enough trails for an epic pilgrimage.

Before you hike, stop by the reception hall in the Central Lodge. The concierge can provide you with a detailed map, directions for reaching the trails, and other pertinent instructions. In addition to standard disclaimers about hiking at your own risk, heed any advisories regarding wildlife, such as bears and mountain lions known to frequent the area, and potential conflicts with the skeet range, near the Yellow Trail. Stay on the easements when crossing private property. Avid birders should also ask for the Bishop's Lodge bird list. Finally, for a less demanding walk, request an art-tour brochure map, featuring outdoor sculptures from a local bronze foundry, or take the short nature walk, which starts in the garden by the chapel.

This hike begins on the east side of the horse stables, about 200 yards north of the Central Lodge. The wranglers there can field any questions about the trails that the concierge couldn't answer. Follow the dirt road around the east side of the big corral and cross a paved driveway to find markers for the Green, Red, and Yellow trails. By now you might be thinking this hike is as much fun as an Easter-egg hunt. The remaining markers, however, are not always so cleverly hidden.

Start on the **Green Trail,** taking the path through an opening in a wooden fence. Follow the horse tracks downhill alongside the paved street (Lodge Road). As it curves left toward the security gate at Bauer Road, stay straight on the horse path and continue north about 100 yards to the Red Trail junction. Stay on the Green Trail as it switches back and climbs southeast. About 0.7 mile into

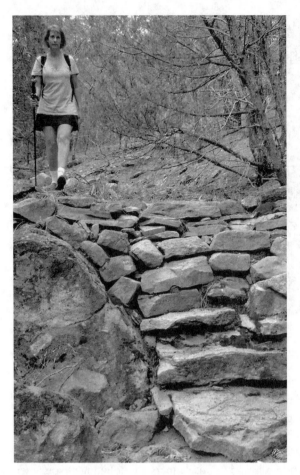

A wooded canyon trail leads to Big Tesuque Creek.

the hike, just past another switchback, you arrive at a Blue Trail junction. From here the Green Trail turns wonky and doesn't quite match up with maps provided by Bishop's Lodge, so turn right onto the Blue Trail.

By now you'll have surmised that an extensive web of informal trails, game paths, and drainages spans these piñon–juniper foothills. Just keep an eye out for subtle signage and stay on the beaten tracks, which over centuries of use have been worn down to a trench in places.

The **Blue Trail** continues climbing southeast alongside a deep arroyo. Over the next 0.5 mile, it passes another Green Trail junction, crosses a road, and climbs up to a signed fork. Residential encroachment along this stretch has been on the rise in recent years, and you may likely hear strains of Stravinsky wafting from these lofty homes.

Signs at the fork indicate that either way leads to the viewpoint at the top end of the loop, about 1.5 miles into the hike. The 7,743-foot summit is the highest point on the Bishop's Lodge property. Peaks exceeding 12,000 feet are lined up behind the ski basin, 8 miles to the northeast. About 45 miles in the opposite direction, the Sandias rise to flank Albuquerque's east side.

Numerous trails converge at the viewpoint, though most have been obscured for rehabilitation. Take the one with the little white sign that indicates the way to Julian's and Little Tesuque trails. It curves southeast, then northeast, all downhill to a signed junction. From here you have three choices for looping back to the lodge. This hike opts for the one on the left.

Head north toward Big Tesuque Creek. Passing through the open gate puts you in **Santa Fe National Forest**. This well-defined singletrack heads north into young but well-shaded coniferous woodland and follows a drainage that cuts deeper as it meanders down the canyon. Mature ponderosa that soon crop up along the path lack the bear-claw scars commonly seen along the Burn Trail (399), which runs roughly parallel less than 0.5 mile to the east.

About 0.4 mile from the gate, or 2.2 miles into the hike, this gentle and shaded trail takes an abrupt turn away from the drainage and climbs east to an exposed ridge. The diversion is necessary to avoid a fenced wildlife refuge downstream, as you'll later notice.

Enjoy the views over the canyon during this brief walk along the ridge. The trail soon declines again, and after a short but steep switchback it arrives on the south side of Big Tesuque Creek.

Winsor National Recreational Trail (254) runs along the north side of the creek. The segment used for this hike is all too short, so if you have the time, consider an upstream detour along this magnificent 10-mile trail. A popular turnaround point is the river crossing at the "big pine," about 0.4 mile upstream. Otherwise, cross the creek here, turn left, and head downstream for 0.4 mile. A left turn at the end of a coyote fence puts you on the road back to Bishop's Lodge. (Look for a dirt/gravel road going uphill from a wooden fence and an open metal gate on the left. If you come to a point where the creek flows through an iron fence, you've gone too far.) From the open metal gate, go uphill and turn right at the water tank. Bauer Road briefly climbs west, then goes 0.5 mile south toward Bishop's Lodge. A left turn just past the small corral leads you straight back to the parking area.

NEARBY ACTIVITIES

The best part about hiking from the **Bishop's Lodge Ranch Resort & Spa** is the opportunity to reward yourself for the effort. The Sunday brunch at Las Fuentes Restaurant is a Santa Fe favorite, and its dessert menu is sinful. For casual fare, try the Sunflower Poolside Bar & Grill. The award-winning ShāNah Spa offers treatments inspired by Native American healing traditions. Other activities available include guided horseback riding and skeet and trap shooting. Call ahead, (505) 983-6377 or (800) 419-0492, or visit **bishopslodge.com.**

34 HYDE MEMORIAL STATE PARK

KEY AT-A-GLANCE INFORMATION

LENGTH: 3.3-mile loop, 0.5-mile spur

DIFFICULTY: Moderate

SCENERY: Campgrounds, views of Santa Fe from 9,400 feet, evergreen, alder, aspen

EXPOSURE: Mostly shaded

TRAIL TRAFFIC: Popular

SHARED USE: Low (no horses, bikes, or motor vehicles)

TRAIL SURFACE: Fine gravel, rock

HIKING TIME: 2 hours

DRIVING DISTANCE: 68 miles

ACCESS: Day-use activities: 6 a.m.– 9 p.m.; gate hours: 8 a.m.–11 p.m.; $5 per vehicle or New Mexico State Parks Annual Pass

LAND STATUS: State park

MAPS: Trail maps available at visitor center and trailhead; USGS McClure Reservoir

FACILITIES: Water, restrooms, campsites, RV hookups, picnic shelters, wheelchair-accessible tables, grills, and restrooms

SPECIAL COMMENTS: Check for maintenance or snow closures by calling (505) 983-7175 or visiting nmparks.com.

GPS TRAILHEAD COORDINATES

Latitude   35° 43' 50"

Longitude   105° 50' 15"

IN BRIEF

An old favorite at the southernmost tip of the Rockies is a short drive from the Santa Fe Plaza. The nostalgic campgrounds in Hyde Memorial State Park attract wildflower enthusiasts in the summer and aspen lovers in the fall, whereas winter crowds come for the sledding, snow-shoeing, and cross-country skiing.

DESCRIPTION

On this loop, the segment on the west side of road boasts the better views, but it's a steep mile up, followed by a steep mile down. For an easier hike, stick to the lower, shadier trails on the east side of the road. Start up the stepped trail near the northeast corner of the visitor center to follow the route counterclockwise. Pressed for time? Enjoy a 1.7-mile out-and-back to the waterfall.

To follow the route clockwise, as described here, start by locating the trailhead directly across Hyde Park Road. The trail starts out deceptively quaint, with a wooden fence by the roadside, a rock border, and a stone bridge over Little Tesuque Creek. On the far side of the bridge are an interpretive sign and a black mailbox that (sometimes) contains trail brochures.

Directions

From I-25 North, take Exit 282 and go 3.6 miles north on Saint Francis Drive (US 84). Turn right on the *second* Paseo de Peralta. (It's a loop.) Go east 1 mile, then turn left on Bishop's Lodge Road. Go north 0.18 mile and turn right on Artists Road, which becomes Hyde Park Road (NM 475). Continue 7.4 miles and turn right at the Hyde Memorial State Park Visitors Center and Lodge. Park near the lodge and pay at the station next to the visitor center.

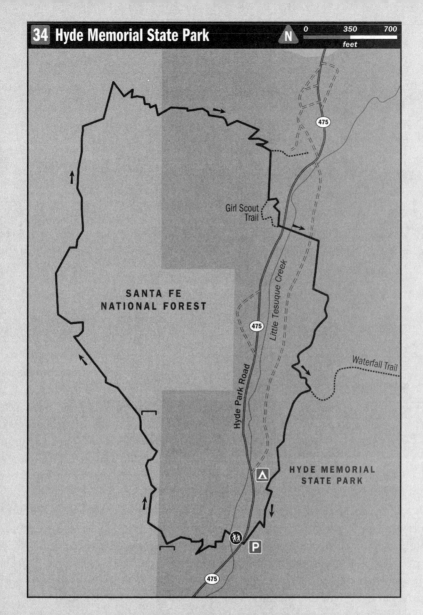

N

0   350   700
feet

SANTA FE
NATIONAL FOREST

Girl Scout
Trail

Little Tesuque Creek

475

475

Hyde Park Road

Waterfall Trail

HYDE MEMORIAL
STATE PARK

P

475

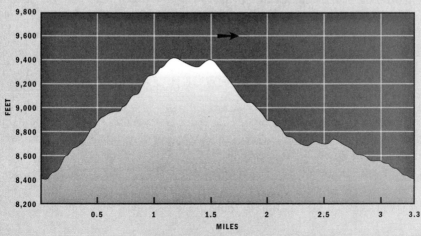

FEET

9,800
9,600
9,400
9,200
9,000
8,800
8,600
8,400
8,200

0.5   1   1.5   2   2.5   3   3.3

MILES

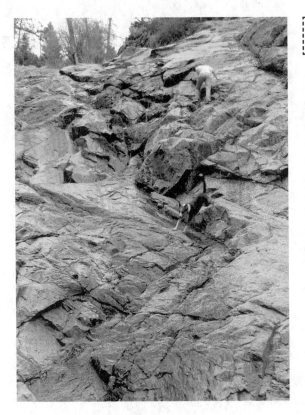

This is not the easy way to the top of the waterfall.

Take a moment here to limber up, giving the calves and hamstrings an extra stretch. The first mile is like a good workout on a Stair-Master, only far more scenic. You ascend from a lush creekside forest to thinner stands of fir and pine as the trail climbs steadily from an elevation of 8,400 to just over 9,400 feet. It seems longer than a mile, and maybe it is if you count backsliding on loose gravel. Multiple switchbacks contribute to the illusion that the top is just around the bend. Park benches near the 0.25- and 0.75-mile marks provide brief respites from exertion.

Keep an eye out for garter snakes and horned lizards prowling through the pine needles. Black bear, mule deer, and porcupine also inhabit the area but are rarely sighted. A favorite among the summer wildflowers is scarlet gilia, or sky-rocket. Oregon grape blooms in the spring and resembles holly with blueberry clusters when it ripens in the late summer. The plant is better known for its medicinal uses than for its snacking value. The berries are edible, though bitter, and children have been known to feel queasy after eating a few. You'd be better off foraging for wild strawberries.

You know you're near the top when the rocks begin to sparkle with mica. When the trail finally does level off, push on just another 0.25 mile. Past an area of storm-felled trees you will find two picnic tables and the best views in the park. Santa Fe sits near to the west, while the Jemez Mountains make up the bulk of the shadowy heaps in the distance.

When you're ready to continue, follow the arrow back down the mountain through another course of switchbacks. Some impatient hikers have trampled shortcuts straight down—refrain from following in their footsteps.

A signpost on an otherwise unmarked fork turns up about 2 miles into the hike. This is *not* the small loop seen on park maps. Instead, the left fork leads to the RV area. Unless you need the shortest route to the restrooms, avoid the detour.

The trail turns south and leads you to a fork with signs indicating that the left branch belongs to the Circle Trail and the right is the Girl Scout Trail. Both paths feature rock borders and labeled plants. They end up in the same place, though the Girl Scout Trail is slightly longer. The history of the Scouts in this area predates the founding of Hyde Park. Benjamin Hyde, affectionately known as "Uncle Bennie," became Santa Fe's scoutmaster shortly after moving to town in 1927. His wife, Helen, bequeathed the land to the state in the year following his untimely death in 1933.

You soon return to Hyde Park Road, about 0.7 mile north of where you began. Cross back over the road and look for a nearby bridge, followed by a staircase in the embankment. At the top of the stairs are an Adirondack shelter and, beyond that, a dirt road. Straight across the road are signs for Circle Trail and the Visitor Center, followed by a map signboard. The trail runs parallel to the campground road and you may be able to spot campsites through the trees, hear campers' songs, and smell what's cooking on the grills. The area is mellower when the main camping loop closes for the winter (November 1–Easter).

About 0.5 mile into East Circle Trail, or 3 miles into the hike, you'll reach a well-signed junction with Piggyback Trail. Veer left to stay on Circle Trail. About 40 yards farther, another sign shows where the Waterfall Trail begins. This 0.25-mile spur is a cool side trip up a shady little canyon. Routed to follow a rocky stream, the riparian path seems a world away from the rest of the park. Though it flows only after rain or snowmelt, it's well worth a 30-minute detour, even when it lacks a waterfall.

To continue on Circle Trail, return to the Waterfall trailhead and cross the wooden footbridge. At 0.25 mile or so past the bridge, a steep clearing begins to show through the trees. That's the sledding area. In the 1940s and 1950s, it was Santa Fe's first and only ski basin, complete with a towrope powered by a Cadillac engine. The structure at the base was built by the Civilian Conservation Corps in 1938 and allegedly used then as a cooking school. You'll recognize it now as Hyde Park Lodge. A couple of switchbacks take you back down to the parking area.

NEARBY ACTIVITIES

Hyde Park is the gateway to endless opportunities for outdoor recreation. Start by driving north 8.4 miles on Hyde Park Road, also known as the Santa Fe National Forest Scenic Byway. It ends at the Santa Fe Ski Area, near the southwest corner of the vast Pecos Wilderness. The Hyde Park Visitors Center has all the information you need for exploring this corner of Santa Fe National Forest.

35 GALISTEO BASIN PRESERVE:
Cowboy Shack

KEY AT-A-GLANCE INFORMATION

LENGTH: 3-mile balloon

DIFFICULTY: Easy–moderate

SCENERY: Ranching remnants, ridgetop views over juniper hills and grasslands, stream corridors, and other scenic erosion features

EXPOSURE: Some canyon shade

TRAIL TRAFFIC: Moderate

SHARED USE: Moderate (mountain bikers, equestrians; popular with dog owners)

TRAIL SURFACE: Dirt

HIKING TIME: 1 hour

DRIVING DISTANCE: 70 miles

ACCESS: Daylight hours, year-round

LAND STATUS: Commonweal Conservancy–Galisteo Basin Preserve

MAPS: USGS Galisteo

FACILITIES: Restroom at trailhead, no water

LAST-CHANCE FOOD/GAS: All services on US 285, about 5 miles from the trailhead.

SPECIAL COMMENTS: Maps and guidelines for hiking at the Galisteo Basin Preserve are posted at trailheads and at galisteobasin preserve.com.

GPS TRAILHEAD COORDINATES

Latitude   35° 28' 25"

Longitude   W105° 55' 35"

IN BRIEF

Progressive planning in residential development led to the creation of a public trail system with unspoiled viewsheds just minutes south of Santa Fe. In choosing just one among the many attractive options, the unanimous decision favored the trail that boasts a little bit of everything.

DESCRIPTION

The Galisteo Basin is packed with remnants from multiple cultural occupations, including the largest pueblo ruins in the United States. San Marcos Pueblo, located a few miles west of the Preserve, boasts 2,000 rooms, a far higher count than settlements in Chaco Culture National Historical Park or Mesa Verde National Park can claim.

Pioneers, ranchers, railroads later left their distinctive marks. The construction of the Atchison, Topeka & Santa Fe (AT&SF) Railway in the 1880s displaced the Galisteo Creek and reduced the width of the floodplain. Overgrazing, coupled with the 1920s Dust Bowl drought, led to increased desertification and continued incision of Galisteo Creek. Before the 1880s, the Galisteo watershed contained an estimated 5,000 acres of wetland, wet meadow, and riparian ecosystems. Today that estimate is down to 1,000 acres.

Directions ————————————————→

From I-25 North, take Exit 290 and go 5.3 miles south on US 285. About 0.5 mile after crossing the railroad tracks, turn right on Astral Valley Road. Go 1.2 miles southwest on Astral Valley Road/Morning Star Ridge and park in the lot by the Cowboy Shack.

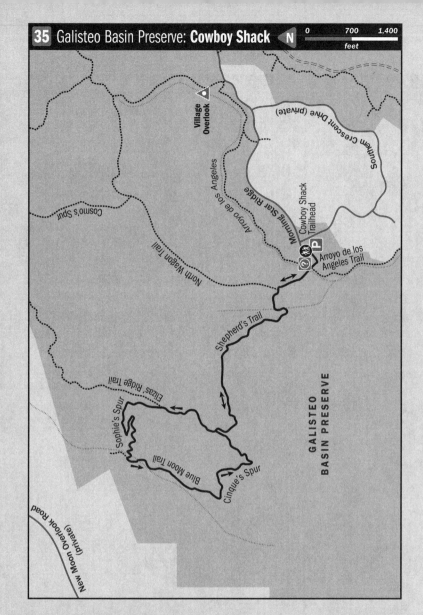

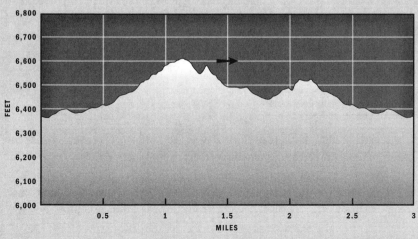

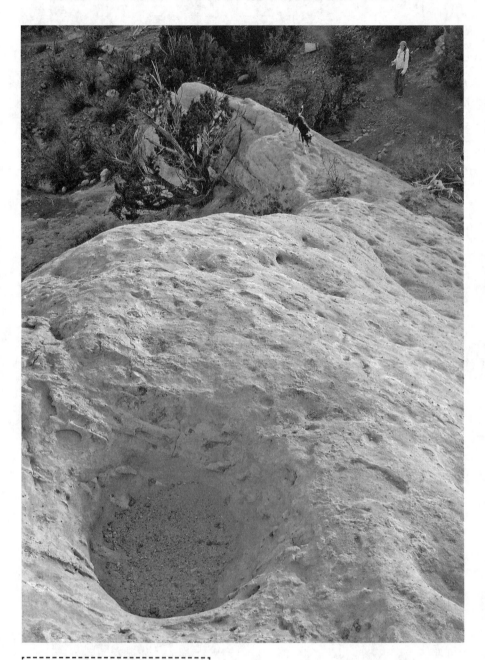

The "blowhole" on the white whale rock

In the early 2000s, both real-estate developers and oil prospectors suddenly took a sharp interest in the basin, sending preservationists scrambling to protect historic and cultural sites throughout the area. In 2004 the U.S. Congress responded by passing the Galisteo Basin Archaeological Sites Protection Act, which identifies 24 archaeological sites worthy of preservation, protection, and interpretation. For years these sites were among the state's best-kept secrets outside of Los Alamos. Then in 2010 the BLM–Taos Field Office released a report that pretty much pinpoints their locations. Several hikes in this book visit lands with protected sites, including Las Huertas de Placitas, Ball Ranch, La Cienega, and Cañada de la Cueva.

If the process of developing these areas for public access and interpretation seems excruciatingly slow, it's a good indication of the level of protection the sites are receiving. True, geologists are still poking around for petrol, and new roads and houses seem to spring up daily throughout the region; but rest assured that when it comes to new hiking trails, the pace of progress is cautionary.

Commonweal Conservancy, a Santa Fe–based nonprofit organization, leads the pack, blazing paths at a rate that exceeds 2 miles per year. Their vision for the 13,522-acre Galisteo Basin Preserve includes 50 miles of hiking, mountain biking, and equestrian trails that connect to trail networks on adjoining federal, state, and Santa Fe County public lands to create a regional open-space area of more than 22,000 acres.

For now, about 15 miles of developed trails wind along the east side of the Preserve. Maps posted at the trailhead and on the Galisteo Basin Preserve website illustrate your hiking options here. (See Special Comments.) After a daylong sampling of these various trails, our test group unanimously agreed upon a favorite route.

The hike begins on the North Wagon Trail. Locate Marker 17 about 200 feet southwest of the Cowboy Shack. Turn right on an old doubletrack to cross a shallow streambed in the Arroyo de los Angeles and pass by the Spring Well windmill. Unlike most stock tanks in cowboy country, the one here is stocked with goldfish. Relics from the bygone era of ranching turn up trailside just ahead: a derelict corral and trough, an array of shooting targets dangling on rusty chains. The Galisteo Basin Preserve is centered on the east side of the Galisteo Basin, on property formerly known as Thornton Ranch, one of the key culprits responsible for the degradation of the Galisteo watershed. If there's a plus side to their legacy, it's that erosion tends to result in interesting landscape features. The scenic value of downcutting and incising is undeniable, as you'll soon see along the trail ahead.

Continue up this brief segment of the North Wagon Trail to Marker 18, then turn left on Shepherd's Trail. This 0.7-mile singletrack starts on an S-curve to cross a large headcut in the upper branch of the arroyo. Sediment layers in the cut range in color from tawny to ocher, with another half-dozen pigments from the Santa Fe palette. Upstream portions of this draw are solid white slots running 20 feet deep and narrowing down from shoulder-width to a hairline fracture.

Shepherd's Trail resumes north, then bends west as it climbs through a gap in a low ridge. The ground soon takes on a candied shade of red, eroded to expose pillowy white rocks. Whatever you see in it, you'll have to admit the quirky shapes and color combinations in the landscape are at least momentarily arresting.

Less than a mile into the hike, the trail hooks around a rock that vaguely resembles a white whale. (Venture up top to check out the blowhole.) It then hooks back to a saddle on the ridge, where you find Junction 19. Bear right on Elizas' Ridge Trail and continue uphill, climbing north to Junction 20. Take a breather here to enjoy the views from the 6,600-foot peak of this route.

Elizas' Ridge Trail continues north from Junction 20, but this short route bears left onto Sophie's Spur, a 0.4-mile corkscrewed path that drops west into an unnamed arroyo. Turn left to follow Blue Moon Trail down the streambed. This shaded 0.3-mile segment terminates at Cinque's Spur, a 0.3-mile segment that meanders up the low end of the ridge to meet the south end of Elizas' Ridge Trail. A left turn here leads back to the saddle where you found Junction 19. Turn right back onto Shepherd's Trail to retrace your steps down to the Cowboy Shack.

NEARBY ACTIVITIES

The Museum of New Mexico Foundation leads field trips to Galisteo Basin sites that are otherwise closed to the public. Check the MNMF Friends of Archaeology events calendar at **museumfoundation.org/calendar,** or call (505) 982-6366. The Museum of Indian Arts & Culture also leads tours in the area. Check **miaclab.org** (click on "Events & Exhibitions") or call (505) 476-1250. Be aware that these tours are often fully booked weeks in advance.

The **Santa Fe Botanical Garden** hosts guided hikes and scheduled events April–October at the Ortiz Mountains Educational Preserve, about 8 miles south of Cerrillos. Visit **santafebotanicalgarden.org** for the OMEP schedule, or call (505) 471-9103. For additional local information, visit **galisteoarcheology.org** and **turquoisetrail.org**.

GLORIETA CANYON GHOST TOWN

IN BRIEF

Take a break from yucca and cacti for a cool hike through aspen and spruce. The shaded canyon route visits relics from the last century, while short side paths lead to abandoned mines. Vintage cars stuck along the trail suggest it was once a horrible road. The traffic now is an intermittent stream of mountain bikers, equestrians, and hikers with pack-mule dogs.

DESCRIPTION

Will Rogers once observed, "Whoever designed the streets in Santa Fe must have been drunk and riding backwards on a mule." Apparently, the same engineering process was applied to a nearby segment of interstate highway. Northbound lanes on I-25 from Santa Fe go directly southeast to the Glorieta Unit of Pecos National Historical Park. This misdirection is temporarily corrected between Cañoncito and Glorieta Pass, but from there it turns southeast again as it skirts the base of Glorieta Mesa.

North and South have been at odds here before. On March 28, 1862, the Union captain Gurdin Chapin (my great-great-grandfather-in-law) led a reconnaissance mission into the

Directions

From I-25 North, take Exit 299 at Glorieta. Turn left to cross the bridge over the interstate, then turn left again, following the signs to the Glorieta Conference Center. The main entrance is less than a mile from the exit. From the front gate, go straight 0.75 mile on Oak. Turn left beneath the "Rancho de Glorieta" sign on Holly and follow the arrows to the hiker's parking lot.

KEY AT-A-GLANCE INFORMATION

LENGTH: 8-mile out-and-back

DIFFICULTY: Moderate

SCENERY: Aspen, mixed conifer, early-20th-century ruins

EXPOSURE: Mostly shaded

TRAIL TRAFFIC: Heavy

SHARED USE: Heavy (mountain bikers, equestrians; popular with dog owners; restricted motor-vehicle access)

TRAIL SURFACE: Dirt, loose rock

HIKING TIME: 3–4 hours

DRIVING DISTANCE: 74 miles

ACCESS: Monday–Saturday, year-round

LAND STATUS: Private trailhead area; Santa Fe National Forest–Pecos/Las Vegas Ranger District

MAPS: Santa Fe National Forest–East Half; USGS Glorieta, McClure Reservoir

FACILITIES: Signed trails; food services and restrooms pending new ownership policy

LAST-CHANCE FOOD/GAS: Gas stations in the town of Glorieta

SPECIAL COMMENTS: This hike starts on private land.

GPS TRAILHEAD COORDINATES

Latitude   35° 35' 57"

Longitude   105° 46' 12"

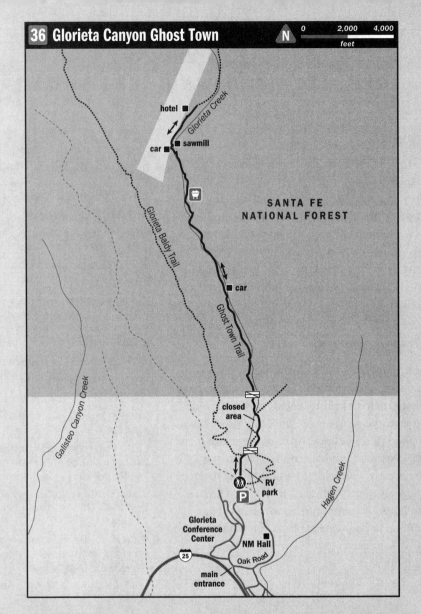

N

0   2,000   4,000
feet

hotel

Glorieta Creek

car   sawmill

SANTA FE NATIONAL FOREST

Glorieta Baldy Trail

car

Ghost Town Trail

Galisteo Canyon Creek

closed area

Hagen Creek

RV park

P

Glorieta Conference Center

NM Hall

25

Oak Road

main entrance

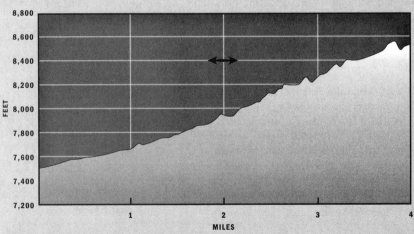

woods at Glorieta Pass. His cavalry unit advanced fewer than 800 yards before spotting Confederate troops in attack position. In the ensuing battle, later to be known as "the Gettysburg of the West," the South's Texan regiments ultimately outgunned the North's Colorado units. Meanwhile, however, the New Mexico Volunteers had scrambled and rappelled down the cliffs of Glorieta Mesa to torch a supply train behind enemy lines. With their provisions incinerated, the Rebs had no choice but to fall back.

Two weeks later, Colonel Gabriel René Paul (Chapin's father-in-law) led attacks on retreating Confederate troops near Peralta, about 10 miles south of Albuquerque. This battle was immortalized (and greatly exaggerated) a century later in Sergio Leone's cinematic masterpiece *The Good, the Bad and the Ugly*. In terms of ending the South's advancements into northern New Mexico and ultimately defeating the Confederate campaign to win the West, the more significant showdown was the Battle of Glorieta Pass.

But the South would rise again. In 1949 the Southern Baptist Convention settled on Glorieta for the site of its western assembly. Construction of the Baptist Conference Center began in 1952, and the venue grew into the resort-like complex that dominates the town today. After 25 years of operating as the LifeWay Glorieta Conference Center, the 2,200-acre facility was sold in 2013 for $1 to Glorieta 2.0, a nondenominational Christian summer camp. How this will affect access to some of the finest trails in the southern Sangre de Cristo Mountains is now uncertain. As of 2014, hiking is not permitted on Sundays, and the upper reaches of this hike have been declared off limits. More about that later.

The most popular destination is the Ghost Town, misspelled in spooky letters on some signs for the campy fun of it. What remains of the neglected settlement near the end of the trail doesn't quite amount to the makings of a very Brady adventure, but natural scenery throughout the canyon is reason enough to hike this route more than once. In May and June, wild iris blooms in watercolor pastels, while scarlet columbine glows as though electric. Look closely at the latter and you'll see how it got its name. (Hint: *Columbine* means "dovelike.") Stands of aspen create pockets of gold in autumn.

The hike: Follow the obvious trail and arrows to a gate at the north end of the RV park. Signs posted just past the gate indicate that the Glorieta Baldy and Broken Arrow trailheads are nearby to the left. The trail to the Ghost Town begins here.

Turn right and head north along the braided road. About 0.7 miles into the hike, veer left at the fork and cross the creek at a partially washed-out dam. (If you miss this turn, you'll end up in the wrong canyon.) You'll soon arrive at a second gate that's identical to the first one. Go through the pedestrian access and continue north.

The trail from here is easy to follow. It slims down as it exits the meadow and enters the narrow, wooded canyon. An arrow at the fork ahead recommends the left branch, but take your pick: low and damp or high and dry. The branches rejoin about 500 feet upstream.

The creek fades in and out along the way, sometimes spilling over the trail, and sometimes withering away. It can get muddy in spots, particularly after a heavy summer rain, or slick with ice in the winter. On the plus side, the predominantly south-facing slope and relatively low altitude help thaw out this trail sooner than most others in northern New Mexico. Smooth horsetail adorns the creekside, as does the body of a Chevy humpback, or maybe a Packard judging by the X-member frame. Apparently a mid-1930s model, the unfortunate vehicle has been stranded 1.5 miles up this former forest road (FR 374) for at least half a century.

Another fork appears 0.8 mile past the car. Again, the diversion is temporary, but cliffs flanking the left branch make it the more scenic way to go. Just past the merge, look for a clearing on the right. A new shelter stands close by on the west side. On the north side, an old miner's cabin has been remodeled into a primitive lean-to. Footpaths lead off to the south and east to weave through clusters of abandoned mines. It's worth a quick detour, but heed the posted warnings.

A half-mile past the clearing, you arrive at a collapsed wooden bridge. Another car is parked ahead on the left side of a meadow. It's in slightly better shape than the last one but still doesn't leave much to identify. A 1939 Plymouth sedan might be a good guess based on its outside door hinges and square headlights. Beyond it on the right, you will come to the site of an old sawmill, as evidenced by a heap of lumber and the scar of a skid trail on the sloping canyon wall. Broken boards and rusty nails are abundant nearby—watch your step. Also heed any valid NO TRESPASSING signage posted in this area, keeping in mind that New Mexico statute requires such notices to include the owner's name and address. The anonymous signage that appeared here in 2014 is unclear on where the boundary lies. However, forest service GIS data indicates that the trail enters private land approximately halfway between the Plymouth and the sawmill, and exits directly south of the hotel mentioned below. Hence, you could stay on forest property by walking several yards east of the trail for the next quarter mile.

This site is generally referred to as the Glorieta Ghost Town, which seems a bit off when you consider that the town of Glorieta is a few miles south and still somewhat alive. A relatively flat 0.25 mile past the sawmill, a two-story hotel once faced the craggy cliffs towering to the east. Built around 1880, the Glorieta House Hotel (sometimes referred to as The Palace Hotel) hosted numerous balls in its early years, the popularity of which seemed to coincide with crackdowns on saloons and brothels in the nearby towns of Glorieta and Las Vegas. The hotel later catered to prospectors and hunters. The building collapsed in the 1950s, and little more remains than a stone foundation no bigger than an economy-motel suite. Behind it, a makeshift wooden cross teeters at the head of a stony grave. Hidden farther back to the right, a narrow shaft tunnels into solid rock. Its depth exceeds the range of pocket flashlights.

The route ends here, but the trail continues northeast. Seasoned hikers can proceed uphill if they wish. At about the point where the creek bends up to the

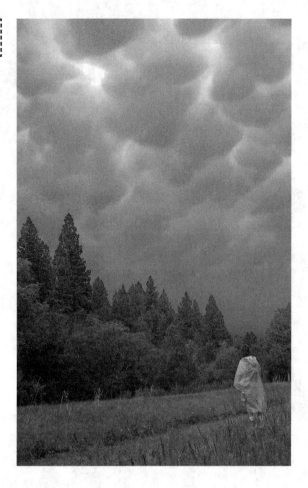

> Always be prepared for sudden changes in weather.

west, the trail turns north. From there it's a steep half-mile up to La Cueva Ridge. Glorieta Baldy is 1.5 miles west. From there, the Glorieta Baldy Trail runs about 5 miles back down to the RV lot, losing 2,700 feet in elevation along the way.

NEARBY ACTIVITIES

Reflect upon the world-renowned iconography at the **Pecos Benedictine Monastery.** The chapel on the 11,000-acre monastic property was originally built as part of a dude ranch for vacationing city slickers more than 50 years ago, and the adobe building that houses the Abbey Gift Shop previously served as a stop on the Pony Express. To get there, drive straight from the main entrance to Pecos, about 6.5 miles east on NM 50. Turn left at the junction with NM 63 and go north about 1.5 miles. The monastery entrance is on the left. For more information, call (505) 757-6600 or visit **pecosmonastery.org**.

Glorieta Battlefield Trail, an interpretive walking trail, is an expertly groomed and tightly coiled path that winds for 2.3 miles along a wooded ridge. To find this hidden bit of history, you'll first need to visit the Pecos National Historic Park Visitor Center, which is also on NM 63, about 2 miles *south* of the NM 50 junction: (505) 757-7241; **nps.gov/peco**.

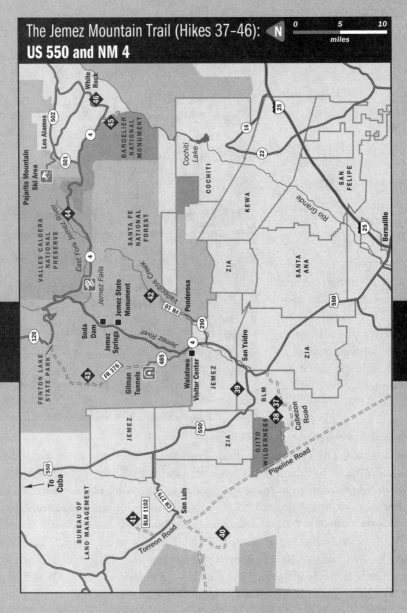

The Jemez Mountain Trail (Hikes 37–46): US 550 and NM 4

N

0   5   10
miles

THE JEMEZ MOUNTAIN TRAIL
(NM 550 AND NM 4)

37 WHITE MESA BIKE TRAILS AREA

KEY AT-A-GLANCE INFORMATION

LENGTH: 5.1-mile loop and spur

DIFFICULTY: Moderate

SCENERY: Gypsum ridges, painted desert, classic anticline, wildlife

EXPOSURE: Minimal shade

TRAIL TRAFFIC: Moderate

SHARED USE: Moderate (mountain bikers, separate horse trail; no motorized vehicles)

TRAIL SURFACE: Sand, dirt, loose rock, gypsum

HIKING TIME: 3 hours

DRIVING DISTANCE: 42 miles

ACCESS: Year-round

LAND STATUS: BLM—Rio Puerco Field Office

MAPS: USGS Sky Village NE (Cerro Conejo), San Ysidro

FACILITIES: Detailed maps at trailhead and trail junctions

LAST-CHANCE FOOD/GAS: Convenience store—gas station in San Ysidro (See Directions)

SPECIAL COMMENTS: For an authoritative briefing on the complex geological features at White Mesa, visit geoinfo.nmt.edu/tour/landmarks/san_ysidro.

GPS TRAILHEAD COORDINATES

Latitude   35° 29' 54"

Longitude   106° 50' 30"

IN BRIEF

Fifteen miles of well-marked trails—open to both biking and hiking—explore a land packed with geological curiosities. Though this hike hits most of the major features, it covers just a fraction of all possible routes on this endlessly fascinating terrain.

DESCRIPTION

A large trail map stands at the trailhead just beyond the green gate. Numbers on the map correspond with trail junctions, where smaller versions of the same map are located. This route follows the numbers in this order: Outbound: 1–3, 21, 22, 12, 11, 10. Return: 10–17, 23, 1. The connecting segment between 17 and 23 is a well-defined dirt road that does not appear on the maps.

Now that you've got the instant overview, follow the doubletrack to Junction 1. Keep to the left along a path on a low ridge. More roads meet at Junction 2 than the maps show, but continue straight.

The first 0.3 mile is on the dull side, but the scenery changes abruptly at Junction 3. Here, on the cusp of a scooped valley, it appears

----

Directions ————————→

From I-25 North, take Exit 242 at Bernalillo. Turn left on US 550 and go northwest 21.2 miles. (San Ysidro is about 2 miles too far.) Turn left on Cabezon Road. (Look for the brown sign for Ojito Wilderness and White Mesa Bike Trails on the right, followed by a green street sign for Cabezon Road on the left.) Go left at the first fork ahead. After 4.4 miles on Cabezon Road, turn right, into a fenced parking lot for the White Mesa Bike Trails Area. The trailhead is at the gate in the northeastern corner of the parking lot.

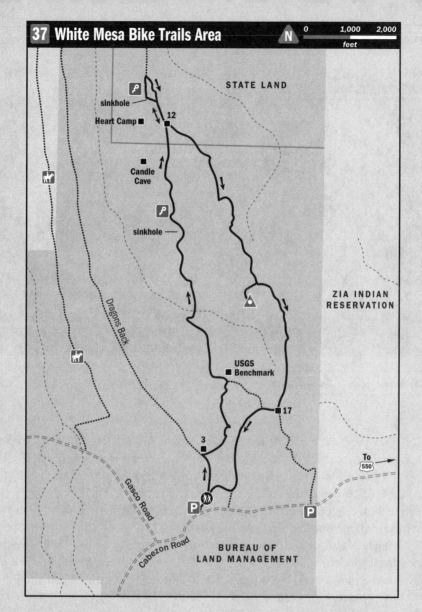

N   0   1,000   2,000
feet

STATE LAND

sinkhole

Heart Camp ■   ■ 12

Candle
Cave ■

sinkhole

ZIA INDIAN
RESERVATION

Dragons Back

USGS
Benchmark ■

■ 17

3 ■

Gasco Road

To
550

P

P

Cabezon Road

BUREAU OF
LAND MANAGEMENT

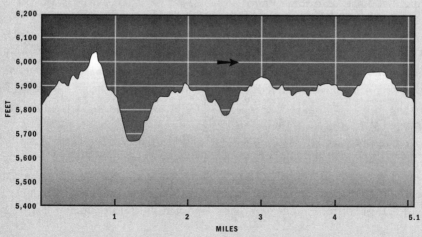

6,200
6,100
6,000
5,900
5,800
5,700
5,600
5,500
5,400

FEET

1   2   3   4   5.1

MILES

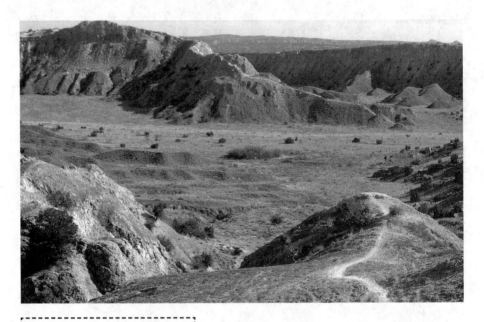

Southwest view near Trail Marker 14

a leviathan took a bite out of the Earth's crust. If such an enormous creature did exist, it might resemble the ridge to the left, aptly named Dragon's Back. The harrowing 3.25-mile bike path along its spine leaves little room for error.

At least two paths run off to the right at Junction 3. The more popular one sticks close to the rim, while the official trail takes the higher ground. Either way, keep the rim on your left until you hit Junction 21.

Straight ahead of 21, the rim rises nearly 100 feet to an overlook. The dark stumplike cylinder at the peak is a USGS benchmark. There, you'll find the best views on the trail system, but watch the kids—the drop on the other side is a sheer 200 feet or more. Many casual hikers are content in making this their destination for an out-and-back that totals up to 1.6 miles, but we're just getting started.

Take a moment to scope out the terrain ahead. The next leg of the hike is the narrow gypsum ridge reaching out on the left like Dragon's Back in miniature. It points toward an elongated dome informally known as Travertine Ridge, which stretches along the floor of the valley. With binoculars or a sharp eye, you can make out the trail curving around it to the right. Now note the yellowish sandstone ridge at the far end of the valley. It extends south for the entire length of the east rim—that's your return route.

Dragon's Back and the sandstone ridge mark the flanks of the Tierra Amarilla Anticline, sometimes called the San Ysidro Anticline. Don't be surprised to find a geology class on a field trip here. This fold in the surface exposes a chronological sequence of rock layers. The oldest rock, at the core of the anticline, is composed of red-to-green siltstones and mudstones deposited on the floodplain of a river system about 210 million years ago. Dinosaur bones and gizzard stones from more recent times occasionally turn up in nearby washes. (Fossil collecting is strictly prohibited here, so leave them where you found them.)

Another landmark worth noting, though it's not on public land, is White Mesa, peeking up about 2 miles to the northeast. B-movie-trivia buffs, take note: much of the sci-fi thriller *Ghosts of Mars* was shot there in 2000. The gypsum mesa required thousands of gallons of food dye before it could pass for the red planet. It took several reapplications because frequent monsoon rains kept washing it back to its natural albino state.

To continue the hike, follow the white ridge down into the valley. The red valley floor can get sloppy after rain or snow, but you'll soon climb out of it as you ascend Travertine Ridge. Once on the ridge, the trail skirts around the right side of a series of domed hills. Sinkholes at the top of any one of them reveal cavernous interiors. These travertine hills sound hollow under a pair of hiking boots, and walking on them may give you the sensation of treading on thin ice. So are any too fragile to support the weight of, say, a hiker? According to one geology expert, that's a good question.

Mineral springs—not fit for drinking—leak out near the trail. A more active one bubbling up on the left is about the diameter of a rain barrel but probably deeper. You may notice the greenery and sulfuric smell before finding the water. Enjoy this unusual little ecosystem from a distance, because the surrounding mud is also deeper than you think.

Past the spring, the path curves around the right side of a hill with conjoined peaks, followed by a larger hill. Just ahead, a pair of signposts indicates that you're entering public land. Consider turning left at the signposts for this off-trail detour: continue around the north base of the mound about 500 feet until you reach the edge of a cliff. To the immediate left, two deep fissures split the west side of the hill wide open. Climb down the cliff for a closer look. The fissures spread south, forming a labyrinth of slots, tunnels, and cracks that could take all day to explore. Poke around enough and you'll find a cave stocked with votive candles.

When you're ready to move on, return to the point where you climbed down, and then follow the base of the cliff north about 500 feet to a low point where it's easier to climb back up. Then follow the dry wash east, back to the main trail. Turn left and you'll soon reach Junction 12. Another sizable hump rises on the left, and another valley opens ahead on the right. In view beyond the valley, US 550 and a white ribbon of the Rio Salado skirt the southern end of Red Mesa.

At Junction 11, turn left and follow a footpath uphill. It soon crosses a fissure that widens to the left. Follow it south to another sinkhole. An opportunity for another off-trail detour begins here. About 400 feet southwest of the sinkhole is a pair of cuts in the rocky slope, each about as wide as a country lane. The upper one is an L-shaped gap. The lower one is rectangular and resembles a small corral; perhaps it was used as one long ago. Its sheltering walls make it an ideal spot to break for lunch on hot days or to pitch a tent on windy nights. Some refer to this

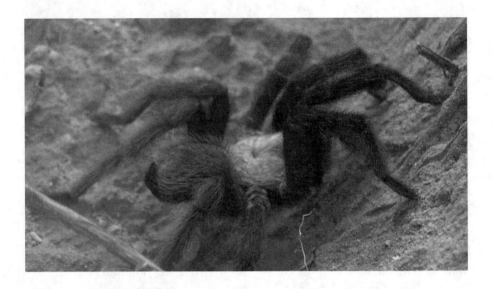

place as Heart Camp because a curious collection of heart-shaped stones has been placed on the walls. As with Candle Cave, no one seems to know when or why the tradition began.

Return to the crack on the ridge and follow it north. Springs seep out and wash over rippled mineral residue. Junction 10 stands at the base below. You could continue south on the trail another 2 miles. Or, to follow this route, turn around here and walk along the east side of the mound, back to Junction 12. Bear left to Junction 13.

From Junction 13, the smaller path on the right is more scenic and less confusing than the road on the left. It also runs closer to the rim, which you'll keep on your right for the next 0.8 mile to Junction 16. There, on the right, you'll find the second of two spurs marked DEAD END. This one is a 0.25-mile (round-trip) detour down a dead-end ridge with breathtaking drop-offs on both sides. It leads to a scenic overlook.

Just under 0.7 mile past Junction 16, the trail splits in at least four directions in a kind of roundabout at Junction 17. From here you have three options for returning to the parking lot. The navigationally challenged might find it easiest to return to the anticline overlook, about 0.25 mile to the northwest via Junction 20, and then backtrack to the parking lot from there. Energetic hikers might head southeast for a steep descent through banded terrain. This 0.55-mile segment leads to the east parking lot on Cabezon Road; turn right and follow the road about 0.5 mile from there back to the west parking lot.

This route follows a marginally shorter way along a dirt road not indicated on the maps. From Junction 17, it heads west about 0.1 mile before bending southwest for another 0.1 mile. There it joins the doubletrack running straight south from Junction 20. After going 0.3 mile south, turn right at the fork to reach Junction 23. Turn left there to reach Junction 1 and the parking lot.

OJITO WILDERNESS:
Querencia Arroyo

IN BRIEF

This freeform route follows ridgelines, drainages, and a dirt road to explore the rim and alcoves of an unnamed mesa on the seldom-visited east side of the Ojito Wilderness.

DESCRIPTION

Since the original Wilderness Act passed in 1964, the National Wilderness Preservation System has grown to include 680 areas nationwide. The first was New Mexico's own Gila Primitive Area, as it was then called. Another 22 followed in about as many years. With nearly 1 percent of New Mexico's public lands designated as wilderness, the state would let it rest at that for the next 18 years. The hiatus finally ended with the Ojito Wilderness Act of 2005, which permanently protects more than 11,000 acres of beautifully rugged land next to the Zia Reservation.

If you've explored the Ojito before, you'll find the scenic value of the route described here is (let's be honest) only slightly above average. The truly photogenic terrain is in the vicinity of Bernalallito Mesa, in the southwest corner of the wilderness (see Nearby Activities, page 215),

KEY AT-A-GLANCE INFORMATION

LENGTH: 6.3-mile loop

DIFFICULTY: Moderate with short, strenuous climbs

SCENERY: Banded cliff formations, sinuous arroyos, ruins

EXPOSURE: Minimal shade

TRAIL TRAFFIC: Low

SHARED USE: Low (equestrians; livestock; primitive camping; target shooting; no vehicles off designated roads)

TRAIL SURFACE: Dirt, rock

HIKING TIME: 3–4 hours

DRIVING DISTANCE: 44 miles

ACCESS: Year-round

LAND STATUS: BLM–Rio Puerco Field Office; Wilderness Area

MAPS: USGS San Ysidro, Ojito Spring

FACILITIES: None

LAST-CHANCE FOOD/GAS: Convenience store–gas station in San Ysidro, about 7 miles from the trailhead (see Directions)

Directions ⟶

From I-25 North, take Exit 242 at Bernalillo. Turn left on US 550 and go northwest 21.2 miles. (San Ysidro is about 2 miles too far.) Turn left on Cabezon Road and go 4.7 miles west, a quarter-mile past the second fenced parking lot for White Mesa Bike Trails. Turn right on Gasco Road (signage missing) and go 1.25 miles northwest. Just after the road bends north (and 100 yards before the gate) turn left on a doubletrack and go 0.3 mile southwest, bearing right at the Y. Park alongside the red-and-white ridgepoint.

GPS TRAILHEAD COORDINATES

Latitude   35° 30' 08"
Longitude   106° 52' 03"

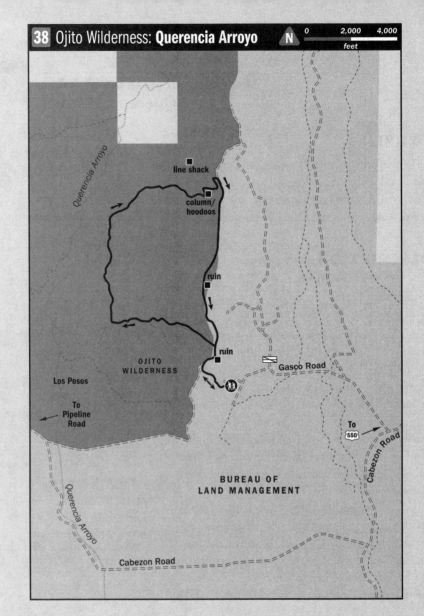

N

0   2,000   4,000
feet

line shack

column/
hoodoos

Querencia Arroyo

ruin

ruin

Gasco Road

OJITO
WILDERNESS

Los Posos

To
Pipeline
Road

To
550

Cabezon Road

BUREAU OF
LAND MANAGEMENT

Querencia Arroyo

Cabezon Road

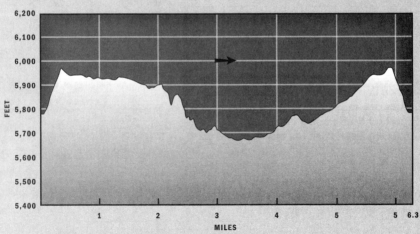

6,200

6,100

6,000

5,900

5,800

5,700

5,600

5,500

5,400

FEET

1   2   3   4   5   6.3

MILES

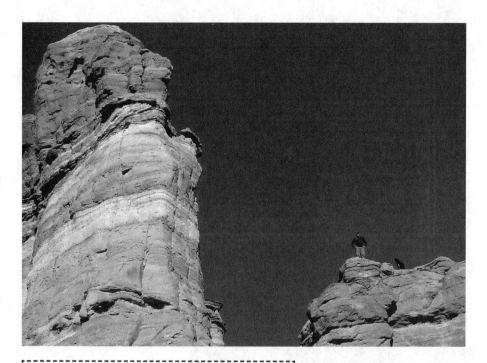

A column of rock stands in the east corner of the last alcove.

and north of the Arroyo Bernalallito (as described in the first edition of this book). Those routes are also better established, making them fairly easy to follow. But reaching their trailheads requires a longer drive on Cabezon Road, which has seen improvements in recent years yet still gets dicey after a little rain—especially if you get caught west of the Querencia Arroyo.

This route was plotted in response to requests for the quickest way into (and out of) the Ojito. It focuses on an unnamed mesa east of the prominent drainage. Querencia Arroyo passes through Los Posos ("the dregs") and parallels the north–south segments of this hike. You won't see much of it along the way. It just happens to be the nearest named landmark—and what an appropriate name it is. *Querencia* is defined as both "homing instinct" and "haunt of wild hearts." Put another way, it's the natural inclination that draws you to the place of your desire.

The hike begins with a challenge. You're facing 200-foot cliffs with no discernible trails to the top. Several ridges offer a ramp up. The nearest one is a possibility but isn't the easiest. Try the one to the immediate south, crossing the mouth of the alcove and a dry wash along the way.

From the ridgepoint, climb 0.3 mile west-northwest. Look for game paths to help guide you along. A few yards beyond the uppermost rim, you'll intercept a well-defined dirt road that designates the east boundary of the Ojito Wilderness. Take a good look around. You'll need to recognize this area to find your way back down later on.

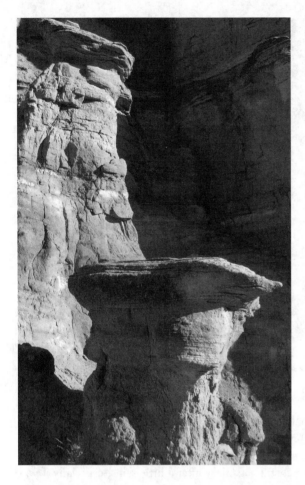

Turn right and follow the road north. About 200 yards ahead on the right is an ancient settlement about the size of a baseball field. Scarcely a cornerstone remains intact, but heed the discreetly posted notice: This site is under the protection of the Archeological Resources Protection Act, the Antiquities Act, and the Native American Grave Protection and Repatriation Act. Leave it the way you found it.

Directly across the road from the site is an expanse of grassland and juniper. Wander off in that direction (northwest) and soon you'll intercept one of several small erosion channels that eventually funnel into a main wash. As you continue downstream, the sinuous wash cuts deeper, sculpting bedrock as it winds west. About a mile from the road (including twists and turns), it passes an orange fencepost and shallows out as it enters a meadow. Turn right to exit the wash.

The next segment is a half-mile, cross-country meander north over a low rise. If you didn't bring a compass, keep the orange fenceposts in sight and on your right to maintain your direction. You might also pick up a cattle trail to make the walk easier. Either way, you'll eventually intercept the rim of a finger canyon. Negotiate one last drop to the floor of the Ojito.

The next mile or so is simply a matter walking alongside the mesa, keeping the wall on your right, and exploring whichever alcoves and niches pique your interest. There's not much in the way of paths to follow, but you will cross multiple channels and two barbwire fences before you reach the main alcove. You'll know it when you see the towering column of rock standing in the easternmost corner.

The east boundary road passes within 200 yards of the rim behind the rock tower, but you won't find a sensible way up in the immediate vicinity. Continue exploring the alcove. A faint path begins at the point of the first ridge north of the tower. It climbs past a pair of hoodoos on the way to the rim.

Once above the rim (where you'll encounter yet another barbwire fence), scan the alcove below for stone ruins of what may have been a homestead or a line shack. (Line shacks were small cabins built on the open range where cowboys could take shelter.) Also take in views that extend well beyond Ojito boundaries: Red Mesa peaks about 5 miles north-northeast. Cucho Mesa rises 2 miles northwest. Cabezon Peak stands 14 miles northwest. The massive formation to its south is Mesa Prieta.

Head east from the rim to locate the east boundary road, then hike it about 1.8 miles south, back to the point you climbed up. You'll pass a few more pueblo mounds along the way. About a mile east, one of the White Mesa bike trails draws a distinct line down the spine of a ridge nicknamed "Dragon's Back." A mile west, the Querencia Arroyo cuts a dark, twisted channel through the valley below.

NEARBY ACTIVITIES

For the two most popular hikes in the Ojito, return to the junction of Gasco and Cabezon roads and turn right. Cabezon Road continues another 4.5 miles (1 mile south, 2.3 miles west, and 2.2 miles northwest) before arriving at the south Ojito boundary. At 5.2 miles from Gasco Road (10 miles from US 550), a parking area on the left and fence on the right mark **Puñi View.** A fabulous full-moon hike in warmer seasons, this easy 2-mile out-and-back starts at the fence. A doubletrack runs north about 1 mile to the edge of a small mesa, where the trail fades. Nearby, though unmarked, is the site where two hikers found unusual bones in 1979. Excavations later revealed the 170-foot skeleton of a "Seismosaurus" (eventually downsized to a 110-foot *Diplodocus*). A replica is on display at the New Mexico Museum of Natural History in Albuquerque.

Another mile west, shortly after crossing Arroyo la Jara, a pulloff on the right and a faded doubletrack heading north mark the trail informally known as **Hoodoo Pines.** This easy out-and-back runs just over 2 miles, leading to everything its names suggests—and more.

39 SAN YSIDRO TRIALS AREA

KEY AT-A-GLANCE INFORMATION

LENGTH: 2.7-mile loop (3.9-mile balloon without gate key)

DIFFICULTY: Easy–moderate

SCENERY: Sinuous canyons, hard-rock desert, sandstone and gypsum mesas

EXPOSURE: Some canyon shade

TRAIL TRAFFIC: Low

SHARED USE: Low–moderate (mountain bikers, equestrians; livestock, primitive camping; motorcycling with special permits)

TRAIL SURFACE: Dirt, sand, rock

HIKING TIME: 2–3 hours (3–4 hours without gate key)

DRIVING DISTANCE: 43 miles

ACCESS: Year-round, but see note at end of Description about gate key and racing events.

LAND STATUS: BLM–Rio Puerco Field Office

MAPS: USGS San Ysidro

FACILITIES: Trailhead parking, marked trails

LAST-CHANCE FOOD/GAS: Convenience store–gas station in San Ysidro

GPS TRAILHEAD COORDINATES

Latitude   35° 34' 06"

Longitude   106° 48' 48"

IN BRIEF

A unique slot canyon area at the southern tip of the Sierra Nacimiento offers a comprehensive lesson in geology—or, for the layperson, just a lot of strange rocks to gawk at.

DESCRIPTION

The Sierra Nacimiento is by far the elder of the two Rocky Mountain ranges that stretch down into the Jemez Pueblo. And since it also has the longer reach, the Sierra Nacimiento has been proclaimed "the southernmost tip of the Rockies." However, they share this distinction with the Sangre de Cristo Mountains, located about 60 miles due east.

The gray-and-pink granite that forms the bulk of the Sierra Nacimiento is getting on in years—around a billion in all. About 220 million years ago, it sat at the bottom of an inland sea and later under deltas and rivers as the sea retreated.

The receding waters left deposits that would later become thick layers of shale and sandstone—the cross bedding seen in the mesa cliffs today from eastern Nevada to the Texas Panhandle. Known as the Chinle sedimentary

---

Directions ――――――――――――――▶

From I-25 North, take Exit 242 at Bernalillo. Turn left on US 550 and go 25 miles to a weigh station on the right (1.5 miles past the town of San Ysidro). The paved turnoff for the San Ysidro Trials Area is at the far end of the weigh station. Drive up to the locked gate on the left side of the parking area. (If you don't have the key, park here and walk through the pedestrian gate.) Follow the rugged dirt road 1.2 miles to the parking area, and park near the signboard.

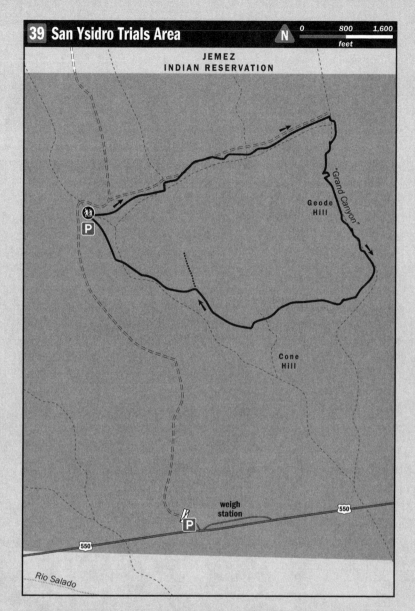

0   800   1,600
feet

N

JEMEZ
INDIAN RESERVATION

"Grand Canyon"

Geode
Hill

Cone
Hill

weigh
station

550

550

Rio Salado

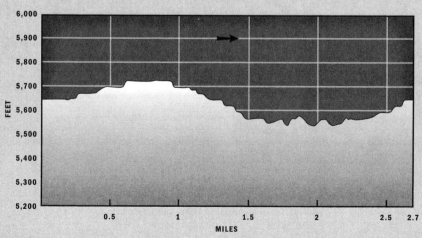

6,000
5,900
5,800
5,700
5,600
5,500
5,400
5,300
5,200

FEET

0.5   1   1.5   2   2.5   2.7

MILES

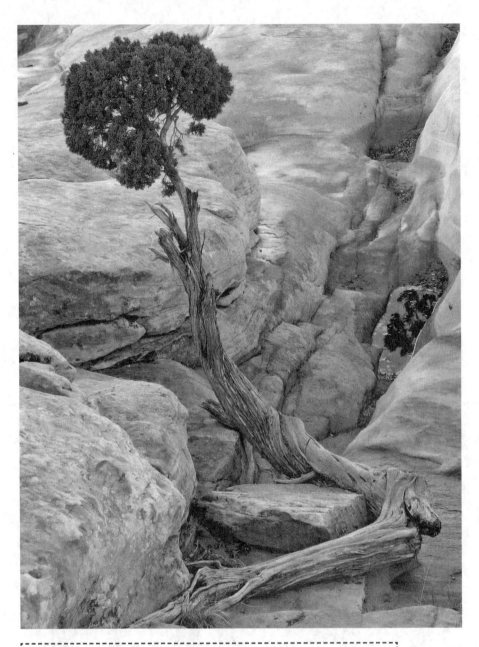

Areas of sandstone pavements north of the parking lot are also well worth exploring.

formation, it's also credited with preserving the logs in Arizona's Petrified Forest National Park.

The old granite reemerged about 75 million years ago in the Laramide Revolution, the same great compressive spasm that thrust up mountains across the American West. The Sierra Nacimiento uplifted along a north–south fault, resulting in a

50-mile range from San Ysidro to Gallina. By contrast, the eastern Jemez Mountains showed up with volcanic eruptions in just the last few million years.

The Sierra Nacimiento ("birth mountains," in reference to the birth of Christ) flank the San Juan Basin. This frontline position allows them to intercept east-bound storms. Average annual precipitation at higher elevations is nearly 3 feet (compared to Albuquerque's 8 inches). The resulting runoff carves small but intricate canyons through the foothills, notably in the San Ysidro Trials Area.

The trials area is closed to off-road motorized vehicles, except during special-use events permitted to the New Mexico Trials Association (NMTA). They were among the first to recognize that the area's unique geologic features—namely "grippy rocks"—would enhance their motorcycle competitions and their practice events.

The NMTA hosts five events here each year. Surprisingly, the dirt bikes haven't shredded the landscape. In terms of Leave No Trace ethics, cows seem to be the worse offenders.

I'm no fan of motoring through nature, but I have to admit the stunts they pull on San Ysidro's colossal rocks are stupefying. And yet if you happen to arrive on a day without a motorbike event, all the better. You'll probably have the whole place to yourself, and the hiking possibilities can be overwhelming. Just look around the parking area, and you'll spot six or seven trailheads, each marked with a dirt-bike icon. These markers appear on trails throughout the area. All signs are identical and hence useless for distinguishing one route from another.

For those in a hurry, the trailheads on the east side of the parking lot are quickest way to access marvelous canyons. You'll also encounter a few protected pueblo sites along the short stroll to this rocky playground. Other nearby slots and sandstone pavements worth exploring begin just 0.2 mile northwest of the parking area and extend north to the Jemez fenceline and west to the "Grand Canyon" mentioned following.

The route described here is a simple combination of prominent paths and waterways in the heart of the trials area. For a quick orientation: the hike traverses a hilly valley bound by Red Mesa to the west, Mesa Cuchilla to the east, and White Mesa on the far side of US 550 to the south. To narrow it down further, it's confined to a triangular space defined by two major drainages that merge before crossing US 550.

Start the hike by walking straight past the left side of the signboard. Hop across a small wash. The wash deepens as you continue east and slightly to the north. You can walk in it or, during wetter seasons, take the track running parallel on the north bank. The wash gets very narrow after about 0.75 mile, so you'll probably opt for the high road anyway.

Maintain a fairly straight path and you'll intersect a canyon just under a mile from the parking area. You can't miss it—some bikers have dubbed it "The Grand Canyon." That's an enormous exaggeration. It's not more than 50 feet across at its widest point, and it narrows to a classic slot in places.

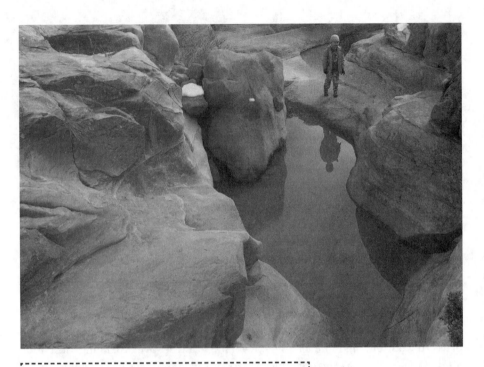

Small pools can become big obstacles deep in narrow canyons.

A cairn near to the right marks an easy entry point, though there are several to choose from. You can also look upstream for easier ways in. Be advised, however, that the Jemez Reservation lies less than 300 yards to the north. Please respect its boundaries. Also, do not enter the canyon if the forecast calls for rain. Pay special attention to the northern skies. Storms up to 10 miles away could send torrents of water and debris through this channel, and emergency exits are few over the next 0.5 mile.

That said, walk down to the canyon floor, and turn right to head downstream. The wide sandy wash narrows into sinuous chutes with polished sandstone walls. Each turn reveals marvelous details. Scoured spillways and basins hint at the furious rapids and whirlpools that follow stormy weather.

You may encounter a few ponds en route. If they're too big to cross, you'll need to backtrack for an exit from the canyon. You can reenter the canyon downstream, but the hard-rock route along the rim is just as interesting, and smaller waterways on either side of the main canyon are worth exploring as well. Also, the hill on the west bank is allegedly littered with geodes and gypsum crystals. (I didn't find any.) Or if you're confident in your sense of direction, wander off to the east—where sandstone hoodoos and ancient petroglyphs populate the ridges and gulches—then return to this canyon to finish the hike.

Once the canyon squeezes past the hill, it shallows out to a stream that trickles through dense stands of willow and tamarisk. Do not follow the stream into this wooded area. Instead, pick up the motorbike trail that curves southwest as it wraps around the base of the hill. It will lead you away from the stream and into an open meadow. Follow the track through a low pass at the far corner of the meadow.

Once you cross the ridge, you'll see two cone-shaped hills on your left, about 100 yards south. Stay on track as the path continues west and slightly to the south through a stand of tamarisk in a small wash. From there, the motorbike trail bends around the base of a ridge on your right and then aims northwest, roughly parallel to a major arroyo about 500 feet to your left. You can't see it from here, but a tree line marks the spot.

At the next fork, stay left. As the trail bends closer toward the arroyo, cross over to walk along its streambed. From here, less than 0.5 mile remains in the hike, but the wavy bedrock makes an impressive finale. As the top end of the drainage curves to your right, exit left and walk uphill about 100 yards to the parking lot.

Note: Pick up a gate key from the BLM office at 435 Montano Road NE in Albuquerque. Though it's not usually necessary, you can also call (505) 761-8700 to reserve a key. To catch or avoid motorcycle competitions, check the events schedule posted on the New Mexico Trials Association website (**nmtrials.org**), keeping in mind that competitors may show up for practice runs up to five days before an event.

NEARBY ACTIVITIES

Perea Nature Trail is a 1-mile loop through restored wetland on the bank of the Rio Salado. Benches, boardwalks, and wildlife blinds enhance enjoyment of this shaded nook. The Perea trailhead is at the end of a paved pulloff near the northwest corner of the Rio Salado bridge on US 550, about 0.8 mile south of the NM 4 junction.

40 CABEZON PEAK

KEY AT-A-GLANCE INFORMATION

LENGTH: 2.4-mile balloon, plus optional summit spur

DIFFICULTY: Strenuous approach, moderate loop, insane spur

SCENERY: Views over mixed grass-land steppe and volcanic fields

EXPOSURE: Mostly sunny

TRAIL TRAFFIC: Low–moderate

SHARED USE: Low (rock climbing)

TRAIL SURFACE: Dirt, rock

HIKING TIME: 2 hours, another 2–3 hours for the summit spur

DRIVING DISTANCE: 74 miles

ACCESS: Year-round

LAND STATUS: BLM–Rio Puerco Field Office, Wilderness Study Area

MAPS: USGS Cabezon Peak

FACILITIES: None

LAST-CHANCE FOOD/GAS: Convenience store–gas station in San Ysidro, about 35 miles from the trailhead.

SPECIAL COMMENTS: The last 7 miles of roads and the trail can turn treacherous in wet conditions. A brochure on the Cabezon Peak Wilderness Study Area can be acquired from the BLM office in Albuquerque, or you can download it from nm.blm.gov.

GPS TRAILHEAD COORDINATES

Latitude   35° 35' 49"

Longitude   107° 06' 19"

IN BRIEF

This loop on the shoulders of a giant volcanic plug offers amazing vistas at every turn. A nontechnical but nonetheless harrowing spur presents the option of climbing to the top of its towering neck.

DESCRIPTION

The pedestal of Cabezon stands well over 1,000 feet high. Jutting up another 800 feet is a ribbed column of basalt that once filled the throat of a great volcano. The cinder cone has long since eroded to expose this monolithic core.

The Navajo name for it is *tse najin,* or "black rock" Their legends tell of the Twin Warrior Gods who decapitated a giant. The blood from the fatal wound spilled to the south and congealed into the lava flow at El Malpais (Hike 59), and its head became what the Spaniards would later call *Cabezón,* which translates as "big head."

Spanish settlement here in the upper Rio Puerco Valley began shortly after the reconquest, but the early ranchos were soon under continual attack from Navajo neighbors to the west. Relations with eastern neighbors were

---

Directions

From I-25 North, take Exit 242 at Bernalillo. Turn left on US 550 and go northwest 23 miles toward San Ysidro. Stay left on US 550 and continue another 18 miles toward Cuba. Turn left on County Road 279 to San Luis. The paved portion ends after 8.5 miles. Continue 3.8 miles straight on the dirt road. Veer left at the Y onto BLM 1114 and go south 2.9 miles. Turn left at the sign for Cabezon Peak and go east 0.9 mile to the parking area at the end of the road.

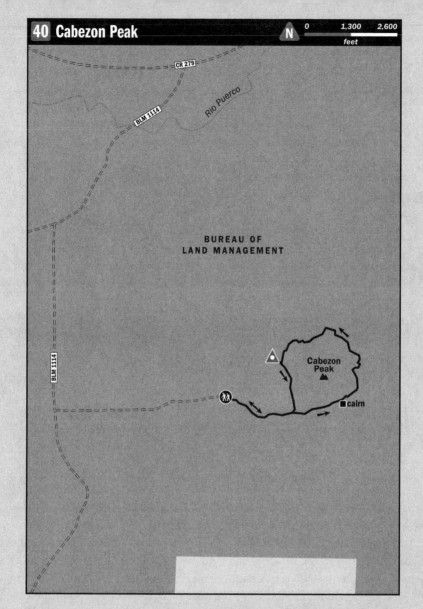

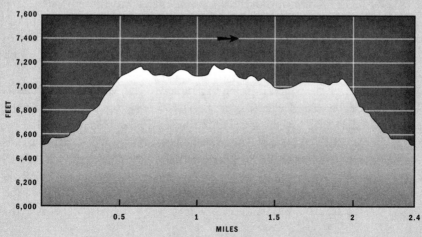

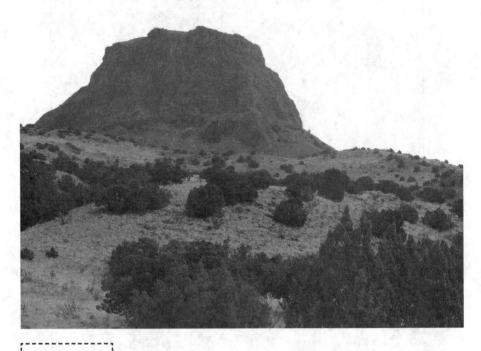

Cabezon Peak

strained in 1815 when the Spanish government awarded tracts of Zia, Jemez, and Santa Ana pueblo lands to Cabeza de Baca. The resulting dispute over this grant, known as the Ojo del Espiritu Santo, lasted well over a century.

Cabezon Peak straddles the western boundary, with its summit just inside the Ojo del Espiritu Santo Grant, though land on both sides is currently administered by the BLM. The property was badly eroded and overgrazed when the U.S. government purchased it in 1934. Over the past 70 years, resource-management programs have brought modest improvements to the upper Rio Puerco Valley. The once-fertile farmlands have yet to return, but the terrain does support an impressive array of wildlife. Common creatures include three toad species, in addition to beaver, badger, bobcat, and porcupine. Golden eagles, great horned owls, and a variety of hawks often nest by the peak.

Cabezon is often described in some variation of New Mexico's little Devils Tower. But check the stats: Devils Tower rises 1,267 feet from the Belle Fourche River to peak at 5,112 feet, whereas Cabezon rises 2,020 feet from the Rio Puerco to peak at 7,785 feet. So why the diminutive comparison? Maybe because Devils Tower, America's first national monument, is a solitary landmark that dwarfs everything else in its empty corner of Wyoming. By contrast, Cabezon stands in the company of about 50 other plugs in the shadow of Mount Taylor, the volcano peaking at 11,301 feet about 35 miles to the southwest. Or maybe because the vertical rock on Devils Tower exceeds Cabezon's by just enough to pose a significantly more challenging climb.

Cabezon's primary summit route is not considered a technical climb, but that doesn't make it easy or particularly safe. A hardhat is well advised (a bike helmet should suffice in a pinch). If the prospect of scrambling through talus and clawing your way up a chimney sounds daunting, don't let it keep you away from Cabezon. You can enjoy a hike here without a trip to the summit.

The hike begins on the eastern side of the parking area, where an aging signboard marks the trailhead. Start up the steep trail toward the volcanic neck. After a steady climb for nearly half a mile, the trail splits. Take your pick—both branches soon cross an old barbwire fence that marks the western boundary of the Ojo del Espiritu Santo Grant.

The branches merge shortly thereafter. Continue around to the south side of the neck. Less than 0.25 mile past the fence, look for the marker for the summit route. Stones arranged into a 10-foot arrow point the way. There's no clear trail through the scree, so aim for the chimney. There you'll find rock ledges adequate for handholds and footholds to pull your way to the rim. A marked path and a few more scrambles will get you to the top. The route is rated third class, but the first and last scrambles feel more like fourth class. Ropes aren't necessary, but helmets are strongly advised. Something to remember before attempting any ascent: descents are invariably more challenging.

After several minutes of contemplating the vertical route, you might wonder if circumnavigating the peak would be more fun than scaling it. Those prone to the slightest fits of acrophobia will certainly enjoy the loop more than the climb. Hearty hikers bent on doing both should do the ascent first, while their legs are still strong. Continuing with the hike, follow the path around to the southeast shoulder. There you'll find what appears to be an easier summit route. Trust me: it isn't. From here the loop path fades as it drops into a boulder field. Few cairns mark the way, but the strategy from this point is obvious: keep the boulder fields on your left and the edge of the shoulder on your right.

Some easy boulder hopping and a short climb are necessary to round the corner to the north side. Drop back down one level to get around the boulder field there. Cross a downed fence and continue around to the west side. An outcrop pointing due west provides a fine overlook of other plugs like Cerro Cuate ("twins hill"), 4 miles west-northwest. And just in case you forgot where you parked, look down to your left.

The final quarter of the loop is across a steep slope. Avoid drifting too far downhill or you'll face more difficulty in crossing the ridge ahead. Once over that last hump, you'll intersect the trail that brought you up here. Turn right, and follow it back down to the parking area.

41

CONTINENTAL DIVIDE TRAIL:
Deadman Peaks

KEY AT-A-GLANCE INFORMATION

LENGTH: 2.8-mile loop, longer options

DIFFICULTY: Easy

SCENERY: Mesa vistas, rock formations, burned-out coal deposits, skittish cows

EXPOSURE: Minimal shade

TRAIL TRAFFIC: Low

SHARED USE: Low (equestrians, livestock; roads are good for mountain biking, but no vehicles are permitted on this portion of the CDT)

TRAIL SURFACE: Rocky trail, dirt road

HIKING TIME: 1 hour (minimum)

DRIVING DISTANCE: 73 miles

ACCESS: Year-round

LAND STATUS: BLM—Rio Puerco Field Office

MAPS: USGS San Luis, Headcut Reservoir

FACILITIES: None

LAST-CHANCE FOOD/GAS: Convenience store—gas station in San Ysidro, about 35 miles from the trailhead

SPECIAL COMMENTS: Driving the dirt road can get tricky in wet conditions. See longer note at the end of the Description.

GPS TRAILHEAD COORDINATES

Latitude   35° 44' 37"

Longitude   107° 04' 28"

IN BRIEF

Hike the Continental Divide National Scenic Trail (CDT)—or at least a small portion of it. Access points closest to Albuquerque allow for extensive walks in Cabezon country. The loop described here uses equal parts dirt road and the CDT to circumnavigate a cluster of red hills known as Deadman Peaks. Of course, you also have the option of following the trail for many miles in either direction.

DESCRIPTION

Upon arrival at the base of Deadman Peaks, first thing everyone wants to do is check out the hoodoos. They're an odd sight, standing out there on the caliche like a colony of giant mushrooms sprouting from snowy-white earth. Next they want to know where the CDT is. Fact is, they're standing right on it.

The Continental Divide National Scenic Trail, more often referred to simply as the CDT, doesn't always follow the Continental Divide. The latter, of course, is the physical ridge separating the watersheds that drain into

- -

Directions ⟶

From I-25 North, take Exit 242 at Bernalillo. Turn left on US 550 and go northwest 23 miles toward San Ysidro. Stay left on US 550 and continue another 18 miles toward Cuba. Turn left on County Road 279 to San Luis. The paved portion ends after 8.5 miles. Turn right here onto Torreon Road (also paved) and go north 3.7 miles. At the top of the hill, turn right onto BLM 1102. (Look for a stop sign and a yellow cattle guard.) You can park here to pick up the CDT, or follow the main dirt road northeast 3.4 miles to the next CDT intersection on the south side of Deadman Peaks. Park roadside in front of the mushroom-shaped hoodoos.

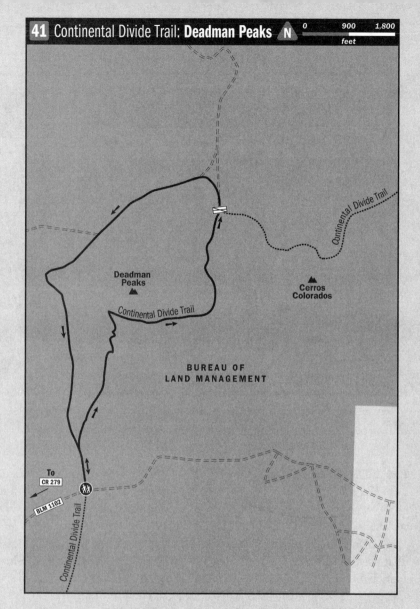
N

0   900   1,800

feet

Continental Divide Trail

Continental Divide Trail

Deadman
Peaks ▲

Cerros
Colorados ▲

Continental Divide Trail

**BUREAU OF
LAND MANAGEMENT**

To
CR 279

BLM 1102

Continental Divide Trail

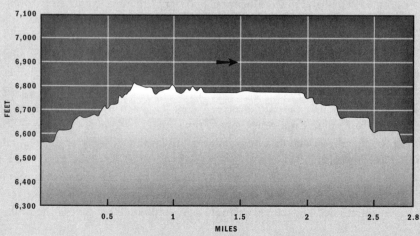

7,100

7,000

6,900

6,800

6,700

6,600

6,500

6,400

6,300

FEET

0.5   1   1.5   2   2.5   2.8

MILES

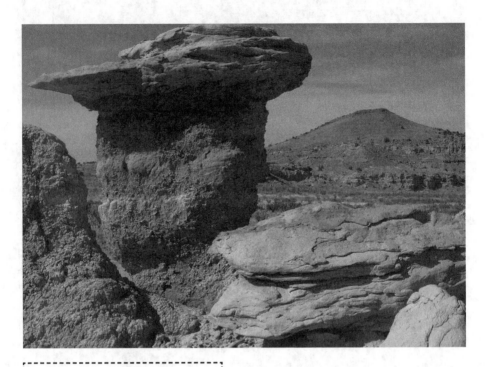

Hoodoos stand in front of Deadman Peaks.

the Pacific Ocean from those flowing to the Atlantic and the Gulf of Mexico. If for some reason you need to be on the actual divide, drive back to US 550 and turn left. From there it's a 35-mile drive to an unremarkable spot on the Continental Divide.

Private land issues are one reason for the CDT's deviation from its namesake, one that has proved to be the trail's biggest obstacle since Congress established it as a National Scenic Trail in 1978. An inexplicable lack of support and enthusiasm also plagued the project for its first two decades. The trail developed in fits and sputters until 1998, when the Continental Divide Trail Alliance launched its ambitious 10-year plan to complete the trail. With one year remaining, the 3,100-mile CDT was still largely a work in progress. In 2007, estimates of its usability ranged from 65 to 70 percent. At the same time, New Mexico's 740-mile portion was about 41 percent finished. By 2011 the state's portion had grown to 770 miles and was 75 percent finished.

The stretch through the Rio Puerco Valley has been operable for several years. You probably didn't notice it the first time you crossed it as you turned off the paved road, and you may not be able to identify it immediately at this second junction. Not to worry.

The hike begins at the hoodoos. Just turn your back to them and walk straight north along the road. You should spot the cairns within a minute. Each is a pyramid stacked about knee-high. Keep them in sight, and you'll never lose the trail.

About 0.2 mile from the hoodoos, the trail deviates east from the road and climbs the side of a ridge pointing south from the pedestal of Deadman Peaks. About 0.25 mile farther up is the first of six switchbacks leading to the biggest of Deadman's three peaks.

At first glance, the peaks appear as ordinary volcanoes capped with the usual rust-red cinders. A closer look reveals a shade of reddish-orange that's not quite as common in these otherwise dun mesa lands, though many roads around Torreon are the same fiery shade. This surfacing material is sometimes referred to as "red dog." Pick up a few scatters along the path, and you'll see it isn't lava. This red rock forms when heat from coal-seam fires cause low-grade metamorphic changes in the mudstones sandwiched between the coals.

The trail levels out for the next 0.6 mile as it follows the rim. On your left, the main peak rises another 200 feet. On your immediate right, the drop from the rim is 100 feet or so. The views south to Cabezon and beyond are wonderful. If you're lucky, the elements will treat you to the spectacle of a thunderstorm rolling across the valley. If you're really lucky, it'll rumble by without chasing you back to your car.

One mile into the hike, the trail turns north along the rim of a canyon that separates Deadman Peaks from the somewhat bulkier Cerros Colorados. Once the trail reaches the back end of the canyon, it turns right and joins a double-track. The old road comes in from the north through a drop gate and heads east into the Cerros Colorados. If you're pressed for time, it's best to leave the trail at this point. Once you turn the corner into the Cerros Colorados, you could easily lose half an hour gawking at rock formations in a 0.25-mile twist of waterways. Then there's always something else to lure you around the next bend—the way it hugs the cusp of Rincon de los Viejos is particularly exhilarating—and before you know it you're standing on the edge of a 500-foot precipice on La Ventana Mesa with 6 miles of trail between you and your car. (Note that if you continue up toward Cuba, white-painted posts and blazes are interspersed with the rock cairns.)

So if you're in this hike for the quick 2.8-mile loop, go through the drop gate, leave it as you found it, and don't look back. Turn left on the dirt road about 200 yards ahead. From there it's about 1.4 miles back to the junction where you parked. Don't be alarmed to find a herd of ominous black cows lurking behind you. They flee like squirrels when approached.

Once back at the hoodoos, you might be tempted to see what lies along the CDT to the southwest. You'll soon run into the same problem: one hyperscenic turn after another lures you farther along the trail, dropping to cross the Arroyo de Los Cerros Colorados and then quickly climbing past the 6,650-foot peak of San Luis. Next you're crossing pavement on Torreon Road and heading out on a high bench on Mesa San Luis. Before you know it, you're standing on the edge of a wind-sculpted sandstone ridge, once again with 6 miles of CDT between you and your car.

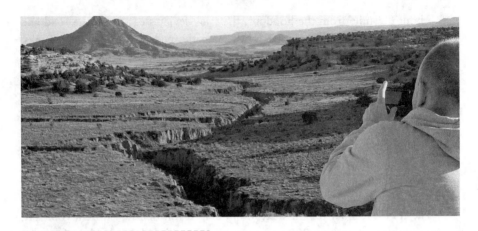

Cerro Cuate, viewed from La Lena WSA

Another reason for the deviation from the physical divide: scenery has a heavy influence on route selection. Though criteria for determining scenic value can be highly subjective, few rational hikers could disagree with the choices here in Cabezon country.

With massive cairns guiding your way, navigating this wild landscape is easy. The difficult part is knowing when to quit. One highly rated daylong hike is the 25-mile segment between Deadman Peaks and the northern end of Forest Road 239. The rescue index is fairly low, so this is not a trek to undertake on a whim. It crosses breathtaking landscapes in the Ignacio Chavez Special Management Area, a rugged and remote swath of gorgeous desert wilderness.

Note: For updates on the Continental Divide National Scenic Trail, visit **continentaldividetrail.org**. Excellent maps of the Rio Puerco segment, which includes Deadman Peaks, can be downloaded from **nm.blm.gov**.

NEARBY ACTIVITIES

La Lena Wilderness Study Area is 10,208 acres of badlands between the CDT and San Luis Road. For a quick peek into one of its better corners, drive back to County Road 279 and turn right onto San Luis Road (the dirt portion of CR 279). Follow it southwest 5.2 miles, passing the turnoff for Cabezon. Immediately after crossing a cattle guard and the bridge over the Cañada Santiago, turn right. This dirt road starts out good but soon deteriorates as it skirts the west bank of the cañada. You should be able to drive it at least 1.3 miles to an open gateway. After another 0.5 mile, look to your left for the first of four parallel gouges in the mesa wall. Each cut extends about 0.2–0.5 mile southwest and runs about 100 feet deep. Exploring them all can be a full-day affair. Entry to the last (and perhaps the best) one is less than a mile past the gateway. Incidentally, if you continue up the road another 2 miles from there, you'll reconnect with the CDT.

PALIZA CANYON GOBLIN COLONY

IN BRIEF

Near the newly renovated Paliza Family Campground, this hike starts on a primitive road alongside a wooded creek, follows it into a ponderosa-shaded canyon to visit an assembly of standing rocks known as hoodoos and goblins, then continues up to a ridgeline viewpoint for a look out over the canyon.

DESCRIPTION

Welcome to the famous Jemez (pronounced HAY-mess), a mountainous land so vast it would take several books to describe half of it. Allow me to recommend a few to get you started: In *Jemez Spring*, the Aztlán literary guru Rudolfo Anaya concocts a plot to blow up Los Alamos National Laboratories for the final installment in the Sonny Baca mysteries. For considerably slimmer and more practical reads, try *Guide to the Jemez Mountain Trail* by Judith Ann Isaacs and the classic *Exploring the Jemez Country* by Roland A. Pettitt.

This hike visits a spot that Pettitt described as "the wildest half-acre in the

Directions

From I-25 North, take Exit 242. Turn left on US 550 and go 23.5 miles to San Ysidro. Turn right on NM 4 (beware of speed traps) and go 6.3 miles to the signs for Ponderosa. Turn right on FR 290 and go 6.9 miles, where it becomes FR 10, a maintained gravel road. Continue straight another 2.5 miles. About 0.5 mile past the paved entrance to Paliza Family Campground, a maintained gravel road (FR 266) starts on the right. Pull over to the left and park in the clearing ahead. The hike begins directly across the road on FR 271 heading north. During seasonal closures on FR 10, park at the gate and walk the remaining 0.8 mile to FR 271.

KEY AT-A-GLANCE INFORMATION

LENGTH: 4-mile out-and-back

DIFFICULTY: Easy, but exploring the goblin area can be strenuous.

SCENERY: Towering ponderosa, riparian habitat, sculpted rock

EXPOSURE: Mostly shaded

TRAIL TRAFFIC: Moderate

SHARED USE: Moderate (target shooting, camping, equestrians, mountain bikers; motorized vehicles)

TRAIL SURFACE: Dirt roads

HIKING TIME: 2 hours

DRIVING DISTANCE: 56 miles

ACCESS: Year-round, but seasonal gate closures will add 0.8 mile to the hike. Though not required for this hike, entry to the Paliza Family Campground is $10 per vehicle.

LAND STATUS: Jemez Ranger District

MAPS: Santa Fe National Forest (West Half); USGS Ponderosa, Bear Springs Peak

FACILITIES: Camping, picnic tables, drinking water at the Paliza Family Campground, wheelchair-accessible restrooms

LAST-CHANCE FOOD/GAS: Bar and grill in Ponderosa, usually open 2 p.m.–late; convenience store, gas station, and visitor center on NM 4, about 2 miles north of the turnoff for Ponderosa

GPS TRAILHEAD COORDINATES

Latitude   35° 42' 32"

Longitude   106° 37' 39"

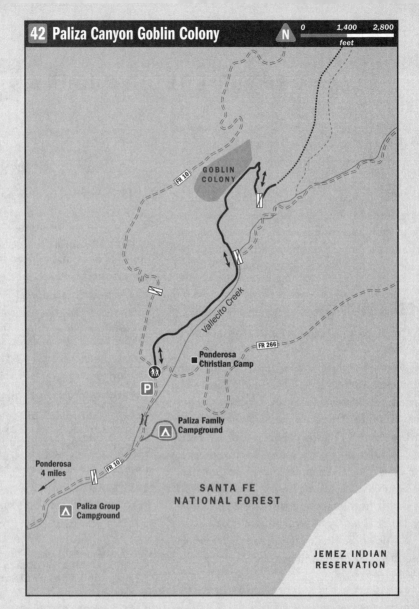

N

0   1,400   2,800
feet

GOBLIN
COLONY

FR 10

Vallecito Creek

FR 266

Ponderosa
Christian Camp

P

Paliza Family
Campground

Ponderosa
4 miles

FR 10

Paliza Group
Campground

SANTA FE
NATIONAL FOREST

JEMEZ INDIAN
RESERVATION

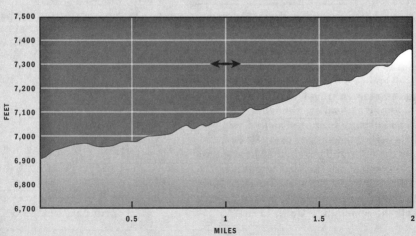

7,500
7,400
7,300
7,200
7,100
7,000
6,900
6,800
6,700

FEET

0.5   1   1.5   2

MILES

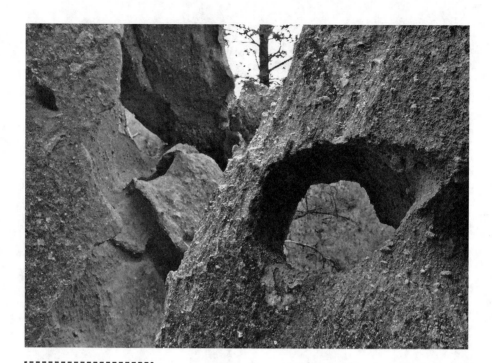

Hoodoos lurk in the pine.

Jemez." His comments were brief and his directions vague, which helps explain why so few people know about it today. He also underestimated the extent of the bizarre features found here: they occupy an area of at least 30 acres. However, he did an admirable job in describing the landscape: "There are gargoyles, Cleopatra's needles, backs of Triceratops and Stegosaurus dinosaurs, tents, haystacks, exploded solidified bubbles, roller coaster rides."

Indeed, these volcanic-rock formations also evoke Swiss cheese, Japanese cemeteries, and Easter Island. Add totem poles and hooded clowns to the inventory, and you begin to get the idea. And as if the rocks weren't naturally odd enough, mysterious images have been carved into some of them. Ancient petroglyphs depict antennaed humanoids and at least one creature resembling an armadillo.

The hike: To see the spectacle for yourself, walk north on the rutted red road. You'll soon cross beneath power lines, which unfortunately follow much of this route. Early in the hike you might catch a glimpse of a tent rock in the distance. It hints at the shape of things to come.

For now the trail crosses a patchwork of vegetation types, moving quickly from grassland to piñon and juniper to ponderosa. There's also a lush riparian habitat along Vallecito Creek and a smattering of Gambel oak for good measure. It's a fair sampling of Jemez Mountain flora, minus the aspen found at higher elevations.

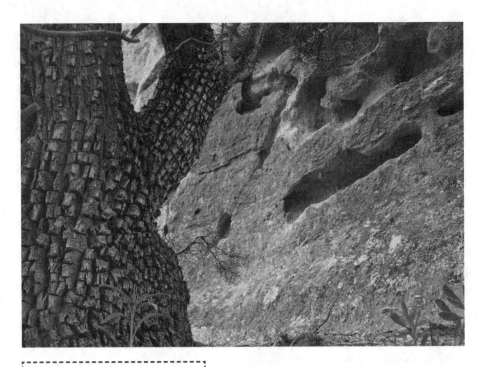

Alligator juniper in the goblin colony

In just less than a mile, the road splits, with the right branch going through an open gateway. Do not go through the gate. Instead, follow the road to the left. A few sandy washes cross the road within the next 0.5 mile. Stay on the road until you spot a cluster of unusual formations a short ways upstream. (You'll know it when you see it.) This is your cue to turn left and begin exploring the goblin colony.

They're not as big as the tent rocks at Kasha-Katuwe (Hike 27) on the east side of the Jemez, nor are they as uniform. Each figure seems to have its own character. In *Dry Rivers and Standing Rocks: A Word Finder for the American West,* Scott Thybony offers no fewer than three dozen names for rocks like this. In New Mexico, *hoodoo* and *goblin* are common terms, and perhaps the most appropriate for the majority of rocks here, but use your imagination when naming these figures.

Some things to keep in mind as you explore the formations: There are no developed trails in this area. Drainages provide the most convenient access corridors. Areas outside of drainages are more sensitive to erosion caused by foot traffic. Tread lightly, and avoid trampling vegetation.

Though rocks are riddled with holes ostensibly well suited for footholds, refrain from climbing on them. Many animals have already taken residence in them, including birds, chipmunks, and probably a few snakes. Also, the rock—

compacted ash, really—is not as solid as it appears. In some cases, a fine balancing act is all that keeps slender goblins from toppling over.

The canyon wall is very steep, rising nearly 300 feet in less than 0.2 mile. Use caution around ledges. If you find it too difficult to return to the road below, keep ascending. FR 10 is just over the ridge. You can follow it downhill back to the parking area, but be aware that trucks from local pumice mines often use this narrow, winding road.

Getting lost in this area is unlikely. With a road above and a road below, finding either one is simply a matter of gravity awareness. However, it's easy to lose track of fellow hikers, particularly the little ones. Consider establishing a nearby meeting point in case you get separated.

Finally, don't let the rocks steal all the attention. The scaly bark of alligator juniper contributes to the variety of textures, while seasonal wildflowers add to the color palette. Petroglyphs are few and far between. It takes a good eye to spot them. (I counted four in 2 hours.)

When you're ready to move on, return to the road below and turn left. That is, if you haven't exhausted yourself racing up and down the arroyos. Stick to the main road as it winds uphill. At the second hairpin turn is another open gateway. Take a moment here to enjoy the view of canyons below to the east and west.

The road levels out somewhat from here for a short but pleasant walk along the ridge. Feel free to turn back anywhere along this stretch. The route ends here, but the road continues. About 0.4 mile from the gateway, it splits around a pueblo mound. You might not recognize the mound as anything of significance; only an obscured sign marks it, explaining that the area is under the protection of the Antiquities Act of 1906. The roads ahead continue to split and proliferate into a network of unauthorized roads and informal tracks. Even with the most detailed maps, it can get a bit confusing. I wouldn't recommend going farther without a GPS unit, keeping in mind that reception is spotty in Paliza Canyon.

Stroll back the way you came, watching for details you may have missed on the way up. Birdlife is abundant. Raven and red-tailed hawk frequently patrol the canyon. With an audacious call and a crest to match, Steller's jay enlivens picnic areas and campsites. The brilliant hues of the Western tanager strike a sharp contrast against the dark conifer. Burrowing owls often stake out roads and trails shortly after dark. If you happen to be out that late, revisit the goblin colony. It's a different world by moonlight.

Note: FR 10 is subject to closures due to fire or snow. Contact the Jemez Ranger District for current conditions at (575) 829-3535 or **www.fs.fed.us/r3/sfe/ districts/jemez**.

43   STABLE MESA

IN BRIEF

The most scenic drive in the Jemez leads to the western base of Schoolhouse Mesa. The hike takes you to the western rim of its southern neighbor, Stable Mesa. From there you can explore windows and shelter caves in a mile-long pumice ridgeline. An optional extension ventures out to the ruins of an ancient pueblo and a historic logging camp.

DESCRIPTION

Pueblo Indians developed at least 40 settlements in the Jemez Province before the Spaniards arrived in 1541. They established many of the larger pueblos upon mesas, some as high as 8,000 feet. Evidence of later settlements in this area includes the town sites, camps, and cabins associated with the railroad logging period of 1922 to 1941. The road you drove up to Porter Landing is the most prominent legacy of this period. It traces the railroad grade of the Santa Fe Northwestern through the Gilman Tunnels and up the cascading Rio Guadalupe. With a population of 300, Porter was the center of operations from 1925 to 1937. Unusually high floods in 1941 washed out tracks and trestles. With the war

----

Directions

From I-25 North, take Exit 242. Turn left on US 550 and go 23.5 miles to San Ysidro. Turn right on NM 4 (beware of speed traps) and go 9.5 miles to Cañon. Turn left on NM 485 and go north 5.7 miles. The road becomes FR 376, a narrow but well-maintained gravel road. Continue north another 7 miles to Porter Landing. A sign on a gate here reads ROAD CLOSED. Park alongside the barrier rail on the left, immediately before the bridge.

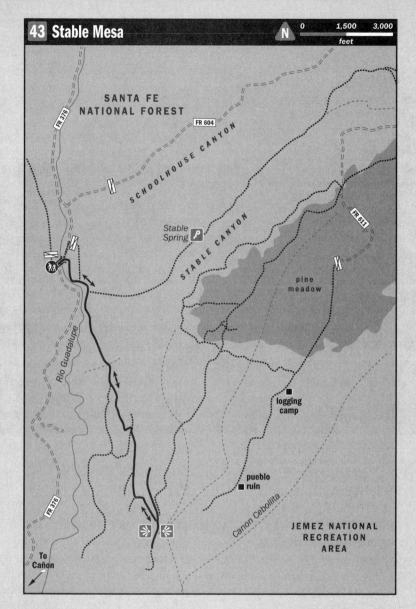

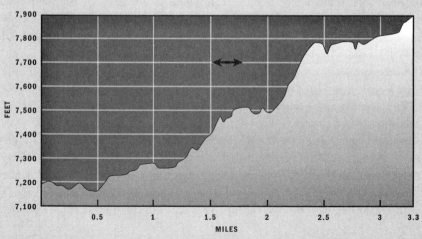

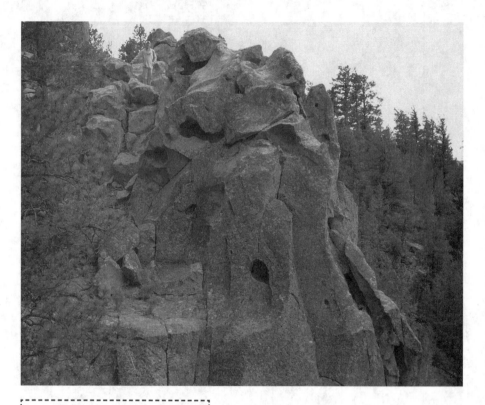

Can you find the author in this picture?

increasing demands for steel, the rail wreckage was quickly salvaged and sold. The last remnant standing in Porter today, a stone hearth in a clearing by the river, is the fireplace from the superintendent's lodge. Other relics remain scattered upon the surrounding mesas and throughout the canyons.

Extensive human activity also left its mark in the form of cow paths, skid trails, and logging roads. Many are permanent scars; some have faded back into the forest. For the purposes of this hike, it helps to keep in mind that the route described below uses the most obvious way to the mesa rim. Hence, if you cross something that kind of resembles a trail, it may very well be one, but it isn't part of this route.

Before setting out on the hike, look above the pines across the river and note a forested peak less than 1 mile southeast. That's the western corner of Stable Mesa. The destination of this hike lies on the rim that seems to dip back behind the treetops.

The hike begins with a short walk up FR 376. Immediately after crossing the bridge, turn right on a footpath through a stand of trees and walk south along the river. (If you miss the path, turn right at the gate 100 yards ahead, and follow the road down to the river.) The path soon intersects a well-defined dirt road that's closed to motor vehicles, though recent tire tracks indicate that it still gets more traffic than it should. About 200 feet ahead on the left is the fireplace from the superintendent's lodge; hidden behind scrub and trees, it's easier to spot coming from the opposite direction.

The road follows the east bank of the river. About 0.4 mile into the hike, Stable Canyon opens up on the left. Stable Spring sometimes keeps the lower canyon fairly damp, and the path is often cluttered with downed trees. Still, it's worth exploring. Marine fossils appear in the limestone cliffs less than 0.5 mile up on the left.

For now, continue south along the main trail to a fork about 200 yards or so past the mouth of Stable Canyon. Bear left and follow the rocky jeep road uphill. (A lesser road stays close to the river.) The terrain soon levels out. About 0.5 mile past the fork, shortly after dipping through an arroyo, the road forks again. Head uphill to the left. The views to the west are astounding as you ascend to the next level.

Another fork is about 1 mile ahead. A fallen tree blocks a faint road going straight. You'll follow the road as it bends left, but first you might want to take a short rest here.

A campfire ring sits in the middle of the faint road. If you're in the habit of leaving trails cleaner than you found them, you could fill a trash bag or two here. Feel free to take all the plastic bottles you can carry, but don't touch any tins, bottles, or other refuse dating to the logging period. If you're not sure whether it's trash or a cultural artifact, leave it alone.

Continue on the road as it bends left, then right, and then up the steepest ascent on this route. About 0.3 mile past the campfire ring, the steep, rocky road ends at the junction with a pronounced doubletrack. Turn right and head over a flat outcrop about 100 yards to the south. Take another break to enjoy the views to the west and get oriented.

Sitting on the western edge of the Jemez Plateau, you're now 2.5 miles into the hike. The narrow north–south trending range to the west is the Sierra Nacimiento, the Laurel companion to the Hardy-shaped Jemez. More specifically, you're sitting on the rim near the southwestern corner of Stable Mesa. A low ridge extends about 0.2 mile south and nearly 1.5 miles north. The backbone of this ridge is volcanic rock, which appears in exposed outcrops all along the western flank. As you can see in the steep outcrop to your left, it's adorned with pocks, holes, grooves, and other intricate details.

Start by exploring the outcrops to the south. If you haven't noticed already, you're on a fingerlike extension of the mesa, with views over a gorge a few yards to the east. When you reach the end of the formations, turn around and head to the north side of the junction to find more outcrops off the left side of the road. The designs become more elaborate, with arches and shelter caves that evoke playful shapes, like grottoes and oversized fishbowl castles. Graffiti etched into the soft rock dates back from a few years to several decades and perhaps many centuries. You could spend hours among these fascinating formations, and then head back the way you came—or consider racking up a few extra miles on the alternate routes outlined on the next page.

THE RUINS AND THE LOOP

The road from the rim junction is relatively flat and easy to follow. As the map indicates, a twin road runs parallel about 0.5 mile to the east. The remains of a logging camp and a pueblo ruin are along that road. Both sites are under the protection of the Federal Antiquities Act. Numerous trees have been felled to prevent vehicles from approaching from the north, but with modest success.

The twin roads are connected by a few east–west trending tracks that are difficult to spot. The first one to stand out noticeably appears on the right, 1.5 miles northeast of the junction on the rim. Two dirt-mound barriers obstruct this former road, which winds 0.7 mile over hills and across drainages to meet the parallel road. The logging camp is about 0.3 mile south of this T-junction. The remains of log cabins are easy to spot on both sides of the road. The pueblo ruin—little more than a mound, really—is another mile south. Hence, a hike from the rim to the pueblo runs about 3.5 miles, one-way. If you intend to shorten your return route by heading east from either the camp or the ruin, be warned that this shortcut can involve considerable bushwhacking, and that the drainages between the two roads become increasingly difficult to cross as they trench south toward the gorge.

Note: FR 376 is subject to closures due to snow or fire. Contact the Jemez Ranger District for current conditions at (575) 829-3535 or **www.fs.fed.us/r3/sfe/districts/jemez.**

NEARBY ACTIVITIES

East Fork Trail (137) features 95°F spring-fed pools at McCauley Warm Springs. The wooded trail starts with a moderate 400-foot ascent, but most of the 2-mile hike is fairly easy. Continue hiking east from the springs another 3 miles to reach the Jemez Falls Group Picnic Area. A popular short spur from there leads to a viewing area above the 70-foot falls. To find the western trailhead of the East Fork Trail, return to NM 4 and drive 13.4 miles north to the Battleship Rock Picnic Area. Visit the ranger station en route for more info. You'll also pass through Jemez Springs, a popular stopover for dining, lodging, and (of course) soaking. Call the Jemez Springs Bath House at (575) 829-3303 or (866) 204-8303, or visit **jemezsprings.org.**

VALLES CALDERA NATIONAL PRESERVE

44

IN BRIEF

The trail takes you up to a midlevel ridge for a glimpse of the landscapes hidden in the Baca. Peaking over 9,100 feet, it's one of the cooler summer hikes. In winter, its modest gain in elevation is ideal for beginner and intermediate snowshoeing.

DESCRIPTION

In 2011 a downed power line to the immediate southwest of the Valles Caldera sparked off what would become the largest wildfire in the history of New Mexico. Burn assessments show low to moderate damage to the Coyote Call and Valle Grande trail areas.

Of course, fire is no stranger here. Remember the 1980 eruption of Mount St. Helens? Multiply that blast by 600, and you get an idea of what the Valles Caldera looked like about 1.2 million years ago, when it ejected 150 cubic miles of rock and sent ash as far as Iowa. This is, in the snappy parlance of telegenic scientists, a supervolcano. New Mexico's sleeping monster hasn't stirred in the past 60,000 years, but nobody knows when it will erupt again.

The giant crater once belonged to the legendary Cabeza de Baca family. In 1860 the U.S. Congress recognized a land debt to the

KEY AT-A-GLANCE INFORMATION

LENGTH: 2.9-mile loop (Coyote Call); 2-mile out-and-back (Valle Grande)

DIFFICULTY: Easy

SCENERY: Aspen, fir, and ponderosa; views across the caldera, possible sightings of bald eagles and elk

EXPOSURE: Mostly shaded

TRAIL TRAFFIC: Popular

SHARED USE: Low (cross-country skiing, snowshoeing; no pets; no vehicles)

TRAIL SURFACE: Grass and dirt, or snow

HIKING TIME: 1–2 hours

DRIVING DISTANCE: 80 miles

ACCESS: Daylight hours

LAND STATUS: National Preserve, private management

MAPS: vallescaldera.gov; USGS Bland

FACILITIES: None

LAST-CHANCE FOOD/GAS: Convenience store and gas station at Jemez Pueblo visitor center on NM 4, about 33 miles before the trailhead; restaurants in Jemez Springs, about 23 miles before the trailhead

SPECIAL COMMENTS: See longer note at the end of the Description.

Directions

From I-25 North, take Exit 242 at Bernalillo. Turn left on US 550 and go 23.5 miles to San Ysidro. Turn right and go 41 miles on NM 4. On the left side of the road, near Mile Marker 41, is a pull-off big enough for four or five cars. Park there, or if it's full, another pull-off is about half a mile ahead. Coyote Call Trail begins at the signed gate across the road from the first pull-off.

GPS TRAILHEAD COORDINATES

Latitude	35° 50' 53"
Longitude	106° 27' 55"

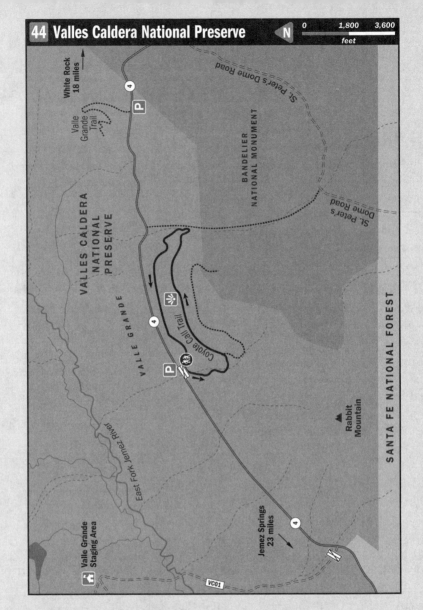

N

0   1,800   3,600
feet

White Rock
18 miles

St. Peter's Dome Road

P

Valle Grande Trail

4

BANDELIER NATIONAL MONUMENT

VALLES CALDERA NATIONAL PRESERVE

St. Peter's Dome Road

Coyote Call Trail

4

VALLE GRANDE

P

SANTA FE NATIONAL FOREST

Rabbit Mountain

East Fork Jemez River

Jemez Springs
23 miles

4

Valle Grande Staging Area

VC01

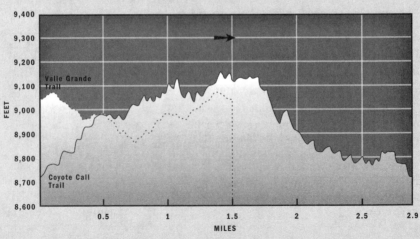

Valle Grande Trail

Coyote Call Trail

FEET

9,400
9,300
9,200
9,100
9,000
8,900
8,800
8,700
8,600

0.5   1   1.5   2   2.5   2.9

MILES

heirs of Don Luis María Cabeza de Baca and offered them the vacant parcel of their choice. Topping their top-five countdown was a 95,000-acre tract in the northern Jemez. The property, which encompasses most of the caldera, is still known locally as Baca Location No. 1, the Baca Ranch, or simply "the Baca."

Ensuing years of livestock grazing, sulfur mining, and extensive logging took a toll on the land. In 1963 a third generation oilman, James "Pat" Dunigan, bought the ravaged property for $2.5 million. A native Texan with a master's degree from New York University, Dunigan is perhaps most fondly remembered for his environmentally balanced ranching and caring stewardship of the Baca. When his sons sold it to the federal government for a cool $101 million in 2000, it was in relatively sparkling condition.

This purchase, made through the Valles Caldera National Preservation Act, would expand New Mexico's already supersized menu of recreational opportunities. But did we really need access to another 40 miles of trout streams, 66,000 acres of conifer forest, 25,000 acres of grassland, Sandoval County's highest peak, and the state's largest herd of elk? Absolutely. The bigger question is how long can we keep it all unsullied?

That challenge falls to the Valles Caldera Trust, a nine-member board of trustees that assumed management in 2002. All seem painfully aware of common recreational practices that amount to ecological mayhem for their neighbors, the Jemez Ranger District of Santa Fe National Forest, and the budget crunches that account for the disrepair occasionally found in adjacent Bandelier National Monument. (To be sure, both the forest supervisor and the monument superintendent serve as voting members on the Valles Caldera board. The remaining seven trustees are appointed by the President of the United States.)

The trustees' approach to recreation has been guarded, to say the least. Their systems of schedules and lotteries seem to be under constant revision, while their policies of nonchangeable reservations and nonrefundable fees are firmly established. In all, they've effectively deterred the masses from swarming the caldera—except for that one weekend in the rainy summer of 2006. In a first-time showcase event that probably won't be repeated, the old ranch roads opened to private vehicles, and more than 1,500 cars showed up to slosh and skid through the preserve.

The lucky few who negotiate passage beyond the barbwire threshold invariably return to describe the caldera experience in superlatives reserved for the Promised Land. The good news is, each year the gates seem to crack open a little wider. Recent additions to the schedule include orienteering, mountain bike tours, fly-fishing clinics, and photography workshops. Most activities, along with the best hikes, tend to book up fast. If you arrived without reservations, you still have two "free spontaneous hiking" opportunities on the southeastern fringe of the preserve: Valle Grande Trail and Coyote Call Trail.

The hike featured here, Coyote Call Trail, begins at the pedestrian gate. There's a wooden box containing a register, a map, and some lost mittens. The

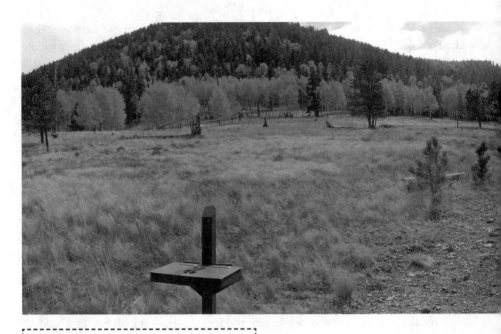

Coyote Call trailhead, before the Las Conchas fire

map shows the trail in more detail than the one in this book does, but it's usually easy enough to follow without either.

The trail is well marked, but markers may get buried under 4 feet of snow. If you came here for a snowshoe hike, take a moment to study the map. Don't rely on a fresh set of tracks for navigation, or you may end up following lost tourists to the far side of Rabbit Mountain.

Start by heading south across the meadow, bearing slightly to the right along an old logging road that climbs up about a half-mile to the eastern side of the domed hill ahead. Midway up the ridge behind the hill, the road turns left.

About 100 yards after rounding the corner, you'll arrive at the junction with Rabbit Ridge Trail on the right. Rabbit Ridge was one of the original free trails. It may or may not reopen in the near future, though there doesn't seem to be anything to discourage anyone from exploring this ridgetop route now. To stay on Coyote Call Trail, continue straight past the junction. The trail conforms to the curvature of the ridge, bowing out and back for the next mile. Near the halfway point, look for a wide break in the woods on the left. It's a good place for a short rest, as the view of the caldera from here is magnificent.

Many visitors mistake the Valle Grande for the Valles Caldera. To clarify, the Valle Grande composes about one-sixth of the Baca Ranch and is the largest of four valleys in the Valles Caldera. The actual caldera, a collapsed volcano, measures 12–15 miles in diameter. The Valle Grande, about 3 miles wide from north to south, is what drivers see from NM 4. In other words, the Valle Grande is merely the crescent, whereas the Valles Caldera is the full moon.

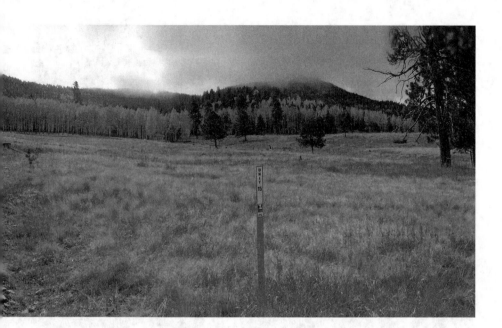

From the overlook, the view stretches clear across to the north rim, but the other valleys remain hidden behind the hills and domes that flank the far side of the Valle Grande. The one on the left is Redondo Peak, the county's highest, at 11,254 feet. The dome on the right is Cerro del Medio. The stream snaking across the meadow in front of it is the East Fork of the Jemez River.

Continue on Coyote Call Trail another 0.5 mile or so to the junction with another old road merging from the right. Take a sharp left here, and head downhill. After another 0.5 mile, NM 4 comes into view. At that point the trail bends to the west and runs roughly parallel to the highway for the remainder of the loop.

Valle Grande Trail begins just west of the boundary to the preserve and Bandelier National Monument. To find it, look for an unmarked pulloff on the south side, between Mile Markers 42 and 43. A tiny wooden sign on the north side marks the trailhead. Cross the road and follow the fence for about 200 feet west to the registration box, then zigzag downhill through a lush forest of fir and aspen. The well-worn mile-long trail takes you to the edge of the meadow in the Valle Grande. It's a short hike, but tack on at least 20 minutes to take in the view.

Note: The Valle Grande Staging Area is the starting point for two more "spontaneous" hikes:

La Jara is a self-interpretive hike begins near a prairie-dog town and crosses the open grassy meadow of the Valle Grande around the base of Cerro La Jara. This easy 1.5-mile route gains a mere 50 feet in elevation, but culminates with a 360-degree view of the Valle Grande.

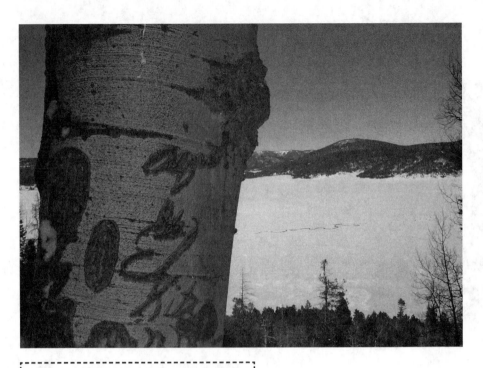

An aspen bears the scars of an unprovoked knifing.

South Mountain Hike travels along service roads on the southwestern edge of the Valle Grande to South Mountain. About a dozen spurs split off the main trail as it approaches the summit. This moderate out-and-back runs 6–8 miles with an elevation range of 8,500–9,400 feet.

Neither hike requires a reservation, but check in advance for hiking fees, shuttle services, and trail closures due to special events or hunting season (September–October). Access to the Valle Grande Staging Area is on the north side of NM 4 near Mile Marker 39. Driving distance from the main gate to the staging area is about 2 miles via a well-maintained gravel road. Plan ahead to take advantage of the wide array of activities throughout the preserve. For an updated schedule of events and trail openings, call (505) 661-3333 or visit **vallescaldera.gov**; for reservations, call (866) 382-5537.

BANDELIER NATIONAL MONUMENT: 45
Falls Trail

IN BRIEF

The extensive trail system in Bandelier National Monument allows for a wide range of hikes, from leisurely strolls among ancient cliff dwellings to weeklong treks into back-country wilderness. Falls Trail is geared for casual hikers, with minor challenges and many rewarding views.

DESCRIPTION

The Las Conchas Fire burned more than 60 percent of the monument in June 2011. Falls Trail dodged the flames but suffered postfire flooding two months later. This major flash-flood event scoured away portions of the trail beyond Upper Frijoles Falls. It wasn't the first flood—and won't be the last—to destroy trails in this section of Frijoles Canyon. With that in mind, I've kept the hike description and map

----

Directions ⟶

Bandelier National Monument is fewer than 40 linear miles from Albuquerque, but there are no reasonable shortcuts to its main entrance. From I-25 North, take Exit 276 to NM 599 (Veterans Memorial Highway). Go north 13.5 miles to its end at US 84. Go north 14 miles to Pojoaque and turn left onto NM 502 (Los Alamos Highway). Go west 11.2 miles and bear left on NM 4 toward White Rock. (Note that the Tsankawi section, on the left 1.4 miles past the junction, features a 1.5-mile self-guided hike through an Ancestral Pueblo village.) Drive 12 miles on NM 4 to the main entrance.
   Alternate route: From I-25 North, take Exit 242 at Bernalillo. Turn left on US 550 and go 23.5 miles to San Ysidro. Turn right on NM 4 and follow it 57 miles to the main entrance. Follow the road down to the Visitor Center. The Falls trailhead is at the south end of the backpacker parking area.

KEY AT-A-GLANCE INFORMATION

LENGTH: 4.8-mile out-and-back

DIFFICULTY: Moderate

SCENERY: Waterfalls, canyon woodland, tent rocks, majestic cliffs

EXPOSURE: Some tree cover and canyon shade

TRAIL TRAFFIC: Heavy

SHARED USE: Low (no pets, no vehicles)

TRAIL SURFACE: Packed dirt

HIKING TIME: 2–3 hours

DRIVING DISTANCE: 98 miles via San Ysidro or 104 miles via Santa Fe

ACCESS: All trails open daily, dawn–dusk, except December 25 and January 1. Day-use fees: $12 per vehicle or $6 per person traveling on foot or bicycle. Federal Recreational Land Passes are accepted.

LAND STATUS: National Park Service

MAPS: Brochure map available at Park Entrance Station; USGS Frijoles

FACILITIES: Visitor center, gift shop, snack bar, restrooms, campgrounds, interpretive exhibits and programs

LAST-CHANCE FOOD/GAS: All services in White Rock (11 miles northeast). Convenience store in La Cueva (32 miles northwest). Gas station in San Ysidro (58 miles southwest).

GPS TRAILHEAD COORDINATES

Latitude   35° 46' 38"
Longitude   106° 16' 12"

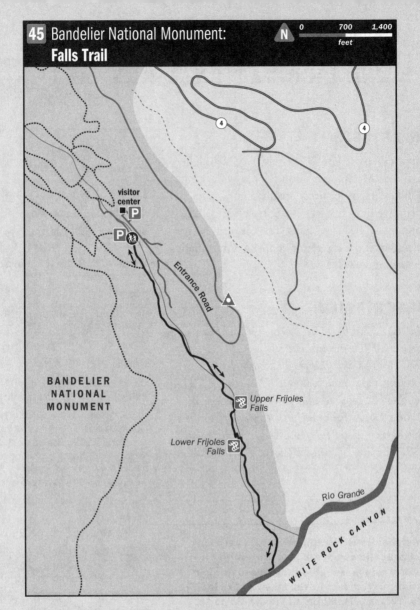

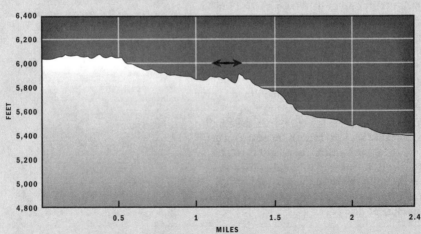

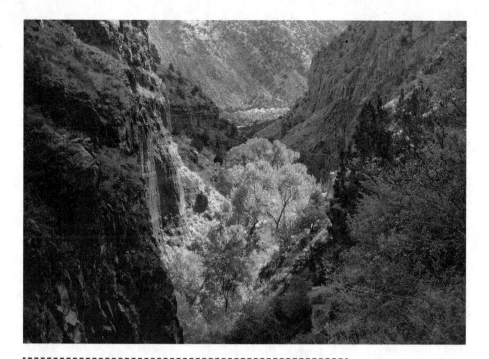

The mouth of an ancient maar volcano resembles a sandstone canyon.

intact. However, it's worth noting that at last check (September 2014) Falls Trail descended a mere 400 vertical feet in 1.5 miles before terminating at the Upper Falls. The area beyond was completely inaccessible. All other trails, which add up to 70+ miles, were open. For updates and park alerts, call the Visitor Center (505) 672-3861 x 517, and visit **nps.gov/band.**

Architectural wonders of the 12th century include the Cathedral of Notre Dame, the Campanile of Pisa, the Citadel of Cairo, and Angkor Wat in Cambodia. During the same time, Ancestral Puebloans were carving the first high-rise condos into sheer cliffs of volcanic tuff on the eastern slopes of the Jemez Mountains. These cliff dwellings are the main attraction at Bandelier National Monument today.

You don't have to wander far from the main loop for wildlife encounters at any time of year. Springtime deer in the area seem indifferent to hikers, as are low-key tarantulas that mosey about in the fall. Summer is prime butterfly season. More than 100 species have been identified in the park. Western tanagers are also summer residents, while golden-crowned kinglets seem popular among the mixed flocks of winter.

With 70 miles of trails to choose from, picking a route in this 33,750-acre monument can be tough. To thoroughly appreciate Bandelier National Monument, you need at least three days—your pass is good for a week. Keep in mind, however, that Bandelier trails are not to be taken lightly. They wind in and out of

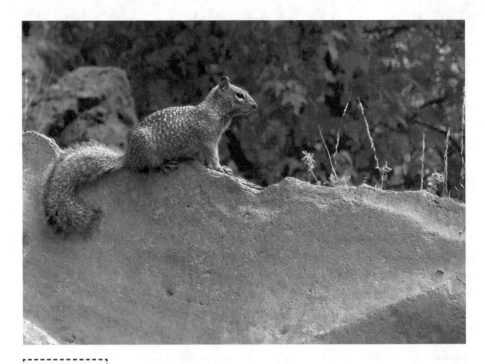

Rock squirrel

numerous canyons cut 500 feet deep into the southernmost Pajarito Plateau. Formed by the ash flow on the eastern flank of the Valles Caldera, this sloping plateau is not as flat as you might have guessed.

The good news is that the trails are easy to follow. Built by the Civilian Conservation Corps in the 1930s, they seem as sturdy today as the day they were constructed. More about that project, and everything else you could possibly want to know about the monument, can be learned in the visitor center. Spend some time with the exhibits and dioramas to prepare for any questions that might pop up on the trail. For this hike, be sure to pick up the 15-page booklet, "A Guide to the Falls Trail."

Weather in the park can be unpredictable. A hike here in May 2007 started in balmy morning sunshine and ended with light snowfall in the afternoon. Another one in October 2010 began the same way and ended in a storm of buckshot-sized hail. Snow and ice buildup add extra challenges in the winter, especially in canyons. Sun exposure and thunderstorms can get fierce in the summer. Park rangers are diligent about monitoring current conditions, so it's worth stopping by the visitor center before hitting the trail.

The hike begins at the south end of the backpacker's parking area, across the stream from the visitor center. The trail descends 700 vertical feet in its 2.4-mile length, passing two impressive waterfalls en route to the Rio Grande. Once you're on the trail, it's impossible to get lost, so we'll dispense with the customary directions in favor of a few interesting details along the way.

Much of the hike is a study in color: Pinkish rocks are volcanic tuff. Outcrops of Upper Bandelier Tuff (approximately 1.2 million years old) form white cliffs. Layers of red soil were produced when one lava flow baked layers formed in previous flows. Basalt is a dark, dense volcanic rock, and it seems to attract bright yellow-orange lichens. A variety of streamside vegetation adds to the palette, including narrowleaf cottonwood, box elder, and canyon grape.

As you follow the stream, you might spot a few minnows. They're descendants of the half-million trout (brook, rainbow, brown, and cutthroat) that were added to Frijoles Creek between 1912 and 1955.

About 1.2 miles into the hike, the Upper Frijoles Falls comes into view, followed by the Lower Falls, about a quarter-mile later. The Upper Falls drops approximately 80 feet, spilling over dense basalt rock from the throat of an ancient volcano. The Lower Falls drops about 45 feet from a basalt ledge. Gorgeous ice sculptures often form at the base in the winter.

You'll cross the creek a few more times before arriving at the Rio Grande. Vegetation grows dense along the trail. Beware of poison ivy and stinging nettle in the summer. The difference in elevations between the canyon bottom and the upper trail translates to a seasonal lag. Down here, wildflowers bloom two weeks earlier in the spring and leaves change color two weeks later in the autumn.

At the trail's end, you arrive at the Rio Grande. The nearest crossings are Otowi Bridge, about 12 miles upstream, and Cochiti Dam, about 12 miles down. In 1985, spring runoff caused Cochiti Lake to backup and flood 200 acres of the monument for well over a year. A layer of nutrient-rich soil emerged in the wake of the flood, and vegetation soon began to flourish along the banks once again. This time, however, native plant species couldn't compete. Nearly everything you see growing in this low, flat land along the river are nonnative species.

The trail officially ends here, though most times of year you can still follow the old trail downstream another 3 miles or so to the mouth of Lummis Canyon. If you decide to venture down that way, keep an eye on your food and water reserves. The hike back up to the parking area takes a bit more energy than the way down.

A Guide to Bandelier National Monument by Dorothy Heard is a portable but comprehensive resource, complete with invaluable 3-D renderings of the trails. The book is available at the visitor center and from the Los Alamos Historical Society: (505) 662-6272; **losalamoshistory.org**.

46 WATER CANYON-POWERLINE MESA

KEY AT-A-GLANCE INFORMATION

LENGTH: 3.5- and 6.4-mile out-and-back options; 7.8-mile balloon

DIFFICULTY: Moderate–strenuous

SCENERY: Wooded canyon, sculpted rock, mesa rim views

EXPOSURE: Half-shaded

TRAIL TRAFFIC: Low

SHARED USE: Low

TRAIL SURFACE: Dirt, rock

HIKING TIME: 2–3 hours (out-and-back); 5 hours (balloon)

DRIVING DISTANCE: 99 miles via San Ysidro or 97 miles via White Rock

ACCESS: Daylight hours

LAND STATUS: U.S. Department of Energy

MAPS: USGS White Rock

FACILITIES: None

LAST-CHANCE FOOD/GAS: All services in White Rock (4 miles northeast). Convenience store in La Cueva (33 miles northwest). Gas station in San Ysidro (60 miles southwest).

SPECIAL COMMENTS: For the latest info on local trails, contact the Los Alamos County Parks Division: (505) 663-1776; losalamosnm.us/parks/trails.

GPS TRAILHEAD COORDINATES

Latitude   35° 48' 13"

Longitude   106° 14' 45"

IN BRIEF

An easy mile down a wooded canyon leads to three options: Bear left or right on trails that climb gently to overlooks and rocky promontories on either rim of Water Canyon. Or head straight for an adventurous hike down the gorge, followed by a 1,000-foot climb to the rim of White Rock Canyon.

DESCRIPTION

Los Alamos County is New Mexico's smallest, with only 109 square miles, 42 of which are occupied by Los Alamos National Laboratory (LANL). Its trail network, however, is not to be taken lightly. Nearly 60 miles of official trails link canyons and mesas on the Pajarito Plateau, a rugged volcanic extension of the Jemez mountain range. Elevations on this tilted landscape range from 5,600 feet at the Rio Grande to 7,800 feet where the plateau meets the Valles Caldera. At the upside of these altitudes, Los Alamos promotes itself as

----

Directions   →

Via San Ysidro: From I-25 North, take Exit 242 toward Bernalillo. Turn left on US 550 and go 23.5 miles to San Ysidro. Turn right onto NM 4 and follow it 60.3 miles. After passing Mile Marker 60, look for an unpaved pulloff on the right. (If you reach the bottom of the hill, you've just missed it.)

    Via White Rock: From I-25 North, take Exit 276 and turn left onto NM 599. Go 13.5 miles north to merge onto US 84. Continue 14 miles north to the Los Alamos exit. Turn left and go 11.6 miles west on NM 502. Merge onto NM 4 toward White Rock and follow it 7.9 miles south. After Mile Marker 61, just past the bottom of the hill, look for an gravel pulloff on the left. It's harder to spot coming from this direction.

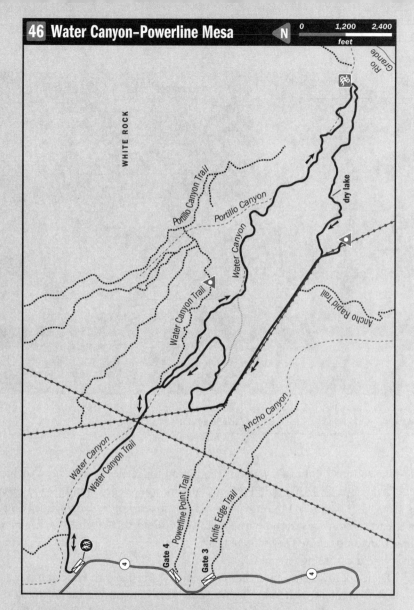

WHITE ROCK

Rio Grande

Portillo Canyon Trail

Portillo Canyon

dry lake

Water Canyon

Water Canyon Trail

Ancho Rapid Trail

Ancho Canyon

Water Canyon

Water Canyon Trail

Powerline Point Trail

Knife Edge Trail

Gate 4

Gate 3

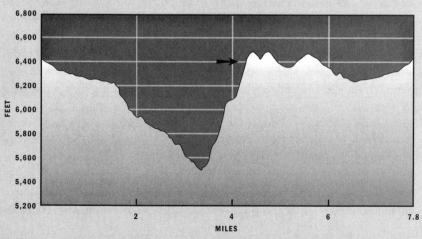

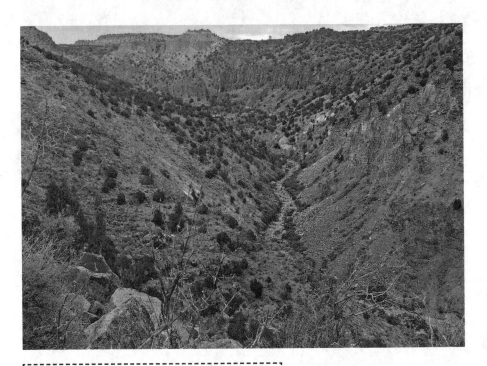

Water Canyon, viewed from the ascent to Powerline Point

"big-pine country" but can't shake its reputation for massive forest fires, including the 48,000-acre Cerro Grande Fire in 2000 and the record-setting 150,000-acre Las Conchas Fire in 2011. Both fires blazed in the upper canyons, leaving the lower east canyons unscathed but vulnerable to flooding. So while the segment of Water Canyon described in the hike below is usually dry, cloudbursts occasionally turn it into a cascading stream.

The best-known attraction on the east side of the Pajarito Plateau is Bandelier National Monument, visited in the previous hike. Canyons to the northeast share many of Bandelier's monumental characteristics, but with a few key differences. For starters, it's LANL territory, so you won't find any welcome centers or nature exhibits. In fact most of it is strictly off-limits and heavily guarded. Areas open to hiking are frequently patrolled and the rules are tight. The list of prohibitions includes motorized vehicles, bicycles, fires, fireworks, weapons, livestock, camping, hunting, trapping, and collecting. Also, don't touch anything that looks like a torpedo. In contrast to the monument, however, dogs are welcome here.

Signs along NM 4 are abundantly clear about where you can and cannot hike. Gate 5 is an exception. It's not visible from the road and its roadside signage went blank years ago, making it tricky to find.

The hike begins at a steep, rutted pulloff on the east side of NM 4. A dirt road starts northeast, almost parallel to the highway. Gate 5 is a few yards downhill, behind overgrown scrub. Informative notices are posted at the gate. A nearby photo display features rockets and hand grenades in a wide choice of fabulous colors. Seems a few undetonated bombs escaped the labs and remain at large.

Continue down the road as it hooks right and runs southeast alongside a shallow streambed. The north side of the canyon, a wall of pocked tuff, soon becomes visible through the pine. You'll get a closer look at Swiss cheese cliffs later. For now take a moment to smell the ponderosa, which have an aroma reminiscent of vanilla and butterscotch. After 1.2 miles on the road, or about 0.3 mile after the road crosses the streambed, you arrive at an unmarked fork that presents three options. Time to make a tough decision.

Water Canyon Trail veers left and climbs away from the rocky streambed. It's the easiest of the three to follow. If you weren't paying attention and missed the fork, you'd probably end up on this route anyway. From the fork it climbs steadily 0.4 mile to a bench, where it begins to level out. The streambed below trenches into a gorge, so 0.5 mile from the fork you've gained only 100 feet in elevation, but you're now about 400 feet above the canyon floor. The trail then starts working northeast to skirt around Portillo Canyon and join up with other trails, creating too many options to list here. You can continue straight to a vertigo-inducing overlook on the rim, where the Rio Grande comes into view. The round-trip distance between Gate 5 and the overlook is about 3.5 miles.

Water Canyon, the streambed itself, is a challenging segment in an unofficial route that should not be attempted on a whim. It's steep, slippery when dry, and treacherous when wet or icy. Flooding is rare but possible, especially from July to September, and emergency exits from the canyon gorge are limited. In the summer, climbing on dark basalt boulders can be almost as uncomfortable as walking barefoot on blacktop. Consider protective gloves. Above all, don't be fooled by the first 1.2 miles of this route, because the next 3 miles are among the toughest in this book. That said, the Water Canyon–Powerline Mesa route is a strong candidate for my favorite of the 60 hikes, its only major drawback being the long drive from Albuquerque.

From the fork, the streambed starts to dive into a darker, narrower canyon. The walls make an abrupt transition from gray and orange tuff to brown, black, and purple basalt. The basalts flowed from the Caja del Rio volcanoes across the Rio Grande and dammed the river several times, pushing river gravels to levels high above the present Rio. These gravel layers sometimes show as bands in the canyon wall, indicating the river's ancient courses.

The basalt blocks form a long series of waterfalls like a giant staircase. Though usually dry, low-porous rock retains water long after the last rain. Pools beneath otherwise dry falls can become challenging obstacles on this course. The streambed winds ever deeper and eventually widens to expose formations that resemble the turrets of white castles. It then braids around an island before Portillo Canyon enters on your left. At this point you're about halfway down the descent. If the day is heating up, take heart that there's shade under mature cottonwoods close ahead. The foliage is brilliant in October.

To the southeast, on the far side of the Rio Grande, cliffs of the Caja del Rio Plateau stand 1,000 feet or higher, but the river isn't as close as you might think. At 3.3 miles into the hike, you encounter one last waterfall, but it's a sheer three-story drop. The river is in plain sight just 250 yards east, but unless you're prepared to rappel, you can't get there by following the streambed.

Take a moment to enjoy the view, then turn your attention to the hill on your right. It's a short push to the ridgeline, where you can get a good look at the next major challenge. From this vantage point just 200 feet southwest of the waterfall, locate the steel tower on the rim of Powerline Mesa, about 0.75 mile due west, and at an elevation nearly 1,000 feet higher than your current position. Take comfort in the fact in spite of appearances, the segment of this hike to the mesa rim isn't as difficult as the canyon descent. It's a mere mile, and the ridgeline makes your approach perfectly clear. As long as you're going uphill, you're moving in the right direction. There isn't much room for deviation, but keep a sharp eye out for cairns and animal tracks to help keep you on the right path.

Midway into the ascent, a dry lake bed provides a brief reprieve from the sharp incline. The narrow gap you passed through to enter this sandy basin is the break that drained it. From here it's obvious that the steepest part remains ahead. The path resumes on the south side of the lake bed and winds northwest as it scales the steep, rocky terrain. If you can't find it, just push west and eventually you'll intercept it. Follow it to the mesa top, then head straight for the power lines ahead. When you reach the dirt road, turn left for a quick detour south to the overlook, just past the steel tower.

Powerline Point Trail is a straight, relatively flat dirt road directly beneath the power lines. If you're daunted by the streambed route described previously, consider this section in reverse for a moderate out-and-back option. The round-trip distance between Gate 5 and the overlook at Powerline Point is 6.4 miles.

From the point, power lines extend over a mile southeast to the next tower, which stands on Chino Mesa. No bridges span the Rio Grande on its 25-mile course through White Rock Canyon. The nearest crossings are Otowi Bridge, about 9 miles upstream, and Cochiti Dam, 16 miles downstream.

To return to Water Canyon, walk the road an easy mile northwest. Along the way, look for narrow grooves worn in the white bedrock road surface. The ruts indicate this was once a wagon road. When you arrive at the fork ahead, bear right and continue on the road beneath the power lines. About 300 yards ahead, just before the road arrives at the last set of utility poles, look for a path on your right. It starts out vague but soon feeds into a drainage that runs east alongside a ridge of exposed tuff.

Path segments worn through exposed tuff are similar to trails used by the Ancestral Pueblo people at the Tsankawi section of Bandelier National Monument. Use these footpaths to explore the ridge north of the drainage for a close look at the pocked walls. Bandelier tuff was created from the slurry of ash and gases that flowed from the caldera eruption. Gas bubbles were trapped inside the

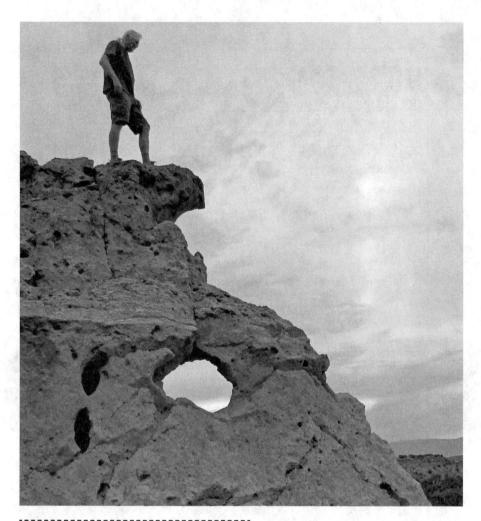

Tuff formation on the north rim of Powerline Mesa

solidifying tuff, which later eroded to form irregular patterns of arches, niches, and windows. Pueblo people modified some of these pockets into *cavates*, or carved rooms. Finding examples of those here takes a little exploring. You could easily tack on an extra mile to your hike with a thorough exploration of the pair of orange-tuff outcrops on this ridge.

To return to Water Canyon Trail, continue down the drainage path. Look for a path on your left that exits the drainage and aims toward the second outcrop of orange tuff. It leads through a break between the orange tuff and the darker outcrop farther down. Once through the break, the path turns northwest and goes downhill 0.4 mile to the canyon floor. Cross the shallow streambed to rejoin Water Canyon Trail at the fork.

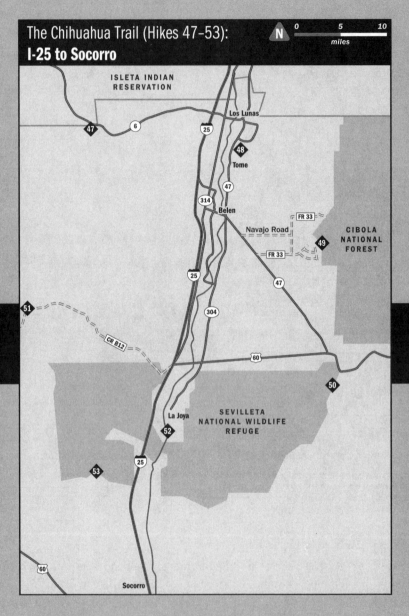

The Chihuahua Trail (Hikes 47–53):
I-25 to Socorro

N   0   5   10
     miles

ISLETA INDIAN
RESERVATION

Los Lunas

47   6   25

48
Tome

47

314   Belen

FR 33

Navajo Road   CIBOLA
NATIONAL
49   FOREST

FR 33

25   47

51   304

CR B12

60

50

SEVILLETA
NATIONAL WILDLIFE
REFUGE

La Joya

52

25

53

60

Socorro

THE CHIHUAHUA TRAIL
(I-25 TO SOCORRO)

47 HIDDEN MOUNTAIN

KEY AT-A-GLANCE INFORMATION

LENGTH: 2.1-mile loop, 1.6-mile out-and-back

DIFFICULTY: Difficult loop, easy out-and-back

SCENERY: Basalt cliffs, petroglyphs, ruins, the Ten Commandments

EXPOSURE: Little shade

TRAIL TRAFFIC: Moderate

SHARED USE: Low (livestock; closed to unauthorized vehicles)

TRAIL SURFACE: Dirt road, rocky arroyos, sand, scree

HIKING TIME: 1.5 hours

DRIVING DISTANCE: 38 miles

ACCESS: Daylight hours; State Land Trust Recreational Permit required

LAND STATUS: State trust land

MAPS: USGS Rio Puerco

FACILITIES: None

LAST-CHANCE FOOD/GAS: Full services at Exit 215. (If you're returning to Albuquerque via I-40, Route 66 Travel Center at exit 140, 32 miles from the trailhead.)

GPS TRAILHEAD COORDINATES

Latitude   34° 47' 36"

Longitude 106° 59' 59"

IN BRIEF

It's got a tough climb and a slippery descent, but the scenic loop reveals there's a lot more to Hidden Mountain than the unsolved riddles inscribed in Mystery Rock, also known as the Decalogue Stone of Los Lunas. But if the stone is all you came to see, then your hike is a whole lot easier.

DESCRIPTION

Hidden Mountain isn't much of a mountain, nor is it very well hidden. The naked cone rises up in full view near the convergence of NM 6, the Rio Puerco, and the BNSF railroad. Aside from the occasional train, it's a quiet junction, and evidence of human activity is nearly absent from sight.

The volcano peaks at 5,507 feet, more than 400 feet above the riverbed, where water seldom flows. The crater on top sits tilted with a chipped rim, like a discarded bowl. A crack spreads down to the north, deepening into a gully cluttered with basalt. Tucked near the bottom of the steep chute is a boulder weighing around 90 tons. In this neighborhood, it looks like an average stone, not the kind that calls attention to itself, except maybe for the way it slumps over a dry wash as though attempting to conceal the one thing that makes it truly remarkable.

Directions

From I-25 South, take Exit 203 at Los Lunas. Turn right and follow NM 6 west and north 14.5 miles. About 0.20 mile after crossing the Rio Puerco, turn left on an access road. Cross the railroad tracks and continue straight out 0.35 mile to the red gates. Park on the side of the road. Do not block any gates. The hike begins at pedestrian gate on the left side of the road.

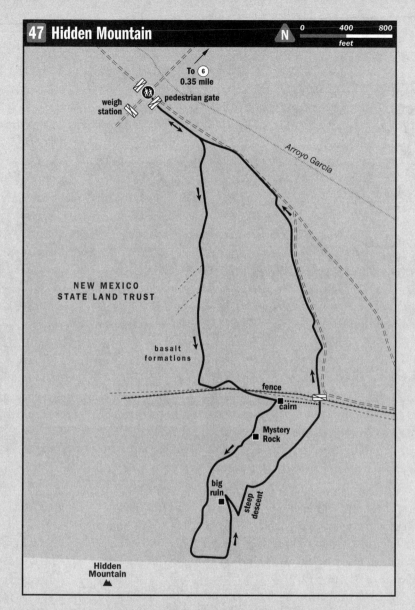

N

0   400   800
feet

To ⑥
0.35 mile

pedestrian gate

weigh
station

Arroyo Garcia

NEW MEXICO
STATE LAND TRUST

basalt
formations

fence

cairn

Mystery
Rock

big
ruin

steep
descent

Hidden
Mountain

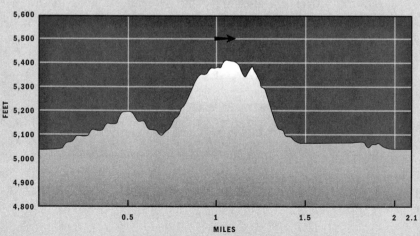

5,600
5,500
5,400
5,300
5,200
5,100
5,000
4,900
4,800

FEET

0.5   1   1.5   2 2.1

MILES

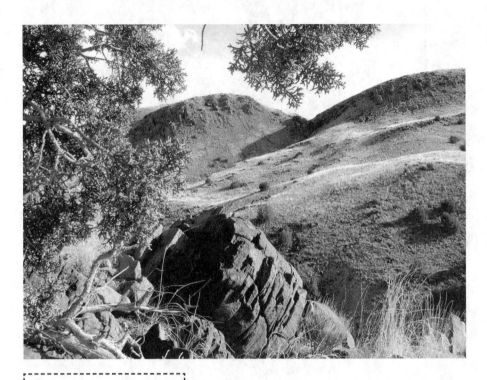

This is *not* the Decalogue Stone.

Pecked into its face is a strange message. Nine lines contain a total of 216 letters from the Old Hebrew alphabet, with a few Greek letters and maybe some Samaritan tossed into the mix. The earliest known documentation of the inscription came in 1936 from Professor Frank Hibben of the University of New Mexico. Since then, every savant with a penchant for cryptograms has attempted to crack the code of Mystery Rock.

In 1949 the Harvard scholar Robert Pfeiffer advanced a Paleo-Hebrew translation that remains inconclusive after decades of academic scrutiny. In 1979 the professional calligrapher Dixie Perkins produced a Canaanite–Phoenician–Greek translation of the rock just four days after learning about it on a local TV special. Her solution also remains open to debate.

To some, the message is a 4,000-year-old memo posted by Navajo ancestors. Or a map to hidden Acoma treasure. Or it's an ancient Samaritan mezuzah, an abridged version of the Decalogue traditionally carved into a large stone slab and placed at the entrance to a synagogue. It's proof that one of the Ten Tribes of Israel passed this way, or it's a propaganda effort by Mormon Battalion soldiers who camped nearby in the 1840s. Others have cited the combination of Hebraic and otherworldly characters as evidence of an intergalactic Wandering Jew. Or maybe it's the incredibly sad story of an unfortunate Greek explorer who sailed up the Rio Puerco 2,500 years ago.

The most commonly accepted explanation: it's a hoax. The likely culprits: Hobe and Eva, a couple of University of New Mexico students armed with chisels and Semitic-language reference books swiped from Zimmerman Library. The evidence: they left their names on another stone not 10 feet away, along with a date (3-19-30) that beats Hibben's initial discovery by three years.

In all the excitement to uncover the truth, the inscription has been scrubbed, chalked, re-etched, and ultimately rendered unsuitable for age-dating analysis. Further, in November 2006, someone gouged out the first line, the one that allegedly read, "I am Jehovah your God who has taken you out of Egypt" or "I have come to this place to stay. The other one met with an untimely death one year ago."

Which one of these translations provoked cryptofascists into censoring the rock? The mysteries never cease.

The easy way to the Decalogue Stone is a mostly flat out-and-back that runs 1.6 miles round-trip. Squeeze through the pedestrian gate and walk southeast along the dirt road. After about 0.3 mile, a doubletrack veers off to the right and runs south 0.3 mile toward a fence. As the doubletrack turns east, continue straight on a footpath to find a small drop gate. Go through the gate, fasten it behind you, and turn right. About 100 yards ahead on the left, you'll find a cairn. Go up the path leading into the gully, following arrows scratched into rocks along the near side of the streambed. You'll find the Decalogue Stone about 130 yards ahead on the left. The inscription faces the streambed at the base of the stone.

The scenic loop also starts at the pedestrian gate but veers right along the *near* side of the first hill. There's no real path here, but stay close to the hill and you'll soon wind up in a sandy wash. Follow it upstream, aiming straight for a gully that cuts through the bigger hill ahead. (Also, notice how the gully points up to a dark cleft in the ridgeline of Hidden Mountain. That will be your passage into its volcanic crater.)

The streambed turns rocky and the channel deepens as you head uphill. Stick to the main channel, bypassing any tributary washes merging on your right. As the channel fades out, aim slightly to the left for a sandy saddle on the ridge ahead. Once at the top, consider taking this short detour: turn right and go about 100 yards up the steep ridgeline to find tilted basalt boulders stacked up in interesting formations.

Continuing from the sandy ridge, follow the cow path curving down to the right. It's an easier descent and won't cause as much damage as trampling straight down the hillside. When you get to an old barbwire fence, turn left, and follow it down to the point where it crosses the wash. Here you can easily duck under it to the other side. Find the cairn about 100 yards downstream; turn right, and head up the path on the left side of the gully, following arrows scratched into rocks along the way.

When you're done examining the rock, continue up the gully, staying in the main channel for about 0.25 mile—but not all the way to the far side of the crater. State land ends about 100 yards shy of the south rim. That's most unfortunate,

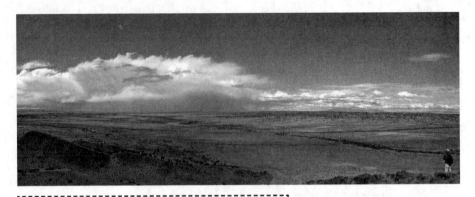

Views from the top of Hidden Mountain are vast and vacant.

because a quaint footpath follows nearly the entire curve of the crater rim, and the view from the top of the sheer black cliffs along the southern side is nothing short of dramatic (or so I'm told).

Though some anarchic hikers evidently cross the invisible boundary, you can stay in fair-play territory by cutting east at a point that seems completely arbitrary. To be more precise: at the point where the channel nearly fades into nothing, turn left. You'll intercept the path on the eastern rim in about 100 yards or so. Turn left again, and follow it north. Look for petroglyphs and shelter ruins along the way. At the fork ahead, take the left branch to check out the largest of the ruins. The circle of rocks, not much bigger than a hot tub, is a good spot to take a breather, watch the trains go by, and enjoy the wide-open views.

To get off the mountain, return to the fork, and take the other branch. The path fades as it drops down through the scree. Tack right, and carefully work your way down into a rocky wash where the terrain is a little more stable. Once the ground levels out, you'll see the gate straight ahead. Go through it, fasten it behind you, and follow the roads north-northwest 0.6 mile back to the parking area.

NEARBY ACTIVITIES

If returning to Albuquerque, consider going north (left) on NM 6 for an 18-mile cruise through the southeastern corner of the **Laguna Indian Reservation**. It adds about 10 miles to your trip, but the scenery is spectacular. (The land is off-limits to the general public, so don't wander.) NM 6 comes out on I-40 near Correo, about 27 miles west of Albuquerque.

If you need another hill to climb, head back down NM 6 to **El Cerro de Los Lunas**. This 1,500-acre open-space preserve, donated by the Huning Land Trust in 2006, contains numerous rugged routes to the 5,955-foot peak. Trailheads are on the south side of NM 6, accessed from West Gate, Jubilee Boulevard, and Huning Ranch Loop.

EL CERRO TOMÉ 48

IN BRIEF

The terminus of New Mexico's most famous pilgrimage, Tomé Hill is also a font of inspiration for great art and literature, both secular and sacred. With views of the Manzano Mountains and over the Rio Grande, the hill has a natural beauty that makes it a great place for a short hike almost any time of year.

DESCRIPTION

In the mid–17th century, Tomé Domínguez, age 90, settled in the Sandia jurisdiction with his wife, Eleña Ramírez de Mendoza. Soon after both passed away, one of their three sons, Tomé Domínguez de Mendoza, moved to Fonclara, a site at the base of this volcanic hill south of Albuquerque. In 1659 he received permission to settle the land, along with the right to "recruit" unpaid laborers from nearby Isleta Pueblo to build a hacienda. The homestead was finished by 1661 but came under attack during the Pueblo Revolt in 1680. Mendoza fled back to Spain and never saw his hacienda again.

In 1739 the Tomé Grant was awarded to the local *genízaros*, a marginalized class of Hispanicized Indians and mixed-blood settlers. Ostracized by both Spanish and Pueblo

---

Directions

From I-25 South, take Exit 203 at Los Lunas and turn left (east) on NM 6 (Historic Route 66). Go 3.5 miles and bear right on Lujan Road. After 0.25 mile on Lujan Road, turn right (south) on NM 47. Go 3.4 miles to Tomé Hill Road. Turn left toward the hill and follow the signs to Tomé Hill Park, 1 mile ahead. Turn right on La Entrada Road, then left into the parking lot.

KEY AT-A-GLANCE INFORMATION

LENGTH: 1.7-mile loop

DIFFICULTY: Moderate

SCENERY: Religious iconography perched atop a solitary volcanic mass; petroglyphs; views of the Manzano Mountains and Sierra Lucero

EXPOSURE: No shade

TRAIL TRAFFIC: Moderate

SHARED USE: Low, though crowded with pilgrims during religious observances. Animals, vehicles, and firearms are not permitted on the hill.

TRAIL SURFACE: Dirt, rock

HIKING TIME: 1 hour

DRIVING DISTANCE: 31 miles

ACCESS: Dawn–dusk

LAND STATUS: Private property

MAPS: Brochure map available (sometimes) at trailhead; USGS Los Lunas

FACILITIES: Interpretive signage, sculpture garden (wheelchair-accessible)

LAST-CHANCE FOOD/GAS: All services in Los Lunas

SPECIAL COMMENTS: See longer note at end of Description.

GPS TRAILHEAD COORDINATES

Latitude   34° 45' 5"

Longitude   106° 42' 21"

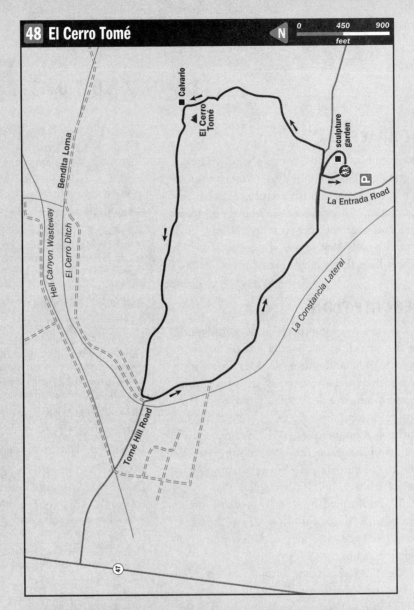

N

| 0 | 450 | 900 |

feet

Calvario

▲ El Cerro Tomé

sculpture garden

La Entrada Road

Bendita Loma

Heil Canyon Wasteway

El Cerro Ditch

La Constancia Lateral

Tomé Hill Road

47

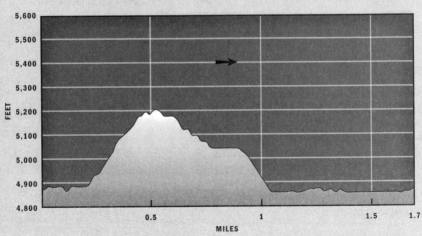

5,600
5,500
5,400
5,300
5,200
5,100
5,000
4,900
4,800

FEET

0.5   1   1.5   1.7

MILES

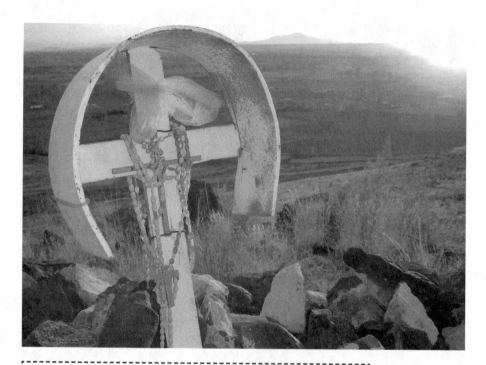

Folk shrines and memorials once adorned the hilltop. They are now prohibited.

societies, many genízaros developed their own customs, including religious practices based largely on native beliefs and Franciscan mysticism. Their unique traditions evolved into the Penitente Brotherhood, noted for acts of mortification,
flagellation, and the Good Friday crucifixion of a Penitente brother.

The annual Passion Play at Tomé Hill today is said to be the same as the
one described by Fray Francisco Domínguez in 1776, with one possible exception. According to a disclaimer posted in Tomé Park: "No actual crucifixion is
carried out."

Credit for organizing the installation of the *calvario* on Tomé Hill in 1947
goes to Edwin Antonio Berry, a World War II veteran and the son of a 19th-
century Penitente leader. Berry also recorded the oral history and songs of his
culture for posterity and remained the steward of Tomé Hill until his death in
2000. A stirring tribute to Tomé's most celebrated citizen can be found in Greg-
ory Candela's locally published poetry collection, *Surfing New Mexico* (Crones
Unlimited, 2001).

The route you walk here is known as Berry's Path. You hardly need a guidebook for this one. Abundant interpretive texts at Tomé Hill Park spell out just
about everything you could want to know about this legendary hill. But to omit
this hike would be a mortal sin, for nothing else encapsulates the essence of New
Mexico quite like El Cerro Tomé. The cultural significance of the hill has earned
it a listing on the National Register of Historic Places.

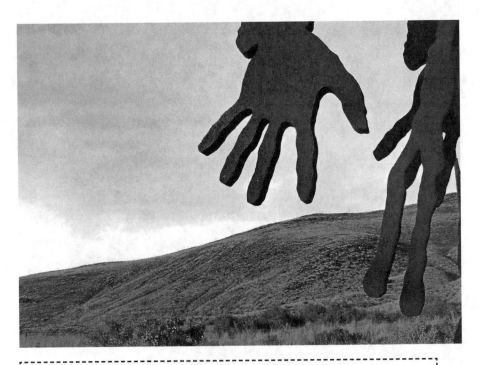

La Puerta del Sol (detail shown) is the steel sculpture in the park on the south side of Tomé Hill.

Park literature depicts the hill as a station at the crossroads of many cultures, but with an interesting slant. For instance, 1846 is recalled as "the year of the U.S. invasion and occupation of New Mexico." By contrast, the Spanish conquistadors are described as mere "explorers." If you don't have time to read all the signs—and unfortunately a few have vanished in recent years—get the equally comprehensive brochure. God willing, you'll find one in the black mailbox.

Begin the hike by walking around *La Puerta del Sol*, the impressive sculptural centerpiece of Tomé Hill Park. The steel-and-rust artwork of the artist Armando Alvarez is a complex vision of the diverse groups who have traveled El Camino Real in the past 400 years. The $100,000 piece features a 25-foot-high gateway and the life-sized likenesses of several historical archetypes. The work is often described as a celebration of cultural diversity; however, bold details evoke darker episodes of cultural conflicts.

Follow the sidewalk around a cable fence and up the road. A crosswalk ahead leads to the start of the steep South Trail. According to a sign back in the park, "The distance to the summit is over a quarter of a mile with an altitude gain of 1,200 feet." Don't worry—it's not quite that severe. The gain is a mere 400 feet. But with only two switchbacks, the rocky path takes some effort. The reward at the top is eternal salvation, along with a lovely view of the valley between the Manzano Mountains and Mesa Gallina.

Though highly discouraged now, leaving a mark on the hill is a custom that dates back 2,000 years or more. As the signs below suggest, petroglyphs appear on every flat slab of basalt on the hill. However, they're not easy to see from the trails, and the literature is a bit murky on how to find them. As a result, visitors often scour the hill in search of pecked rocks. With a good eye and better patience, you can spot a few petroglyphs from designated (though unmarked) spurs off South Trail near the top of the hill.

The calvario at the summit consists of three wood-and-metal crosses, each 16 feet high. A tin shrine sits at the base of the central cross, along with countless votive candles, rosaries, photographs, and handwritten prayers. It is at once a place of profound grief, joy, and hope. In addition to the permanent installation, temporary folk memorials and devotional artworks often crop up at various stations around the hilltop. There's always something new and fascinating on Tomé Hill.

Continue past the calvario on West Trail, also called Via Cruces (Crosses Way). Just over 0.25 mile downhill, a sign on the right indicates a path to the chapel. Stay on West Trail another 0.25 mile or so until it reaches the base of the hill. Turn left, and follow the road 0.6 mile back to the parking lot at Tomé Park. Or for the scenic route, turn right, and follow the road about 3 miles clockwise around the hill.

For an enlightening and entertaining perspective on contemporary life in Tomé, read Ana Castillo's widely acclaimed novel *So Far from God*.

Note: Tomeans (Toméseños?) are generally friendly, if somewhat reserved toward outsiders. Despite their ongoing efforts to preserve their traditional community, growth and development throughout the area has led to an escalating crime rate in recent years. Don't get too lulled in the pastoral setting—use the same common sense as you would when walking in an urban area.

NEARBY ACTIVITIES

Tomé Plaza features the Immaculate Conception Church and Museum. A two-story courthouse once stood on the southwest corner of this historic plaza, but all that remains is the old Tomé jail. The walls are 4 feet thick and built of black igneous rock. To get to Tomé Plaza from Tomé Hill Park, return to NM 47 via Tomé Hill Road, turn left, and drive south 1.3 miles. Turn right on Church Loop and go about 0.1 mile to the small community park on plaza.

49 MONTE LARGO CANYON

KEY AT-A-GLANCE INFORMATION

LENGTH: 5-mile out-and-back

DIFFICULTY: Moderate

SCENERY: Broadleaf and pine forest, wildlife, caves

EXPOSURE: Mostly shade

TRAIL TRAFFIC: Low

SHARED USE: Low (equestrians, livestock; closed to motorized vehicles)

TRAIL SURFACE: Packed dirt, loose rock

HIKING TIME: 2–3 hours

DRIVING DISTANCE: 55 miles

ACCESS: Year-round

LAND STATUS: Cibola National Forest–Mountainair Ranger District; Manzano Mountain Wilderness

MAPS: USGS Manzano Peak

FACILITIES: None

LAST-CHANCE FOOD/GAS: All services available in Belen, about 20 miles from the trailhead

SPECIAL COMMENTS: The last 4 miles of dirt road can get rough, especially after snow or heavy rain. Four-wheel drive is not necessary in dry conditions, but a little extra clearance might help. For current conditions, check with the Mountainair Ranger District: (505) 847-2990; fs.usda.gov/cibola.

GPS TRAILHEAD COORDINATES

Latitude   34° 36' 03"

Longitude   106° 29' 54"

IN BRIEF

Though designated as a trailhead on Forest Service maps, Monte Largo lacks a designated trail. No problem—well-worn paths facilitate hiking along its primary drainage. The lush wooded corridor is a near-perfect environment for hikes throughout most of the year.

DESCRIPTION

Don't let the approach fool you. Though the Manzanos appear as barren scarps of granite and scrub, you'll find long stretches of shaded woodland hidden behind its stark facade. Monte Largo Canyon contains a lush mix of oak and pine. A good supply of acorns keeps squirrels and turkeys well fed, and summer bounties of currants attract birds and bears.

The state's only species of bear is *Ursus americanus,* the black bear, which often appears

----

Directions

From I-25 South, take Exit 195 toward Belen and go 4.6 miles on I-25 Bus/North Main Street. Turn left onto Reinken Avenue (NM 309). Go 2.4 miles east, crossing the railroad tracks and the river. Take a right onto Rio Communities Boulevard (NM 47). Go southeast 5.8 miles and turn left on the dirt road formerly known as FR 33 (now signed on the right as S Navajo Loop). Go east 6 miles and cross a cattle guard. The road jogs slightly to the right and turns to gravel. Stay on it for the next 2.3 miles to the second intersection, marked with a small cairn on the left. (Along this stretch, you'll pass a ranch house with a rail tanker in the yard. The road then bends northeast and becomes rocky.) The second intersection is marked with a small cairn on the left. Turn right (southeast) and go 2.5 miles, cross the cattle guard, and park on the west side of the fenced lot.

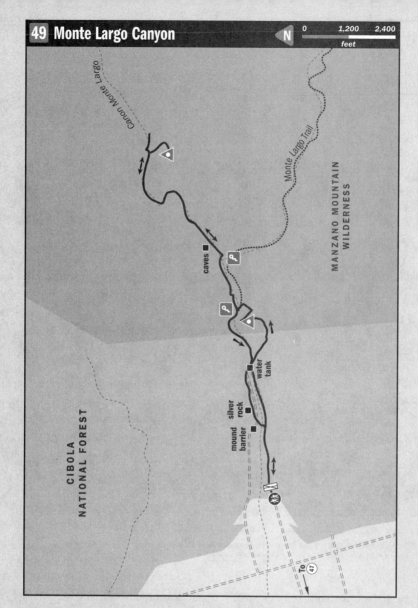

N

0   1,200   2,400
feet

Cañon Monte Largo

Monte Largo Trail

MANZANO MOUNTAIN WILDERNESS

caves

CIBOLA NATIONAL FOREST

water tank

silver rock

mound barrier

To 47

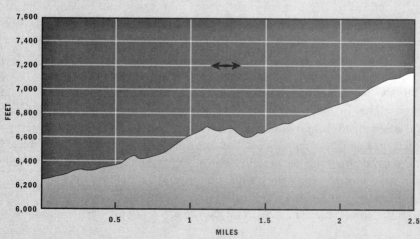

7,600
7,400
7,200
7,000
6,800
6,600
6,400
6,200
6,000

FEET

0.5   1   1.5   2   2.5

MILES

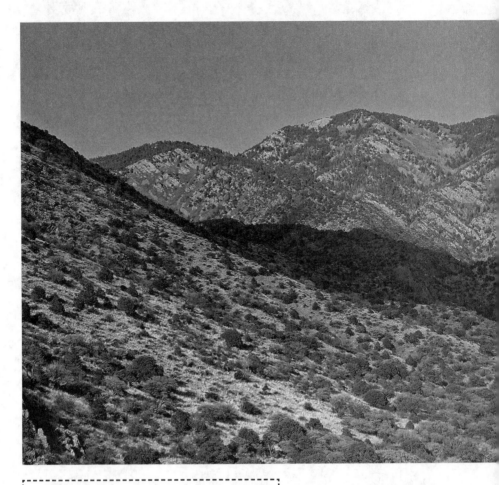

The view northeast from the lower overlook (6,640 feet)

more a shade of cinnamon brown. Its predilection for verdant mountain forests keeps it confined (usually) to wooded "islands" throughout the American Southwest. Black bears may seem cute and clumsy but can charge at speeds up to 30 mph. With that in mind, review the safety tips for hiking in bear country (page 12) before entering Monte Largo Canyon. Most importantly, never try to outrun a bear. You need only run faster than the other hikers.

The hike begins at the gateway. Walk straight east along a path worn through rocky grassland. In about 0.25 mile, it bends downhill to the left. A black water line crosses the path here. Both the line and the path descend closer to the arroyo and then turn east into the canyon. You can follow the line for a more shaded path, though dense scrub ahead will eventually coax you to cross the arroyo. Or you can cross sooner to pick up a sunny doubletrack on the north bank.

Either way, you'll pass a water tower on the north bank. About 500 feet east of the water tower, the trail splits. For a great preview of the route ahead, veer

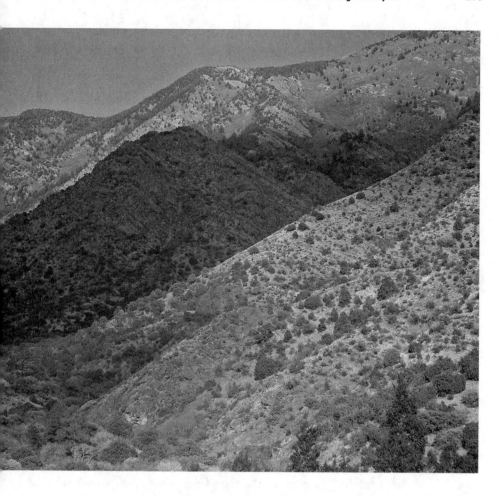

right on the more prominent branch uphill. About 0.2 mile ahead, a steel sign marks the boundary of the Manzano Mountain Wilderness. Continue uphill another 200 yards or so. The object is to reach a rocky outcrop on the nearest ridge to your left, so just aim in that direction if the path fades or seems to stray elsewhere. When you reach the crest of the ridge, turn left and walk out to the point. Cuts in the exposed rock suggest minor quarrying or mining may have occurred up here.

The Monte Largo Spring is directly below to the north, but it may be difficult to spot when foliage is full. Animals frequent the water source, making this overlook the perfect perch for watching birds and wildlife. I've seen fox and mule deer trotting below, apparently oblivious to my presence. Bring binoculars to scope out broader terrain. Dense woods stretch for about 1 mile to the northeast before disappearing into the V of the canyon. Manzano Peak, the highest in the range, stands 2 miles to the southeast.

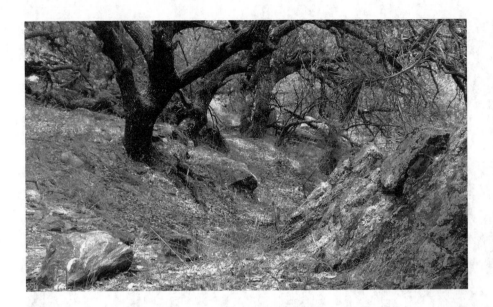

Note that Monte Largo Canyon is one of several in a basin that spans about 2.5 miles north to south. For navigational purposes, it helps to know that all waterways in this basin eventually merge to exit through the bottleneck to the west, the way you just came in. So as long as you don't cross any major ridges, you can follow any drainage downstream to return to the trailhead.

Numerous trails are easier to spot when the trees are bare. A couple of routes that might be more suitable in wet or icy conditions are on the arid slopes a few yards above the streambed. Geared for the rest of the year, this hike sticks to the shaded paths close to the main arroyo.

Return to the canyon floor by going down the side opposite the way you came up, then turn right to continue following the waterline upstream. In 0.25 mile, you'll arrive at a second fork. Stay left. (For reference: the waterline goes right to the Upper Monte Largo Spring, about a minute's walk south. From there the old Monte Largo Trail, a steeper, sunnier path marked with cairns, continues southeast, then climbs east on a strenuous route to meet the Crest Trail 170 about a half-mile north of Manzano Peak.)

As you continue northeast from the second fork, brown cliffs form vertical walls above to your left. Small caves can be seen in the sedimentary rock; pungent odors suggest that some are occupied and probably best left undisturbed. You can get a good view of them by reaching slightly higher ground on your right and looking across the arroyo.

The drainage deepens ahead, and the trail seems to split off in different directions. You may find traces of an old jeep road or a well-worn game path meandering through towering ponderosa. You can usually switch from one to another by running a short lateral. Either way, keep the main channel nearby, usually on your right. If you find yourself bushwhacking, wandering over a barren hill, or struggling up a ridiculously steep drainage, you've undoubtedly strayed off course.

About 2 miles into the hike, the drainage curves around a bulging outcrop on the left. Immediately afterward, it hooks around a towering outcrop on the right. The trail becomes a little steeper along this S-curve.

The incline lessens as the trail runs due east for the next 0.3 mile. Primitive campsites with sturdy shelter frames and fire rings can be found at the beginning of this stretch, along with a flourish of poison ivy. For an optional detour, look for narrow switchbacks on the steep slope to your right. A short but strenuous ascent to the south may require a bit of scrambling, but it puts you atop a ridge with a commanding view of the canyon. To return to the canyon floor this time, go the same way you came up. Bushwhacking down the other side isn't worth the trouble.

You can continue up the canyon, but the campsites seem as good a place as any to turn around, particularly when certain members in your group start getting jittery over signs of bear activity. Follow the drainage 1 mile downstream, until you locate the water line snaking out from the upper spring. Follow the line out of the canyon. As you approach the lower spring, the next 0.25 mile may suddenly seem unfamiliar; this is the part you bypassed on the way up when you climbed over the ridge. Continue down to the water tower, and stay on the old road. About 250 yards ahead is a large silver-painted rock. Just ahead on the left is a cairn. Turn left at the cairn to cross the arroyo. (If you encounter dirt-mound barriers on the road, you've gone about 100 yards past the cairn. Also note that the road does not lead back to the parking lot.) Once across the arroyo, continue on the trail another 0.4 mile back to your car.

NEARBY ACTIVITIES

There are a few good opportunities for **geocaching** in the area. One of my favorites leads to the Lone Wolf Mine near Ojo Barreras, about 1.5 miles south of the Monte Largo trailhead. To prepare for the hunt, log on to **geocaching.com** and search for GC2FARW on the home page. (*Note:* A free site account is needed to view the specific location of the cache.)

For local history, and collections related to the Santa Fe Railroad, visit the Valencia County Historical Society's **Belen Harvey House Museum,** in the Harvey House Dining Room, which is listed on the National Register of Historic Places. En route back to I-25, after crossing the bridge over the railroad tracks, turn left on Third Street. Go two blocks south and turn left on Becker Street. Another two blocks and another left puts you on First Street. The museum is on the right at 104 N. 1st St. Open Tuesday–Saturday, 12:30–3:30 p.m., Sunday, 1–3 p.m., and available for tours (to be safe, call before you visit to make sure it's open). (505) 861-0581; **belenharveyhouse.com.**

50 CERRO MONTOSO

KEY AT-A-GLANCE INFORMATION

LENGTH: 5.2-mile out-and-back

DIFFICULTY: Partially strenuous

SCENERY: Piñon–juniper hills, panoramic mountain views, marine fossils

EXPOSURE: Some canyon and forest shade

TRAIL TRAFFIC: Low

SHARED USE: Low (equestrians, livestock)

TRAIL SURFACE: Sandy washes, rocky hills

HIKING TIME: 3 hours

DRIVING DISTANCE: 74 miles

ACCESS: Year-round

LAND STATUS: BLM–Socorro Field Office

MAPS: USGS Cerro Montoso

FACILITIES: None

LAST-CHANCE FOOD/GAS: All services in Belen, about 40 miles from the trailhead.

SPECIAL COMMENTS: Despite obvious landmarks, navigating the return route can get tricky in places. A compass is helpful. A GPS unit with tracking features is optimal.

GPS TRAILHEAD COORDINATES

Latitude   34° 22' 42"

Longitude   106° 31' 20"

IN BRIEF

You won't find any trails in these lonely hills. This undesignated route begins with a short stroll up a pleasant arroyo. A quick push up a hillside brings you to the first of two overlooks on the boundary of the Sevilleta National Wildlife Refuge. From there you can preview the challenge ahead: a moderate descent into the valley below followed by a steep climb to the top of Cerro Montoso. It's not as hard as it looks, and the rewards are unmatched views of southern mountain ranges and a rare peek at otherwise inaccessible lands.

DESCRIPTION

The Los Pinos Mountains might be small, but don't take them lightly. They're like a scrappy little version of the Manzanos—shorter, yes, but steeper and more rugged. Colorado piñon and one-seed juniper are the dominant vegetation, with a diverse shrub component that includes scrub live oak and mountain mahogany in addition to broom snakeweed, Apache

----

Directions _____→

From I-25 South, take Exit 175 at Bernardo and go 20.3 miles east on US 60. (*Note:* NM 47 from Belen to US 60 is 10 miles shorter but adds at least as many minutes.) After Abó Pass, as US 60 starts east again, look for an asphalt turnoff about 100 yards past the end of the guardrail on the right. Take a sharp right there and go through the gate, being sure to latch it behind you. The road shows up on some maps as B115, but a nearby sign indicates you're now on CR-115/Augie Ranch Road. Veer left at the Y immediately ahead and drive 2 miles south on the main dirt road. Watch for an intersecting wash that's about as wide as the road itself. Turn right and park on the sandy streambed.

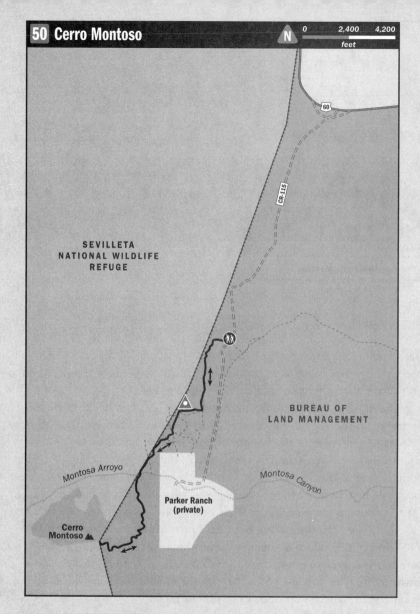

SEVILLETA
NATIONAL WILDLIFE
REFUGE

CR-115

60

BUREAU OF
LAND MANAGEMENT

Montosa Arroyo

Montosa Canyon

Parker Ranch
(private)

Cerro
Montoso

0   2,400   4,200
feet
N

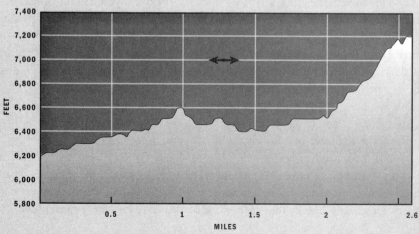

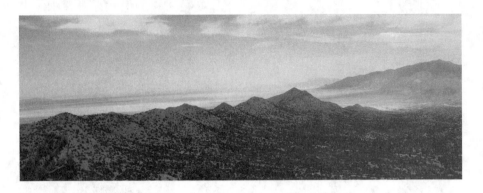

The view from Cerro Montoso

plume, tree cholla, and banana yucca. And then there's the usual smattering of New Mexico thistle and globemallow. Bird species include bald eagle, peregrine falcon, red-tailed hawk, kestrel, and burrowing owl. Mule deer, desert bighorn sheep, pronghorn, mountain lion, and bear make up the local animal life. Largely absent from this otherwise familiar landscape: people.

The oft-overlooked mountains are the last in a line of uplifted fault blocks that make up the Sandia, Manzanita, and Manzano ranges. Nearly the entire Los Pinos range falls within the boundaries of Sevilleta National Wildlife Refuge, a 228,000-acre research area that's largely off-limits to the public. Only the eastern foothills extend into public land. Oddly enough, one foothill ranks among the range's highest peaks. At 7,259 feet, Cerro Montoso ("wooded hill") stands just 271 feet short of the pinnacle of Whiteface Mountain.

There are no trails leading to or up Cerro Montoso, at least not on this side of it. Most of the hill stands behind the Sevilleta fence line, ruling out access from the west. The approach is further complicated by private-ranch boundaries on its northeastern side. Fortunately, a strip of public land between the refuge and the ranch creates an access corridor from the north.

Begin the hike by heading west into a small, rocky canyon. About 200 yards upstream, the wash turns to the south. Continue along the streambed another 0.6 mile. Along the way, numerous drainages enter on the right. The one you're looking for is equal in size to the one you're in. At this point, both are trenched about 4 feet deep, and the divider between them should be pointing straight at you. A couple of cairns on the banks also mark the spot.

This is where you exit the arroyo and begin a 0.1-mile push to the first overlook, so turn right and climb west, keeping the drainage on your left. You'll lose sight of it as it shallows out, so just continue straight up to the top of the hill. There you'll meet a fence and a U.S. General Land Office Survey marker from 1934. You'll also get a radiant 360-degree view that includes the Sevilleta, the southern Manzanos, and the task ahead of you: Cerro Montoso. A clear-cut boundary line neatly bisects the steep wooded hill, giving it the appearance of a zippered jacket. The fenceline illustrates a direct route to the top, but it's harder than it looks.

Take a moment to visualize the hike ahead. For the descent into the valley: if you keep the fence within 100 yards, drainage crossings below will be a little easier. It'll also keep you from straying onto private property. For the ascent, you have two options: follow the fence straight up or veer left to climb up the hill's eastern shoulder. Note the dense vegetation in what might be called the clavicle area. Steer wide to the left to avoid getting snagged in thick juniper. From the shoulder, it's a short walk to the top.

Now that you've got the route in your head, it's time to put it under your feet. Start downhill, stepping over veins and outcroppings of glistening white quartz. You'll soon encounter two to four narrow cuts, depending on whether you cross upstream or downstream of the nearby forks. Continue following the fence over two low ridges (more like humps, really) to find a wide, sandy wash on the far side of each one.

The ascent of Cerro Montoso begins from the second wash, which shows up on some maps as Montosa Canyon. At this point, you're about 1.5 miles into the hike, and you have two options for climbing the hill ahead of you. The easiest way to navigate your way up and back is to stick to the fence. It's daunting, but doable. The other option is to begin veering away from the fence, aiming roughly south for just under 0.5 mile. The idea on this segment is to cross two humps at the base of the hill before turning in for the steep ascent. If you turn uphill too soon, you'll end up in one of two difficult ravines, both of which lead into the thickly wooded clavicle area.

On the steep mid- to upper slopes, limestone outcroppings and scree are loaded with marine fossils. Widespread imprints of bivalve and nautilus shells range in size from fingernails to silver dollars. The BLM does not discourage visitors from picking up common fossils, but you might want to wait until you're heading back downhill before filling your pockets with rocks.

As the grade lessens, start aiming for the peak. The true summit, Parker Peak, is about 150 feet west of the fence, but you can still legally squeak above the 7,200-foot contour line and peer into the Sevilleta. Somewhere down there, researchers might be coaching Mexican gray wolves for release into the wild, discovering a cure for plague in Gunnison's prairie dogs, or analyzing trophic cascades among banner-tailed kangaroo rats. The scientific possibilities are as broad as the land itself.

Views to the north and east include the Manzano and Gallinas mountains, respectively. These two ranges comprise the Mountainair Ranger District of Cibola National Forest. Fewer than 50 miles south, Oscura ("dark") Peak stands at 8,732 feet. The Trinity Site, ground zero for the first atomic bomb, lies 2.75 miles to the west of it. Had you been standing here on Cerro Montoso at dawn on July 16, 1945, you would've seen a mushroom cloud reaching six times higher than the rise of Oscura Peak.

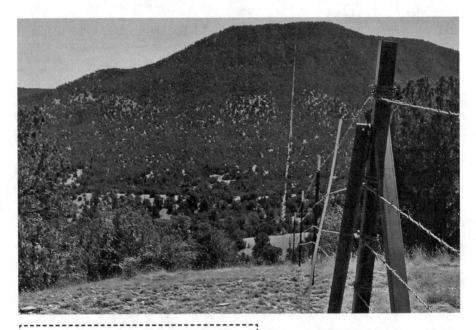

Cerro Montoso, viewed from the USGS survey marker

To return to the car, bolder hikers bent on creating a loop might try circling around the eastern side of the ranch and revisiting Montosa Canyon along the way. (Note that east of the ranch, the canyon runs about 100 feet deep. Erosional features make it an attractive little hike on its own. The exchange between the canyon and CR-115 is easy and does not cross the ranch boundary. You'll come close to the gate, and folks at the ranch might ask what you're doing, but they don't seem to mind hikers. They're just keeping a sharp eye out for poachers.)

Otherwise, follow the directions in reverse—that includes revisiting the first overlook. Any shortcuts will likely send you into a wash that leads to the Parker Ranch. On the plus side, you can't get too lost. All drainages eventually flow to the road, CR-115, so a wrong turn would add no more than 2 miles to the overall hike.

NEARBY ACTIVITIES

Abó Ruins–Salinas Pueblo Missions National Monument: The unique buttressed walls of the Franciscan mission church of San Gregorio de Abó still dominate the Tompiro Pueblo of Abó. To visit this remarkable site, return to US 60, turn right, and drive 8 miles east. Turn left on NM 513 and go 0.5 mile north. Open daily, 9 a.m.–6 p.m., Memorial Day–Labor Day, and 9 a.m.–5 p.m. the rest of the year. (505) 847-2400; **nps.gov/sapu.**

SIERRA LADRONES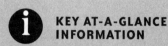

IN BRIEF

Following a game path on a long, undulating uplift, this straightforward route provides a friendly introduction to an isolated mountain range with a mean reputation. Peaks along the way allow for great views down to the foothills and canyons, and up to the toothy ridges of the Sierra Ladrones.

DESCRIPTION

Sierra Ladrones, or "thieves mountains," earned their name as a hideout for Navajo raiders who, having relieved local ranches of their stock, spirited them across the *jaral* (chaparral or scrubland) to untraceable retreats. Later banditos and rustlers continued the tradition by holing up in the range's deep canyons. Few were known to reemerge, and speculation of lost loot continues to this day.

Also called Los Ladrones, the dark mountains figure into local lore as the setting for Apache ambushes, disastrous treasure hunts, and encounters with ghostly white werewolves. Sightings of *brazas*—fireballs wheeling in the night—are not uncommon, and a few known meteor-impact sites in the area do not

---

Directions

From I-25 South, take Exit 175 at Bernardo. Take the first left off the exit ramp and head toward the RV park. Go southwest on Old Highway 85 and cross the Rio Puerco Bridge. A half-mile past the bridge, turn right on County Road B12 and reset your odometer. (B12 is a long, bumpy road, but passable for most vehicles in dry conditions.) Go northwest on the main road, following signs toward Riley and Magdalena. At 18.8 miles, park at the junction. The hike begins at the tip of the ridge on your left. See Description for a shuttle option.

KEY AT-A-GLANCE INFORMATION

LENGTH: 7-mile out-and-back, 5-mile shuttle option

DIFFICULTY: Moderate–strenuous

SCENERY: Desert scrub, cacti, raptors, expansive views

EXPOSURE: Full sun

TRAIL TRAFFIC: Low

SHARED USE: Low (livestock)

TRAIL SURFACE: Sand, limestone pavements, loose rock

HIKING TIME: 3–4 hours

DRIVING DISTANCE: 72 miles

ACCESS: Year-round

LAND STATUS: BLM–Socorro, Wilderness Study Area

MAPS: USGS Riley, Ladron Peak

FACILITIES: None

LAST-CHANCE FOOD/GAS: All services available at Exit 191 in Belen, 38 miles from the trailhead

SPECIAL COMMENTS: The hike featured here does *not* reach Ladron Peak. The elevation profile describes the shuttle option.

GPS TRAILHEAD COORDINATES

Latitude   34° 29' 45"

Longitude   107° 07' 56"

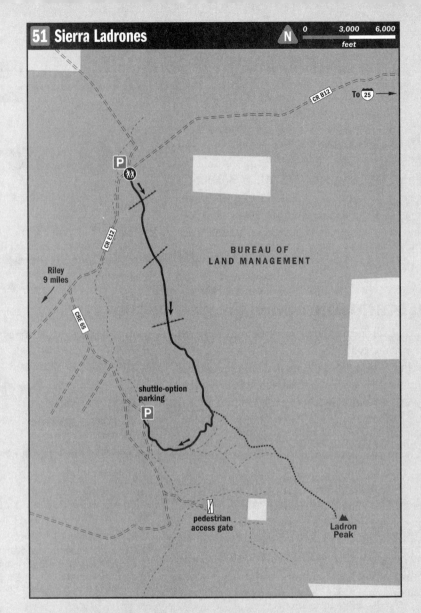

N

0   3,000   6,000
feet

P

CR B12

To 25 →

BUREAU OF
LAND MANAGEMENT

CR E12

Riley
9 miles

CRE 68

shuttle-option
parking

P

pedestrian
access gate

Ladron
Peak

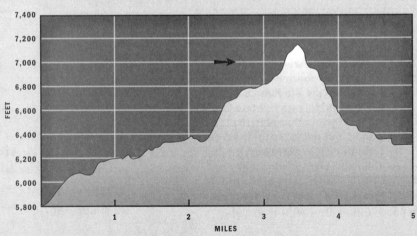

7,400

7,200

7,000

6,800

6,600

6,400

6,200

6,000

5,800

FEET

1   2   3   4   5

MILES

About 3.5 miles up the ridge, you've gained 1,300 feet in elevation ...

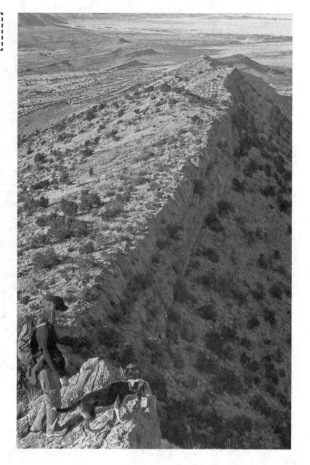

adequately explain the strange phenomenon.

The remote granite massif rises 4,500 feet above the Rio Puerco. It stands alone on a plain too prone to erosion to sustain reliable roads. A checkerboard of private ranchland further complicates the approach from the northeast, whereas its southeast quadrant falls in the strictly off-limits Sevilleta National Wildlife Refuge.

More than 45,300 acres in the Ladrones have been designated as a BLM Wilderness Study Area. The local wildlife population includes mule deer, black bear, mountain lion, and pronghorn. Desert bighorn sheep were reintroduced in 1992. Grasses and scrub sum up the vegetation on the lower slopes; ponderosa pine, aspen, and Douglas-fir grow near the twin summits. The eastern summit, Ladron Peak, is the only named peak in the range, but the summit less than a half-mile to its west is the taller of the two.

Looming on Albuquerque's southwest horizon, the range appears monolithic. Its complexity becomes more apparent up close. It has a longstanding reputation as one of the last places you'd want to hike alone. A local fireman who knows the peak well summed it up best: "It will kick your butt."

Don't let that deter you. Navigationally, this route is foolproof. You just follow a ridgeline from bottom to top or however far you want to go. Climbing becomes more difficult with distance. Each new mile begins with an incremental challenge. How far you get depends entirely on how hard you want to hike. Elevation enhances the views, of course, but you don't have to go far for wide-open vistas in all directions. So pack a lunch and plenty to drink. Above all, gringos, remember the sunscreen.

Start the hike at the side of the road by climbing south up the point of the ridge. This elongated uplift runs parallel to Cañon del Norte, but like most features in the

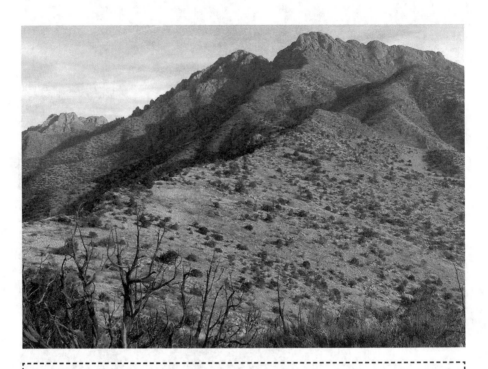

... but you're not quite halfway to Ladron Peak. To follow this route, turn back here or begin your descent to the shuttle.

Ladrones, lacks a name for itself. Creative christening suggestions include: El Cuchillo de la Viuda, Lomo del Vaquero, and Rustlers' Ramp—each appropriate in its own way. For now it remains unnamed.

Juniper, creosote, and cacti do their best to green the otherwise barren slopes. Limestone pavements keep the vegetation spread out, and narrow paths seem to show up wherever grasses take hold. Your only obstacles in the first 2 miles are a few barbwire fences, all easily crossed or circumvented.

The fence at 2 miles into the hike crosses near a peak (elevation 6,398 feet). It's a good spot for a quick breather because the climb is about to become somewhat more difficult. Now instead of marching directly up the backbone, you might find it easier to veer slightly to your right and aim for the saddle ahead. Once you reach that, angle back to your left for a short but steep push back up to the crest. A short rest on the 6,780-foot peak just ahead might be warranted as well.

The next mile skirts the edge of the sheer east-facing cliffs. The drop to your left is a good 300 feet in places. Your next challenge comes roughly 3.2 miles into the hike with a steep 0.25-mile push to the next peak (7,155 feet). From this vantage point, you should be able to make out the giant fir trees growing at the collar of Ladron Peak, in addition to the rows of enormous tiger-tooth rocks standing on its left shoulder. Also take a moment to scout out the trail ahead. The ridgeline bends to your left and assumes a relatively gentle temperament for the next 0.5 mile or so. But then, as you can see, the mountain reddens and becomes fiercely steep. That was my goal, but my group turned mutinous at the sight of it and refused to ascend the ridge any higher. In their defense, temperatures had hit 107, and our perch at 7,155 feet now seemed like a satisfactory accomplishment. Later group hikes stalled out here despite significantly lower temperatures. In that sense, the 7,155-foot mark seems a natural point to turn around or head for the shuttle.

The shuttle option is a bit more complicated and shaves off a couple of miles at best, but it dispenses with the backtracking and varies the scenery. From the trailhead, take two vehicles 1.7 miles southwest on CR 12. A junction here should be marked with a sign for Riley and another for CR E-65. Turn left and go southeast for about 1 mile. At this point, the road bends south (right) to briefly parallel a prominent arroyo. Continue another 0.6 mile and turn left. In another 0.25 mile, the road returns to the arroyo and heads south again. It also gets narrow and rocky, so pull over and park anywhere you can without blocking the road. If you have a GPS unit, you might later find it useful to have taken a waypoint now. However, it's more helpful to know that all drainages on the west side of the ridge eventually lead to this arroyo. Take a moment to inspect it before leaving the vehicle so it'll seem familiar when you return this way.

From the ridge, just past the 7,155-foot peak, descend south about 300 yards, then veer down toward the drainage on your right. Now just follow it downstream for about 1 mile. You might find walking easier on what appears to be traces of an old jeep road near the right bank. Outside the drainage, vegetation remains fairly sparse so there's no need for bushwhacking.

The road leads into the drainage as it widens near the base. After you enter the main arroyo, climb out on the west side (your left) and turn right on the dirt road. If you parked near the second bend to the south, you'll find your car about 0.25 mile down the road.

NEARBY ACTIVITIES

The Bernardo Waterfowl Area (BWA) is the second largest of the four wildlife-management areas that make up the Ladd S. Gordon Waterfowl Complex. (The biggest is La Joya, briefly explored in Sevilleta [Hike 52].) From November to February, about 15,000 sandhill cranes commute along the Rio Grande, with throngs of bird-watchers keeping pace on I-25. Up to 5,000 winged creatures may drop in at once on the BWA. The spectacle culminates in November with the Festival of the Cranes at the Bosque del Apache National Wildlife Refuge. But then that's a 100-mile drive south of Albuquerque, making the Gordon Complex an attractive compromise for its proximity.

Best enjoyed from November through February, the BWA features three observation decks along a 2.8-mile dirt road. To get there from Exit 175, turn left on the frontage road immediately after the northbound ramp. Drive north 1.7 miles and turn right at the sign for the Bernardo unit. For more information, call (505) 864-9187 or visit **wildlife.state.nm.us.**

52 SEVILLETA NATIONAL WILDLIFE REFUGE

KEY AT-A-GLANCE INFORMATION

LENGTH: 7-mile out-and-back; shorter and longer options

DIFFICULTY: Easy

SCENERY: Birds and wildlife along irrigation canals and seasonal wetlands

EXPOSURE: Mostly sunny

TRAIL TRAFFIC: Low

SHARED USE: Moderate (mountain bikers, equestrians, motor vehicles, hunting; dogs must be leashed)

TRAIL SURFACE: Dirt and gravel roads

HIKING TIME: 2–3 hours

DRIVING DISTANCE: 60 miles

ACCESS: Year-round, 1 hour before sunrise–1 hour past sunset

LAND STATUS: U.S. Fish and Wildlife Service, New Mexico Department of Fish and Game

MAPS: Brochure map at visitor center; Sevilleta NWR Hunting Areas; USGS La Joya

FACILITIES: Interpretive exhibits, restrooms, water at visitor center, limited wheelchair accessibility in Unit A

LAST-CHANCE FOOD/GAS: All services at Exit 191 in Belen, 26 miles from the trailhead

SPECIAL COMMENTS: See longer note at the end of the Description.

GPS TRAILHEAD COORDINATES

Latitude   34° 18' 17"

Longitude   106° 51' 07"

IN BRIEF

An overlooked jewel in the south, Sevilleta National Wildlife Refuge contains miles of seldom-traveled dirt roads that meander along an irrigation ditch between the BNSF Railroad and the Rio Grande. Even in the height of winter migrations, most birders bypass the wetlands here for the Bosque del Apache Wildlife Refuge farther south, allowing for secluded walks and bicycle rides most of the year.

DESCRIPTION

The refuge gets its name from a military post established nearby in the 16th century. "New Seville" was later included in the Sevilleta de

----

Directions ⟶

From I-25 South, take Exit 169. At the bottom of the off-ramp, pull a U-turn around the fence to the right and proceed 0.4 mile, following signs to the Sevilleta NWR Visitor Center.

A brochure at the visitor center details directions for the 4-mile drive to Unit A. If the center is not open when you arrive, look for the brochure in the Plexiglas box to the left of the front entry. If it's empty, head to Unit A by driving back down toward I-25 and through the underpass. Immediately after the northbound off-ramp, reset your odometer and turn right. Drive south 0.4 mile. The road curves east and becomes dirt. Area regulations are posted ahead at 0.7 mile. Continue straight east to a T-junction at 1.2 miles. Turn right and go south to a junction at 2.3 miles. Turn left, using caution on the steep crossing at the railroad tracks, and go to the junction at 2.4 miles. Take the first right and drive south along the west side of the ditch. The parking area is on the right at 4.0 miles. The sign there reads NO PARKING FOR NEXT MILE. About 200 yards beyond that is a parking area for physically challenged hunters.

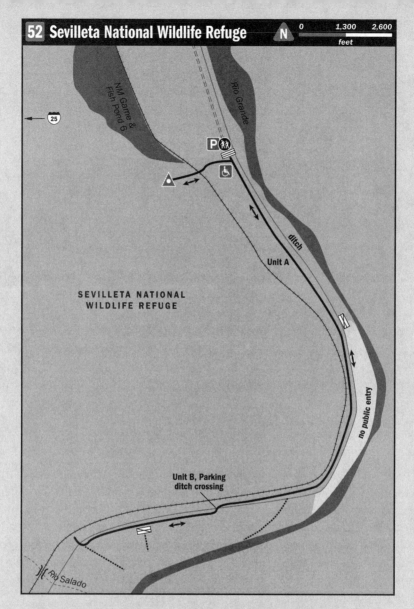

N

0   1,300   2,600

feet

25

NM Game & Fish Pond 6

Rio Grande

ditch

Unit A

SEVILLETA NATIONAL
WILDLIFE REFUGE

no public entry

Unit B, Parking
ditch crossing

Rio Salado

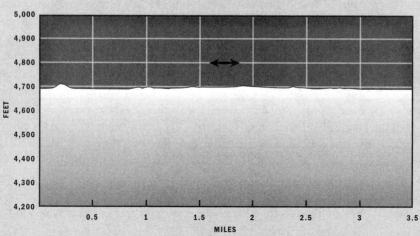

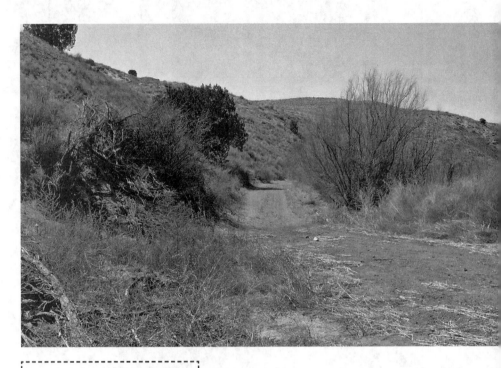

The roads of La Joya, freshly mowed

la Joya Land Grant, awarded by the governor of the New Mexico Province to the community of Sevilleta in 1819. A century later, the State of New Mexico accepted the land from the community heirs in lieu of taxes. The land later served a 30-year stint as the Campbell Ranch before achieving national-refuge status in 1973.

Several major biotic zones meet within Sevilleta NWR, including conifer woodland, Colorado Plateau shrub steppe, and Great Plains grassland. This hike skirts a bosque riparian forest within a finger of Chihuahuan desert that extends north to Albuquerque.

Sevilleta National Wildlife Refuge is managed primarily for the study of natural processes such as flood and fire, but it is perhaps best known for its role in the Mexican Gray Wolf Reintroduction Program. Aside from special tours and guided hikes offered one to three times a year, most of the 360-square-mile ecological research facility is strictly off-limits. However, two areas in the heart of the refuge remain open to the general public. Add to those the adjacent La Joya Waterfowl Area, and you have about 4,000 acres where you're usually free to roam.

Start the hike by walking south from the first parking area. Cross a cattle guard and turn right on the old dirt road before the second parking area; this is the entrance to Unit A, the Cornerstone Marsh. As in most of the Rio Grande floodplain, water here is controlled through a system of irrigation ditches, or acequias. Wheel valves, such as the one that bridges the ditch ahead, are opened in the late fall, creating ponds for a variety of waterfowl and shorebirds, including

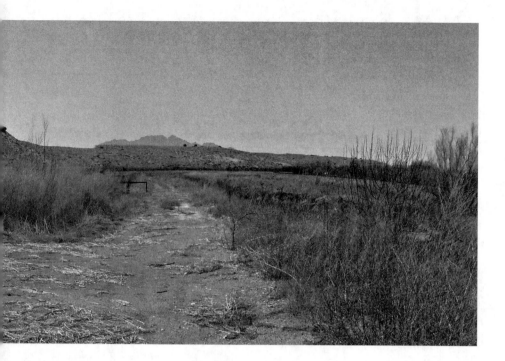

pintails, herons, pelicans, and sandpipers. In all, 225 species of birds have been sighted in the refuge. The ponds are drained in January, allowing weedy fields to overtake the wetlands for the remainder of the year. Pronghorn, elk, bighorn sheep, bobcat, and mountain lion are known to frequent the area.

Continuing along the road as it bends left, you'll find the Unit A boundary ends at the railroad tracks. Walk across the tracks and into the La Joya Waterfowl Area, open to hiking March 15–August 31. Just before a triangle barrier gate, a path to the left leads up a hill. It's a short climb, but as the highest point in the hike, it offers the only overlook of the area. You'll also get a great view of the BNSF as it comes around the bend and thunders down the tracks below.

Beyond the gate, the road tends to get choked with pigweed as it continues between a ditch full of cattails on the right and a series of ponds on the left, which are also subject to seasonal flooding.

When you're done with La Joya, cross back through Unit A, and turn right on the main road. (Or, if pressed for time, you can drive to the next parking area.) From here the way is pretty straightforward. The ditch is on the left; thick vegetation is on the right.

Though beautiful, particularly when blazing autumnal colors, tamarisk releases salt into the soil, killing off native plants. Many attempts to rid it from Sevilleta have failed, but one program launched in the spring of 2006 shows promise. Armed with chainsaws and herbicides, inmate work crews from the Central New Mexico

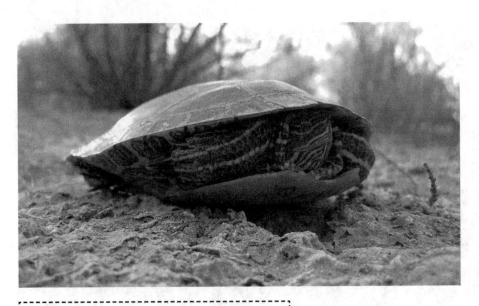

A shy slider in Unit A's seasonally dry Cornerstone Marsh

Correction Facility managed to eradicate the tree from two acres of Unit A in as many months.

Unit B begins just over 2 miles downstream from the Unit A parking area. The road bends west before widening into a gravel lot. You'll find a low railroad trestle on the north side and a parking area on the south. It's also your first opportunity on this hike to cross the ditch.

On the east side, two roads run parallel to the ditch. If you want to wander down to the Rio Grande, see the map for access trails. Whether they're open or closed depends on the nesting whims of certain protected species. Roadside signage tends to be both current and clear on the matter of places you can't go.

The road ends at a wire fence about 0.8 mile past the Unit B parking area. Beyond the fence is the Rio Salado ("salty river"). Its shallow bed spans more than 600 feet and is usually dust-dry. In this barren expanse the only exceptional feature is the old iron railroad bridge, which creates a stunning image when cast in silhouette against a Technicolor sunset.

Note: Access varies by season. Call Sevilleta NWR for details on Units A and B; (505) 864-4021. Call the New Mexico Department of Fish and Game Albuquerque office for details on the La Joya Waterfowl Area; (505) 222-4700. Birders can get a comprehensive checklist from the visitor center. Also, Sheryl Mayfield's *Sevilleta National Wildlife Refuge Field Guide to Flowers,* an outstanding primer on local plant life, is available as a free download from **fws.gov/southwest/refuges/newmex/sevilleta.**

SAN LORENZO CANYON 53

IN BRIEF

Here's the challenge: hike 2 miles of San Lorenzo Canyon without getting lured into any caves, slots, or scrambles to the rim. To accomplish such a task would require a dead-ened sense of natural curiosity or perhaps the unwavering determination of San Lorenzo (Saint Lawrence to the Anglos) himself.

DESCRIPTION

First, if you managed the drive to the mouth of the canyon, you may notice that the road continues around the bend. In fact, the road ends in a box about 1 mile up. Sure, you could drive to it, but then you'd be a nuisance to those here for the canyon's serenity—and besides, you'd miss the best details.

San Lorenzo Canyon thrives with life typical of Chihuahuan desert: fourwing saltbush, rabbitbrush, yucca, tree cholla, and prickly pear cacti. In the warmer months, collared lizards run amok—on their hind legs, when frightened. Cattle sometimes saunter up to the box and stare in bewilderment at the apparent dead end.

The canyon also contains arches, pillars, springs, caves, hoodoos, and other classic

----

Directions

From I-25 South, take Exit 163 at San Acacia. Turn left, cross over the interstate, then turn right and go 2.3 miles south on the frontage road. Turn right onto C94, or B90 on some maps. (Either way, it's unmarked, so just turn right before a small trailer park and drive through a narrow underpass.) When the pavement ends, continue straight west 2 miles on the main dirt road. Bear right at the Y and follow the road up the streambed 2.5 miles northwest to the mouth of the canyon.

KEY AT-A-GLANCE INFORMATION

LENGTH: 4-mile out-and-back

DIFFICULTY: Easy

SCENERY: Sandstone canyon, slots, caves, hoodoos, springs

EXPOSURE: Some canyon shade

TRAIL TRAFFIC: Moderate

SHARED USE: Moderate (mountain bikers; hunting; livestock; equestrians; stagecoaches, motor vehicles permitted in lower canyon)

TRAIL SURFACE: Sand, rock

HIKING TIME: 2–4 hours

DRIVING DISTANCE: 70 miles

ACCESS: Year-round

LAND STATUS: BLM–Socorro Field Office; Sevilleta National Wildlife Refuge

MAPS: USGS Lemitar, San Lorenzo Spring

FACILITIES: None

LAST-CHANCE FOOD/GAS: Exit 191 in Belen, 36 miles from trailhead

SPECIAL COMMENTS: Depending on recent weather conditions, a four-wheel-drive vehicle with high clearance may be necessary for the last 2 miles of the approach to the canyon. Do not attempt to drive the arroyo when heavy rains are expected. For local conditions and other info, contact the BLM Socorro Field Office at (575) 835-0412.

GPS TRAILHEAD COORDINATES

Latitude   34° 14' 38"

Longitude   106° 59' 27"

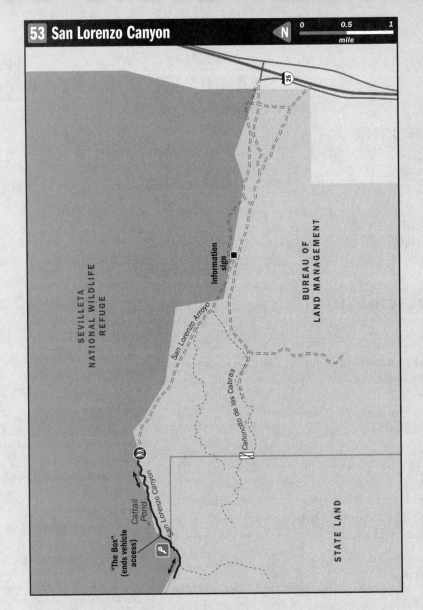

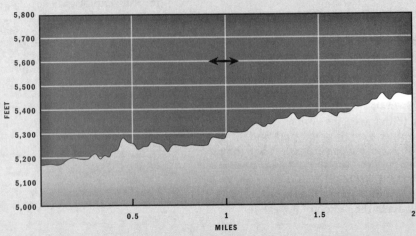

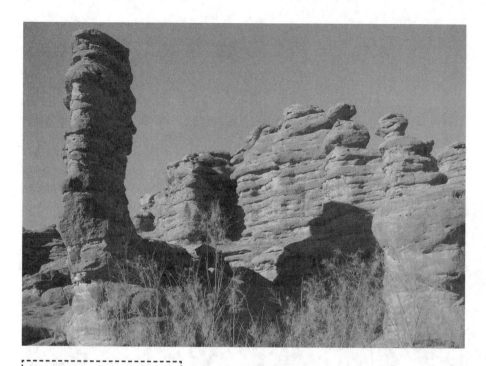

Formations in the lower canyon

Western features. It's the kind of landscape you'd expect to see in an old cowboy flick. A stagecoach would fit right in with the scenery, and you just might see one careening around an outcropping. The road is a favorite haunt of the New Mexico Carriage Club and the Rio Grande Mule and Donkey Association. Both seem to favor the coldest months for rides in the canyon. Lorenzo, or Lawrence of Rome, achieved martyrdom by roasting on a gridiron. Summertime in his canyon can feel the same way.

Aside from the obvious route up the throat of the main canyon, there are many side canyons, slots, niches, and crevices begging for exploration. Possible detours are too numerous to list, so my best advice is this: hike the route as outlined here and explore the most alluring side options on your return. If you start by wandering into every crevice that catches your eye, you'll never make it halfway through this hike.

Some detours are apparent before entering the canyon. If you can't resist wandering off in another direction, be aware that the fenced land to the north is closed to the public. (For more about that area, refer to the previous hike at Sevilleta National Wildlife Refuge.) Technically, the refuge boundary runs down the center of the arroyo, but the entire canyon is open to the public. Also, while the area directly south of San Lorenzo Canyon is popular with hikers, most of it is state land, with some leased parcels. NO TRESPASSING signs are rare but should be observed when encountered.

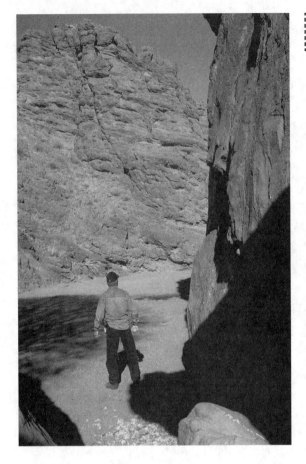

Start hiking up the canyon. Sculpted formations are nearby and impossible to miss. Look closely for the small details as well. For example, the canyon walls seem to be leaking in places. The water source is not exactly certain, but a few plump cottonwoods farther up the canyon suggest it was more plentiful in past years.

The largest of the shelter caves shows up on the right about 0.5 mile into the hike. One potential side hike involves scrambling up through a narrow passage on the west side of the cave and traversing the cliff above it to a point on the outcropping on the east side. After enjoying the view from there, head for the back of the alcove farther east and choose carefully among a number of steep ways down. This roughly M-shaped detour, noted on the map, requires modest climbing abilities.

Note: In 2007 a university student on a stargazing hike slipped off a cliff and fell to his death. The BLM now discourages climbing on the cliffs because of their loose composition.

At 1 mile into the hike, the canyon narrows again and seems to end in a box. Algae-laden water trickles from the rock only to vanish into the sand. A second spring is just around the corner, next to a cave about the size of a broom closet. This cave has a kind of sunroof but remains sufficiently dark to hide a recess big enough to crawl through. No telling how far back it goes because it's soaking wet inside and the smell is horrendous.

Climb over the boulders on the left side of the box at the lowest point and follow the emerald spring. The narrow canyon soon opens to a wide, sandy wash. The upper canyon ahead is chock-full of grand features similar to those in the first half, but here's where the small details get fascinating. Look closely at the porous basalt boulders, particularly those that have tumbled away from the canyon walls

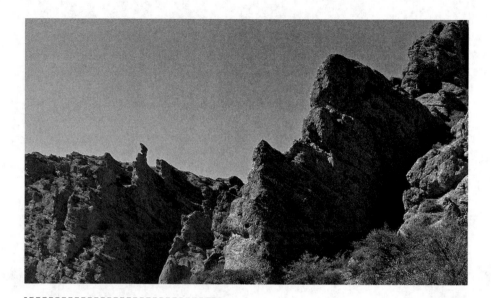

The entrance to Cañoncito de las Cabras

on the right side. At first glance, some appear as though caught in the crossfire of a multicolored paintball battle. These red, white, and green splotches are agate veins that have filled joints and other types of pore spaces in the basalt. Fine-crystalline forms of silica (quartz) mixed with various impurities show up in striking colors. Iron and copper impurities, for example, produce green colorations. Although it's obvious that amateur rock hounds have chipped away their own souvenirs, much still remains for other visitors to enjoy.

Continue following the spring's sinuous route. At 1.4 miles into the hike, the canyon takes a right. A prominent arroyo opens up just past the outer corner of the turn. It flows from Red Mountain, about a 2.5-mile hike to the south, but it contains several steep pour-offs, some about 30 feet high. Proceed with caution if you venture up in that direction.

About 0.5 mile past the big arroyo opening on the left, a downed boundary fence marks the official turnaround point for this hike—or so I'm told. In truth, I've never made it that far. My personal best for resisting diversions along the way currently stands at 1.5 miles—considerably better than past efforts that fell short of the box.

NEARBY ACTIVITIES

For more sandstone cliffs, hoodoos and slickenside walls, visit **Cañoncito de las Cabras** ("little canyon of the goats"). To drive there, return to the Y and head 1.7 miles west to the mouth of the canyon. As before, you can continue driving up canyon, but again, it's far better on foot.

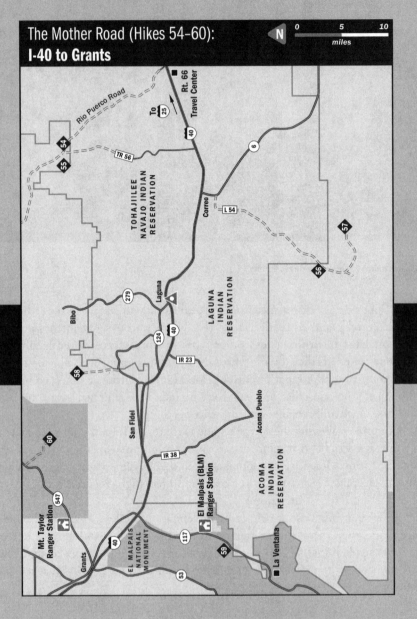

The Mother Road (Hikes 54–60): I-40 to Grants

N

0   5   10
miles

Rt. 66 Travel Center

To 25

Rio Puerco Road

TR 56

40

6

54

55

TOHAJIILEE NAVAJO INDIAN RESERVATION

Correo

L 54

57

56

279

Laguna

LAGUNA INDIAN RESERVATION

Bibo

124

40

58

IR 23

San Fidel

Acoma Pueblo

IR 38

60

El Malpais (BLM) Ranger Station

ACOMA INDIAN RESERVATION

547

Mt. Taylor Ranger Station

40

117

59

La Ventana

Grants

EL MALPAIS NATIONAL MONUMENT

53

THE MOTHER ROAD
(I-40 TO GRANTS)

54   OH MY GOD

KEY AT-A-GLANCE INFORMATION

LENGTH: 6.3-mile balloon

DIFFICULTY: Easy–moderate

SCENERY: Sculpted sandstone domes, bluffs, dunes, slot canyon

EXPOSURE: Mostly sunny

TRAIL TRAFFIC: Low

SHARED USE: Low (livestock; equestrians, mountain bikers; motorized vehicles)

TRAIL SURFACE: Rugged dirt roads, sand, rock

HIKING TIME: 2–3 hours

DRIVING DISTANCE: 33 miles

ACCESS: Year-round

LAND STATUS: BLM–Rio Puerco Field Office

MAPS: USGS Herrera

FACILITIES: None

LAST-CHANCE FOOD/GAS: Convenience store–gas station at Exit 140, 15 miles from the trailhead

SPECIAL COMMENTS: It's a rough dirt road, but most cars can handle the 14.5-mile stretch between Exit 140 and the gate if they take it slowly.

GPS TRAILHEAD COORDINATES

Latitude   35° 11' 24"

Longitude   107° 05' 10"

IN BRIEF

Navigate arroyos and abandoned dirt roads to explore a seldom-visited landscape tucked between the Navajo and Laguna reservations. This hike takes you to one corner full of mystical formations, but plenty more await rediscovery by those prepared to wander.

DESCRIPTION

If you think the road coming out here was rough, try driving beyond the gate. On second thought—don't. Only in the broadest sense of the word do these rutted imprints qualify as "roads." A few years ago, Southwest Off-Road Enterprises used them for an annual dirt-bike rally called the Oh My God 100. Oddly, contenders didn't find the course challenging enough, so SORE moved the rally to a locale near Cuba, New Mexico.

Aside from the near-complete disintegration of the old racecourse, very little has since happened on this land, which is why those who know of it (and few do) still refer to it as the Oh My God. The name seems most appropriate. It's also known as T-11, in reference to its township, but that doesn't quite capture the magnificence of the place.

Directions

From I-40 West, take Exit 140 and follow the frontage road 0.6 mile. Turn right at the intersection ahead to go northwest on Rio Puerco Road (CR 334). After 14.5 miles on this rugged dirt road, cross a cattle guard and pull off to the right where the road bends to the left. Don't block the road or the gate entrance on the right. Driving beyond the gate is allowed but not recommended for most vehicles.

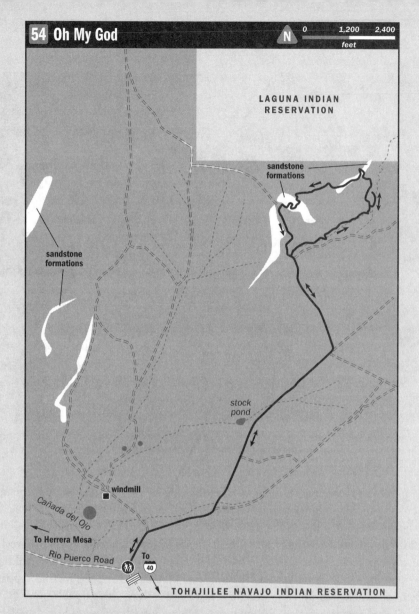

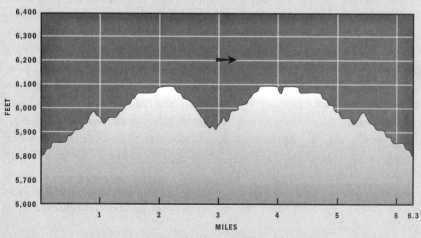

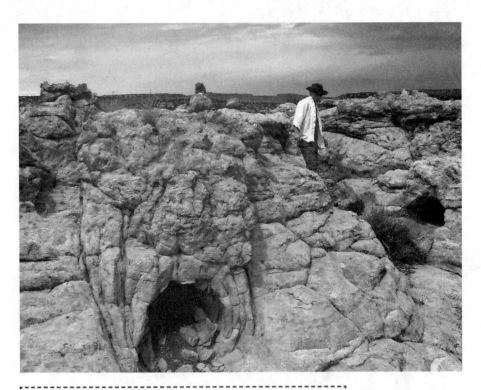

These sandstone formations are at the northernmost section of this hike.

The road to the loop, as described following, is neither the shortest nor the most scenic—it merely follows the most reliable track. Start from the drop gate—be sure to latch it behind you—and head northwest along the road. At the first Y, less than 0.25 mile ahead, bear right. Alternately, those with an unerring sense of direction can attempt to maintain a straight line for a slightly shorter and more colorful route to the loop, while those with a GPS unit can wander at their leisure and report at their convenience to these coordinates: N 35° 12' 43"; W 107° 04' 16".

Those sticking to the road will pass a stock pond hidden down on the left at the end of the first mile. From there the road bends slightly right. Follow it another 0.6 mile to a well-defined junction, where you'll turn left. Continue 0.5 mile to another junction. The road to the right follows the edge of a cliff. Go straight past it, heading downhill to the drainage that runs along the base of the cliff.

The loop starts where the drainage meets the road. Turn right off the road and follow the arroyo northeast. At first glance it seems perilously littered with broken glass. These frosty shards are acicular gypsum crystals. No point in collecting them; they'll just crumble in your pockets. But try this scientific demonstration: expose a piece to a flame. The crystal turns opaque white as it loses moisture. Now it is essentially a fragment of drywall.

As you continue downstream, the cliffs on your right don't rise higher so much as the arroyo runs deeper. Evidence of churning floodwaters reveals itself as washtub-sized potholes in the exposed bedrock. About 0.5 mile from the road, the arroyo drops away in a dry waterfall. It's not too difficult to climb down here, but you'll find an easier way down from the bank ahead. Angle down to the stream-bed, and continue another 200 feet or so, until you see a narrow canyon merging from the left. Follow it upstream to an impressive little slot canyon.

Those with limited climbing abilities might need a boost to get into the slot—and more importantly, a trusted spotter to help them down later. The reward for the effort is a brief passage between sinuously sculpted walls, some just barely shoulder-width apart. You can explore the slot from end to end in less than 10 minutes, but allow more time to appreciate the details. Evidence of past visitors appears on the walls as black smudges from campfire smoke, and as cattle brands etched into the sandstone. (Incidentally, flash-flooding hazards make slot canyons unwise spots to pitch your camp.)

Climbing out of the back end of the canyon is difficult and potentially dangerous. Instead, return to the arroyo and climb out at the point through which you came in. Once on the upper bank, head north, passing the back end of the slot on your right. About 200 yards ahead you'll see the first of many spectacular sandstone formations, namely big cliffs, small caves, and various hoodoos. In early spring, snake tracks follow mouse prints over a sugary dune. Nearby domes appear to be constructed from the hides of white elephants. Other formations take the shape of giant monteras, chupacabras, and other oddities.

The main road is less than 0.5 mile west of the easternmost formations, so your best strategy for exploring this amazing terrain is to meander predominantly in that direction. Steep cliffs and the Laguna boundary fence should keep you from straying too far off-course. Once you reach the road, turn left and follow it south about 0.3 mile to close the loop—or wander off the west side of the road to explore more formations. When you get back to the junction with the cliff-line road, continue south-southeast to return to the gate by the way you came. Or if you're feeling adventurous, try exploring other areas of this BLM unit. Try the drainages feeding Cañada del Ojo, about 2 miles west of the loop. The escarpment about 2 miles due east of the gate is another great place to poke around. A word of caution: there are far more roads and arroyos on site than I could fit on a map, so keep your bearings. A GPS unit and topo map wouldn't hurt either.

55 HERRERA MESA

KEY AT-A-GLANCE INFORMATION

LENGTH: 3-mile out-and-back; 4 miles if walking from the main road

DIFFICULTY: Moderate

SCENERY: Jurassic rock formations, grasslands, homestead ruins, views

EXPOSURE: Mostly sunny, though shaded by midafternoon

TRAIL TRAFFIC: Low

SHARED USE: Low (livestock, equestrians, mountain bikers; closed to all motorized vehicles)

TRAIL SURFACE: Rugged dirt roads, sand, loose rock

HIKING TIME: 2 hours

DRIVING DISTANCE: 44 miles

ACCESS: Year-round

LAND STATUS: BLM–Rio Puerco Field Office

MAPS: USGS Herrera

FACILITIES: None

LAST-CHANCE FOOD/GAS: Convenience store–gas station on BIA-56, about 13 miles from the trailhead.

GPS TRAILHEAD COORDINATES

Latitude   35° 11' 56"

Longitude   107° 07' 02"

IN BRIEF

Near a lonely corner of the Tohajiilee Navajo Reservation, a forgotten trail scraped into rocky ledges presents one of the few routes to the upper tiers of Herrera Mesa. Views along the way overlook equally impressive mesas, outcrops, and canyons.

DESCRIPTION

Most of the approximately 12-square-mile Herrera Mesa stands on Navajo land. Formerly known as the Cañoncito, the Tohajiilee are one of three Navajo bands outside the Big Rez farther west. Their reclaimed name translates to "water dippers," referring to their ancestors' renowned survival strategy of harvesting water from catch basins in the rocks.

The ranch at the base of Herrera Mesa is privately owned and remains active. Even though the house and barn evoke a sense of

----

Directions

From I-40 West, take Exit 131 and go north toward Tohajiilee on BIA-56/Cañoncito School Road. At 7.8 miles, BIA-56 jogs right and becomes a dirt road. Continue north another 3.3 miles and bear right at the Y. Go another 4.6 miles north and look for a dirt road on the left. (It's 0.9 mile past the junction with Rio Puerco Road. If you pass through a wire fence, you've gone about 50 yards too far.) Park nearby, being sure not to block either road. Alternately, you can drive on the dirt road, but be aware that it gets bumpy and there's room enough ahead to park only one vehicle. Follow it as it crosses a shadow road and curves south. After 0.4 mile, it reaches a T-junction. A green gate blocks the road on the right and a dirt barrier blocks the shadow road on the left. Pull up to the barrier and park there. The hike begins at the gate.

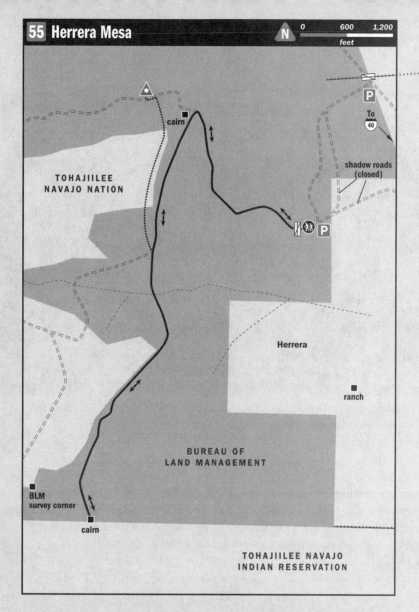

55 Herrera Mesa

N

0   600   1,200

feet

TOHAJIILEE
NAVAJO NATION

cairn

To
40

shadow roads
(closed)

P

Herrera

ranch

BUREAU OF
LAND MANAGEMENT

BLM
survey corner

cairn

TOHAJIILEE NAVAJO
INDIAN RESERVATION

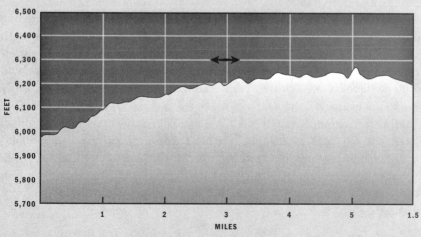

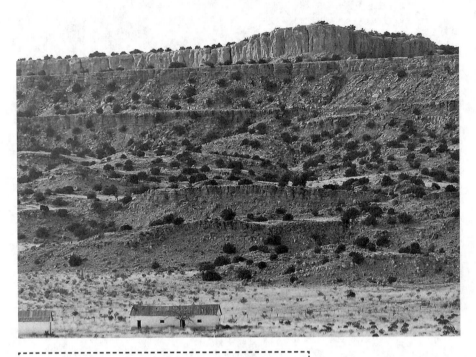

A ranch stands on the old town site at the foot of Herrera Mesa.

hopeless abandonment, and ruts and cacti have rendered their long driveway impassible, the corrals and stock tanks are still in good use. Decades ago, the ranch was simply known as *Ojo,* and some 300 whiteface cattle roamed its 10 sections (6,400 acres). Estevan Herrera sold the ranch in 1985 and passed away three years later.

Ranch boundaries aren't always apparent on the ground, but for a general idea, the shadow road mentioned earlier is on the ranch, whereas the corrected route to the gate is on public land.

Herrera Mesa displays the distinctive banding of the Morrison Formation, a group of sedimentary rock layers of the late Jurassic (161–145 million years ago). From a distance, the eastern face appears as an insurmountable wall. Closer inspection reveals that the wall is stepped. Think of it somewhat like a tiered cake. Old trails follow the edge of each tier, each leading to a point where you can easily walk up to the next level.

Information about these old roads is scant. They may have started as Indian trails, later used by ranchers leading livestock to mesa-top pastures, and perhaps still later enhanced by uranium prospectors. All that's certain is that someone put a tremendous amount of effort into clearing rocks and stacking them into walls to create a semblance of roads that don't seem to lead to anything but wonderful views.

The uranium prospector Rod Peterson came to Herrera Mesa in the 1960s. His search led him to a quarry of dinosaur bones, which contain uranium. Since then, well over 100 bones have been pulled from the site, including several from a large tyrannosaur and some from an allosaurus; additionally, the partial skeleton of a 40-foot sauropod has been uncovered.

The Peterson Quarry is New Mexico's first Morrison Formation dinosaur-bone bed and likely the state's most prolific source of Jurassic material. Volunteers trained by the New Mexico Museum of Natural History assist in the digs, and increasing public interest has the BLM evaluating the potential for site tours.

In the meantime, preservation efforts include discouraging people from visiting. It seems that excavation and collection by amateur boneheads elsewhere have ruined a considerable volume of scientific research and resources. Fossils without contextual data have no value, yet people still collect them. Though the bones at the Peterson Quarry are too big to steal, all it takes to destroy potentially significant remains is one souvenir hunter with a garden spade and a pathological affection for *Jurassic Park*. Maybe he'll score a bone fragment or a rock that looks like one. And then maybe he'll find an agitated mob of paleontologists armed with shovels and picks. In these rugged and remote lands, Nature has a way of striking a balance.

To summarize: avoid the quarry until the BLM says it's ready for visitors.

The hike begins at the gate. In contrast to the ledge trails, the road from the BLM gate is clearly defined. Follow it uphill for less than 0.5 mile to a fireplug-sized cairn on the left. But before making the turn onto an ill-defined trail, consider staying on the main road another 200 yards or so. As the road begins to curve around an outcrop and lead into a wide canyon, fantastic vistas open up to the north. Unusual formations in the valley below might be described (albeit inadequately) as a series of small mesas tilted at a 45-degree angle. Also just around the bend, a steep, faded path starts on the left and follows a ledge above the trail that begins at the cairn. The two run parallel for about 0.25 mile before the lower trail rises to merge with the high one. Keep it in mind as an option on the return route.

Now go back to the cairn and head south up the old trail. It may be little more than a slight indentation, but it becomes clearer as its rock edges stack up higher and it gradually climbs to the next tier. After 0.25 mile or so, the decrepit remains of a wire fence lean over the trail. The ranch can be seen far below to the left. At this point, you have little choice but to step up to the next level. A short climb to the right puts you in a sunken portion of the mesa top, a kind of triangular cove. The walls ahead and on your right delineate the boundary between public land and the Navajo reservation. From this perspective, it may seem as though only the top tiers of the mesa belong to the Navajo. Actually, aside from a few small bits of the northern and eastern sides, it's all theirs.

The upper path mentioned earlier merges in from the north. Again, keep it in mind for the return route. Do not follow it in either direction now. (For reference: It curves west, toward the back of the cove to cross a shallow point in the arroyo ahead. It then cuts back southeast to climb through a cleft in the wall.

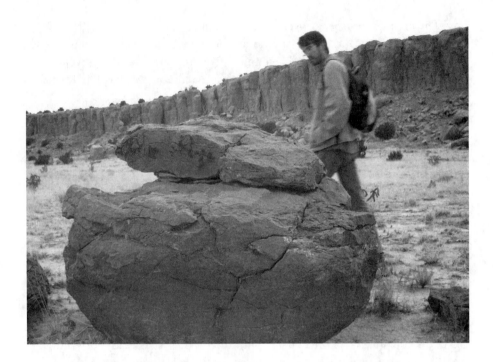

From there it joins up with a doubletrack that looks as though it serves more mule-drawn wagons than motorized vehicles. Overall, it's a long hike you might enjoy another day.)

For this hike, continue south, keeping the mesa rim on your left. Cross the arroyo and pass the eastern end of the cove wall to pick up the old trail. It squeezes along a narrow ledge for about 0.25 mile before arriving at a fence much like the last one. Again, step up to a slightly higher level. This upper ledge soon widens, giving acrophobes a bit more breathing room. At this point you're directly behind the ranch on the old Herrera town site, and about 400 feet above it.

Continue south along the rim to a small cairn. It marks the Navajo boundary, as does a fence below, which stretches due east to the horizon. You're now in the southwesternmost corner of public land on Herrera Mesa. At this juncture, it helps to know that Tohajiilee officials neither encourage nor discourage visitors from hiking on the reservation. Accordingly, the route description ends here, indecisively, at an otherwise arbitrary spot. A more natural terminus might be the mesa point in plain view just 0.25 mile ahead. Whether you proceed to that lovely overlook or turn back at the cairn is up to you.

VOLCANO HILL 56

IN BRIEF

It's a volcano. It's a hill. It's Volcano Hill. This improvised route climbs the southern flank and circumnavigates the crater rim to provide an overview of immense but little-known public lands in the lower Rio Puerco Valley. An additional spur down a scenic drainage leads you to homesteading ruins.

DESCRIPTION

In 2003 the New Mexico Wilderness Alliance completed a four-year study of public wildlands throughout the state to assess their suitability for Wilderness designations. One major focus area was Greater Petaca Pinta, a 74,000-acre confederation of public lands about 40 miles southwest of Albuquerque.

With Laguna Pueblo to the west, Acoma Pueblo to the north, and a checkerboard of private, BLM, and state lands to the east and south, access to the complex can get a bit perplexing. Rugged roads pose further challenges to traveling its interior. But what seems to keep most outdoors enthusiasts away is the fact that few are aware it even exists. Such a vast playground won't likely remain hidden much longer.

- -

Directions

From I-40 West, take Exit 126 and go 2 miles south on NM 6. Turn right on Old US 66 and go 1.5 miles west (over the railroad). Turn left on the road signed Alamo Road, L 54, and CR 81 (it shows up as Utah Road and IR 55 on some maps) and drive 13.8 miles south-southwest to the cattle guard with Laguna signage facing south and/or Cerro Verde Ranch signage facing north. Continue about 200 yards and park roadside.

KEY AT-A-GLANCE INFORMATION

LENGTH: 8-mile loop with spurs

DIFFICULTY: Moderate

SCENERY: Grasslands, cinder cones, mesas, homestead ruins

EXPOSURE: Mostly sunny, some canyon shade

TRAIL TRAFFIC: Low

TRAIL SURFACE: Lava rock, sand

SHARED USE: Low (livestock)

HIKING TIME: 4 hours

DRIVING DISTANCE: 51 miles

ACCESS: Year-round

LAND STATUS: BLM–Rio Puerco Field Office

MAPS: USGS Cerro Verde

FACILITIES: None

LAST-CHANCE FOOD/GAS: Route 66 Travel Center at I-40 exit 140, 32 miles from the trailhead

GPS TRAILHEAD COORDINATES

Latitude   34° 47' 31"
Longitude   107° 18' 35"

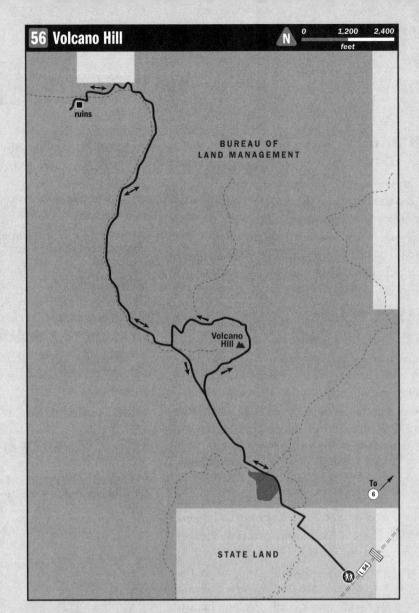

N

0   1,200   2,400

feet

BUREAU OF
LAND MANAGEMENT

ruins

Volcano
Hill ▲

To
6

STATE LAND

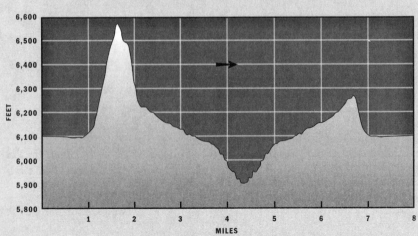

FEET

6,600
6,500
6,400
6,300
6,200
6,100
6,000
5,900
5,800

1   2   3   4   5   6   7   8

MILES

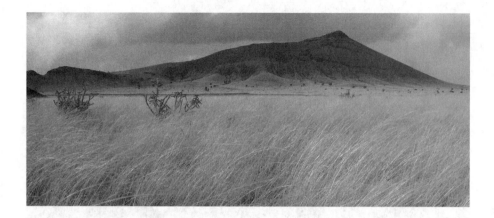

The approach to Volcano Hill

The Petaca Pinta Complex comprises three units: Petaca Pinta, Volcano Hill, and Sierra Lucero. The most easily accessed is the 27,000-acre Volcano Hill unit. Its namesake cinder cone rises 500 feet above a basalt lava flow and nearly 800 feet above the grasslands at the base of the escarpment to the immediate northwest.

The route set for this hike is fairly simple, and there's no particular reason to follow it precisely. There are no formal trails, and it would take a far longer hike to fully appreciate just the centerpiece feature of this vast unit.

The hike previously started by the stock ponds, those earthen mounds you see about halfway between the road and Volcano Hill. The road to the ponds vanished in 2014, though you may find traces of it as you walk the extra half-mile each way. Aim for the right side of the ponds. The high embankments make a clear path through the tall grass. Cross the arroyo that feeds into it. As you approach the volcano, larger chunks of lava rock make walking somewhat tricky. It can be a real ankle-twister, so watch your step. A couple of junipers ahead indicate a small black-sand wash, which creates another clear path toward the volcano. Note two points rising on the left flank, and aim for the base beneath the one on the right. From there, the remnants of a constructed path cut a relatively clean diagonal track up to the low end of the ridge.

The view from the ridge reveals that Volcano Hill is shaped more like a croissant than a cone. When it erupted about 3 million years ago, the blast opened up the west side. The hike goes northeast from here, climbing up to the peak. The brick-red lava is more exposed at higher elevations. Orange, green, and yellow lichens thrive on the craggy rock, which is pocked with all sizes of vesicles, cavities that were formed by expanding steam and gas bubbles as the lava cooled. The lava solidified quickly, resulting in jagged edges, and it'll cut you up pretty good if you're not careful.

Because Volcano Hill is the central unit, its peak offers an excellent vantage point for a quick survey of the surrounding complex. In the western portion, Pet-

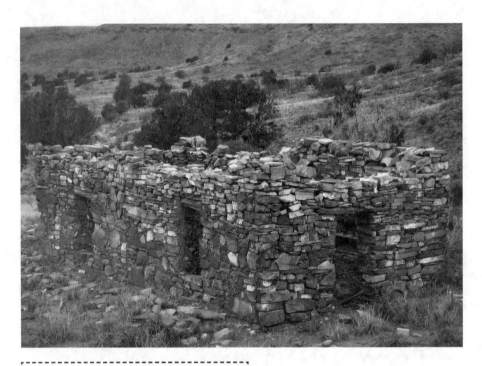

One of several ruins near the low end of the arroyo

aca Pinta is the smallest, though arguably the most scenic, of the three units. Likewise, it is by far the most difficult to access. Driving to that unit via BIA 541 requires permission from both the Laguna and Acoma pueblos.

The namesake feature of Petaca Pinta is an isolated fingerlike extension from Blue Water Mesa at the southern end of the escarpment—the 1,000-foot cliffs on the far side of the plains—though it's difficult to distinguish one monumental feature from the other at this distance. If you're facing due west, Petaca Pinta is at 11 o'clock, about 10 miles out. The colorful escarpment exposes almost the entire 180 million years of the Mesozoic era. The basalt lava that caps the Mesozoic rocks is relatively fresh, having flowed from Cerro del Oro just 3 million years ago.

Nearly the mirror image of Volcano Hill, Cerro del Oro stands at ten o'clock, 14 miles out. Eye-catching features located outside the complex include Badger Butte, the lone plug at one o'clock, 4.5 miles out, and the 11,301-foot summit of Mount Taylor at two o'clock, 35 miles out.

The Petaca Pinta unit also includes juniper-dotted foothills and canyons that drop down to badlands and lava-capped mesas. Pronghorn, prairie dogs, and badgers inhabit the grasslands in the area. The unit's eastern boundary falls a few miles shy of the Arroyo Colorado—the dark scar that cuts through the plains below. It flows (sometimes) to the north to meet the Rio San Jose. Everything that drains out of this area goes into the Rio Puerco, which in turns runs south to join the Rio Grande.

On the near side of the arroyo, a vague road marks the Volcano Hill unit's western boundary. Closer in, scattered springs and numerous natural depressions that retain water are located in the lava flow around Volcano Hill. Though not easy to find, both petroglyphs and cave shelters have been noted around Volcano Hill. The caves are now home to several species of bats, including big-eared bats. You can help protect their health, and your own, by staying out of the caves.

Although the name "Volcano Hill" sounds uninspired, the caves' names read like the premise for an Abbot and Costello routine: Who Cave, What Cave, Which Cave, That Cave, This Ain't That Cave, and so on. Collectively they compose the Pronoun Cave Complex, designated as an Area of Critical Environmental Concern. Fossils found in the caves provide a rare record of species that no longer range in New Mexico. The cave complex extends through the Sierra Lucero unit to Cerro del Oro.

The closest major feature in the neighboring Sierra Lucero unit is Cerro Verde. Peaking at 7,132 feet just 3 miles to the southeast, the "green hill" nearly doubles the climbing challenge of Volcano Hill. Directly behind it are the conjoined mesas, Cimarron and Gallina. Featured in the next hike, Gallina boasts the highest elevation in the complex: 7,855 feet. The high caps on this and other prominent rises catch enough moisture to support dense piñon–juniper woodlands, making Sierra Lucero not only the largest of the three units but also the most ecologically diverse.

Resuming the hike at hand, follow the ridge as it curves around to the west. Use caution: it narrows to the width of a sidewalk, and winds strong enough to knock you off balance are not uncommon. As you approach the end of the northern flank, continue west down hill until you run into a drainage. Turn right and follow it downstream. You'll soon cross under a fence. The wide, sandy wash eventually narrows, turning steep and sinuous. Striking rock features crop up as it winds west. After a few spilloffs, it reaches the valley floor. Ruins of a homesteading operation stand near the south bank. When you're done exploring the area, follow the drainage back up and continue straight southeast to cut across the mouth of the crater. Climb straight up the ridge ahead. Backtrack southeast from here to Alamo Road.

NEARBY ACTIVITIES

Cerro Verde is the volcano standing between Volcano Hill and Mesa Gallina. It also ranks squarely between them in degrees of difficulty. One approach to its 7,132-foot summit begins less than a mile south of the starting point for this hike. Drive to the next cattle guard, continue 0.15 mile south, and look on the left for an old dirt road. Walk it southeast. You'll find stock ponds at 0.7 mile and 1.2 miles. From the second pond, follow the drainage south then east about a mile to the top. Depending on your final approach, some scrambling may be necessary to reach the peak. The overall elevation gain is about 970 feet.

57 MESA GALLINA

KEY AT-A-GLANCE INFORMATION

LENGTH: 7.2-mile out-and-back, 8.7-mile balloon

DIFFICULTY: Strenuous

SCENERY: Piñon–juniper forest, geologic features, wildlife, views

EXPOSURE: Some canyon and woodland shade

TRAIL TRAFFIC: Low

SHARED USE: Low

TRAIL SURFACE: Sand, gravel, loose stone, bedrock

HIKING TIME: 5 hours

DRIVING DISTANCE: 62 miles

ACCESS: Year-round

LAND STATUS: BLM–Rio Puerco Field Office

MAPS: USGS White Ridge, Mesa Gallina

FACILITIES: None

LAST-CHANCE FOOD/GAS: Route 66 Travel Center at I-40 exit 140, 43 miles from the trailhead

GPS TRAILHEAD COORDINATES

Latitude   34° 45' 11."

Longitude   107° 14' 31"

IN BRIEF

As a basic out-and-back, the round-trip hike would be a mere 7.2 miles, almost all of it in a deep, rocky arroyo. Extra miles add up fast when you explore the top of Mesa Gallina, the highest point in the Petaca Pinta Complex. From the top, survey a fascinating landscape where the Rio Grande Rift meets the Colorado Plateau.

DESCRIPTION

Locked gates and stern NO TRESPASSING signs now block the traditional approach to this hike.

Directions ———————————————⟶

From I-40 West, take Exit 126. Turn left and drive 2 miles south on NM 6. Turn right on Old US 66 and go west (over the railroad) 1.5 miles. Turn left on the road signed Alamo Road, L 54 and CR 81, and drive 17.3 miles south-southwest to the south-facing sign for Cerro Verde Ranch. Stop just before the cattle guard and look left for a drop gate marked with a yellow sign about the size of a license plate. Go through that gate and close it behind you. Note: Your vehicle needs at least 10-inch clearance for the roads ahead. Drive about a mile and bear left at the first fork. Continue another 1.2 miles to a subtle fork. Turn left and follow the tilted doubletrack over the hillside west of the dam. The tracks end near the stock ponds on the north side of the dam, but resume about a quarter-mile northeast at 34° 43' 31", 107° 18' 06". Caution: It takes very little rain to turn this flat into an impassible mud bog. Follow the doubletrack another 1.2 miles to the next drop gate, crossing three cuts along the way. Turn right, go 1.4 miles east-northeast, and veer right at the fork. Continue another 2 miles east. Veer right at the next fork and park off-road just before it crosses the Arroyo Lucero streambed.

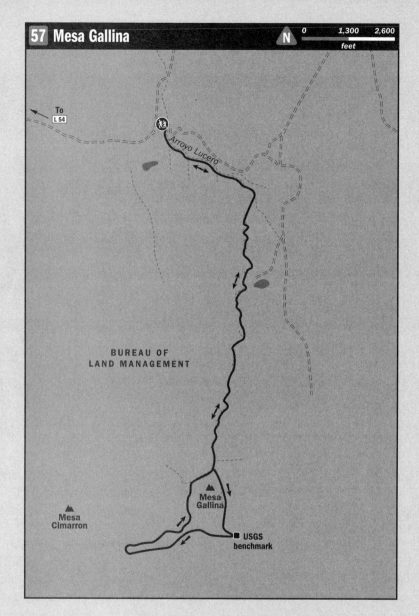

N

0   1,300   2,600
                    feet

To
L 54

Arroyo Lucero

BUREAU OF
LAND MANAGEMENT

Mesa
Gallina

Mesa
Cimarron

■ USGS
benchmark

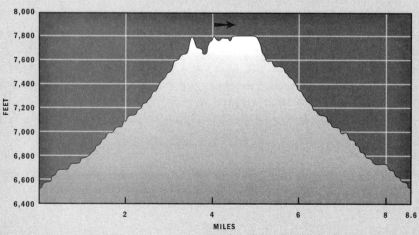

8,000

7,800

7,600

7,400

7,200

7,000

6,800

6,600

6,400

FEET

2   4   6   8   8.6

MILES

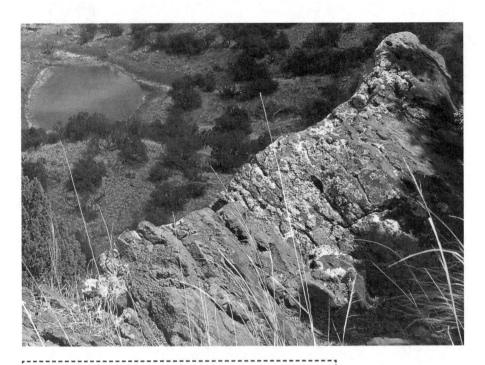

Overlooking the Arroyo Lucero, after an impromptu scramble west

The only legal access (that I know of) requires driving on roads that are ephemeral at best and, in places, can be outright treacherous. Read the driving directions below, keeping in mind that I cannot recommend any attempt to follow them beyond the dam. For more details, visit **restlesstribes.com/57**.

As for the hike here, it's a straight shot south—road to rim in just 3.6 miles. What could be easier? But in retrospect, I'd say this route easily ranks among the top five most difficult hikes in the book. Maybe it was the 1,300-foot gain in elevation over loose rock and sand, or maybe it was the extra 2 miles of wandering the mesa top, but my hiking buddy and I returned from the hike feeling inexplicably fatigued.

Was it worth it? Absolutely. The deep Arroyo Lucero provided ample shade on an otherwise sizzling spring afternoon, and storms brewing over the badlands to the west sent cool breezes to the mesa top. Hawks keened above. Paintbrush, yucca, and cacti bloomed in electric colors. And every so often, crystals sparkled from geodes in the charcoal-colored sand. We were also treated to a rattlesnake encounter—my first in nearly a decade. This three-foot pit viper was a black-tailed rattlesnake, *Crotalus molossus*, one of the least aggressive species. Cornered against a solid rock wall, it gave us ample warning. Its steady buzz seemed to indicate that it preferred a good 15 feet of personal space. We respectfully obliged and passed without incident the first time—but we didn't count on crossing the same snake twice.

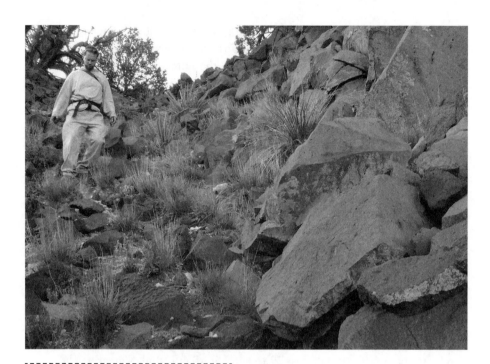

Scial negotiates the south side of the mesa.

That's just a small sampling of the wondrous assortment of animals, plants, and minerals to watch for as you climb Mesa Gallina. Also keep in mind that since the majority of this hike traverses a steep waterway and the mesa is just high enough to snag rain clouds rolling off the Colorado Plateau, you should pay special attention to weather conditions.

The hike begins where the road crosses a rocky and relatively shallow streambed. Follow the wash south-southwest upstream. The arroyo quickly trenches, making it easy to cross under the fence ahead, and leaving little doubt as to which drainage to follow. (One potential point of confusion is a fork 2 miles upstream. The arroyo merely splits around an island—take your pick.)

A mile past the island, a channel comes in on your left, followed by another on your right—go up the middle. The Lucero benchmark is less than a half-mile straight ahead. However, you'll probably drift slightly west as the terrain levels out in that direction. In that case, when you reach the rim, turn left and follow it to the southeastern corner of the mesa.

A standard U.S. Geological benchmark, stamped LUCERO 1952, is set in outcropping bedrock about 50 feet north of the mesa's highest point and 14 feet west of a bluff. Two reference marks from a 1958 survey are nearby.

You can go back the way you came or explore the mesa. Unless you have an unerring sense of direction, do not stray far from the rim. The inner meadows and wooded areas can be somewhat disorienting.

About 0.25 mile west of the benchmark, on the far side of a few low hills, the rim is a jumble of boulders with gaps that form seemingly bottomless shafts. Take an extra measure of caution in this area. To the immediate west and down one level, a shelf affords unobstructed views of ranges to the south. The nearest major peak is Ladron, about 20 miles to the southeast.

Climb back to the upper rim and go to the mesa's southwestern corner for views over the Petaca Pinta Complex. As mentioned in the previous hike at Volcano Hill, this area is composed of three units: Petaca Pinta, Volcano Hill, and Sierra Lucero. Mesa Gallina stands in the easternmost unit, roughly in the center of a north-to-south-trending escarpment known as the Sierra Lucero.

Approximately 30 place names in New Mexico honor Pedro Lucero de Godoy and his descendants. The Mexico City native arrived in Santa Fe in the early 1600s and became an established religious and political figure before the Pueblo Revolt in 1680. His sons and grandsons were prominent in the reconquest of 1692, and many residents of New Mexico and Colorado today embrace their Lucero lineage.

By comparison, about 45 place names in New Mexico pay tribute to *gallina*, which means "chicken," though it more often refers to *gallina de la tierra*, or "wild turkey." A point of slight distinction: Chicken Mountain, the 7,826-foot peak 5 miles to the southwest, falls just 29 feet shy of Mesa Gallina's great height.

When you're ready to return to the road, aim east-northeast. All drains flow into the basin that forms the head of Arroyo Lucero. It's all downhill from there.

As for the rattlesnake, it was where we left it when we returned several hours later and well past dark. We'd forgotten about it, and it didn't bother to remind us of its presence until we passed within a step or two of its rattle. Had it been a Mojave rattler, I might be missing a hiking buddy right now. But then you won't find snakes that mean within 60 miles of Albuquerque.

NEARBY ACTIVITIES

Roads in the **Sierra Lucera unit** are perfect for beginner to intermediate levels of mountain biking. Starting 1 mile past the Laguna/Cerro Verde Ranch cattle guard, contiguous sections of Public Land stretch 5 miles south and 7 miles east—excepting Section 18, a square mile that belongs to ranchers from the Republic of Texas. The remaining 40,000 acres of American land is free for anyone to enjoy. The first drop gate mentioned in the directions above is the best place to start a cycling exploration of the unit. The Acoma Pueblo Surface Management map from the BLM and a GPS receiver with tracking functions are recommended.

WATER CANYON WILDLIFE AREA 58

IN BRIEF

With no trails to follow, hiking options are wide open within the wildlife area boundaries. A gentle streamside stroll turns into a steep climb for those determined to view the Rio Puerco Valley from 8,000 feet.

DESCRIPTION

The Water Canyon Wildlife Area is a narrow 2,840-acre property in the Game and Fish Department's inventory. For Albuquerqueans, it's the quickest access to Mount Taylor, the 11,305-foot volcanic bulge on our western horizon. It holds a sacred status among 30 Native American tribes, and its archaeological, cultural, and historical features number in the hundreds of thousands. Unfortunately, the mountain sits atop the Grants Uranium Belt, a rich reserve that spawned mining booms in the 1950s and the 1970s, the scars of which are still obvious today. Renewed interest in uranium has threatened further degradation and sparked action for Mount Taylor's protection.

In 2009, the National Trust for Historic Preservation named Mount Taylor to its 2009 List of America's 11 Most Endangered Historic Places. The same year, the New Mexico

---

Directions

From I-40 West, take Exit 104. Turn right off the ramp, then left onto NM 124, and go about a mile northwest toward Budville. (Heed the notice regarding the Cubero Land Grant.) Turn right onto CR 7 and go 0.9 mile north. Turn right onto Water Canyon Road and go 0.2 mile northeast. Bear left onto CR 8 and go 2.1 miles to a Y-junction. Bear left onto Picacho Peak Road and go 5 miles north. (It should be suitable for most cars, but can get rugged with bad weather.) Park in the pulloff by the stream.

KEY AT-A-GLANCE INFORMATION

LENGTH: 3.2 miles

DIFFICULTY: Strenuous

SCENERY: Forest, stream, canyon, grassland, expansive views

EXPOSURE: Shaded along the stream; full sun at higher elevations

TRAIL TRAFFIC: Low

SHARED USE: Low (hunting, equestrians, primitive camping; no motorized vehicles or bicycles off the established road)

TRAIL SURFACE: Pine straw, rock, scree

HIKING TIME: 2 hours

DRIVING DISTANCE: 64 miles

ACCESS: Year-round, except during established deer and elk hunts. Access permits are required. (See Special Comments.)

LAND STATUS: New Mexico Department of Game and Fish

MAPS: USGS Mount Taylor

FACILITIES: None

LAST-CHANCE FOOD/GAS: All services at Exit 108, 13 miles from the trailhead. Package store in Budville, 8 miles from the trailhead.

SPECIAL COMMENTS: Purchase a GAIN Permit from the New Mexico Department of Game and Fish: (505) 222-4700; wildlife.state.nm.us.

GPS TRAILHEAD COORDINATES

Latitude   35° 10' 38"
Longitude   107° 30' 38"

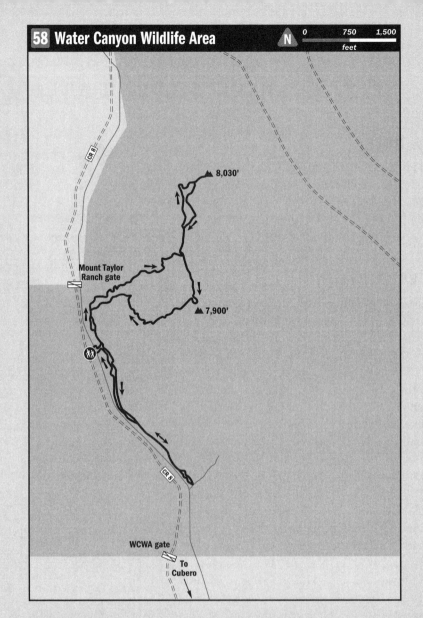

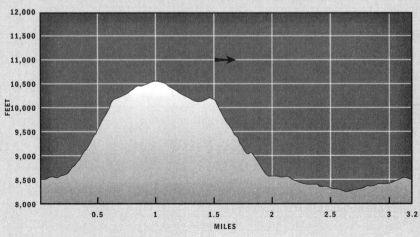

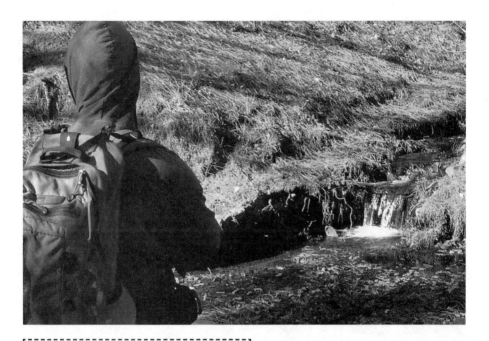

The stream is less impressive in times of drought.

Cultural Properties Review Committee unanimously voted to list Mount Taylor on the State Register of Cultural Properties. The latter designation includes the summit, slopes, and the adjacent mesas of San Mateo, Jesus, La Jara, Horace, Chivato and Bibo—in all 344,729 acres, making Mount Taylor one of the largest properties ever listed in a state or national register.

Water Canyon is a major drainage that spills east from Mount Taylor's caldera and turns south to flow down to the Cubero Land Grant. Its total length runs about 8 miles, 7 of which cross strictly off-limits Pueblo and private lands. In 1953 the state purchased the property that would become the Water Canyon Wildlife Area to provide public access to big game hunting. Deer, elk, bear, and turkey are common targets on the hunters' hit list. Exotic species include Barbary sheep (an African import), and Himalayan Tahr, shaggy mountain goats with rubbery hooves that are well adapted to climbing rocks.

Although the area is a popular destination for hunting and drinking, hikers are also welcome now that the Department of Game and Fish added WCWA to its Gaining Access Into Nature inventory. The GAIN program allows for wildlife viewing and other activities on State Game Commission–owned Wildlife Management Areas (that is, lands that normally are open mainly for hunting and fishing). As elsewhere, dawn and dusk are your best chances for spotting wildlife in the WCWA. Bring binoculars, a hefty zoom lens, and lots of patience.

Several old roads and trails cross the property, but they're not easy to come by. You'll quickly notice the obstacles to long hikes here. The road section through the

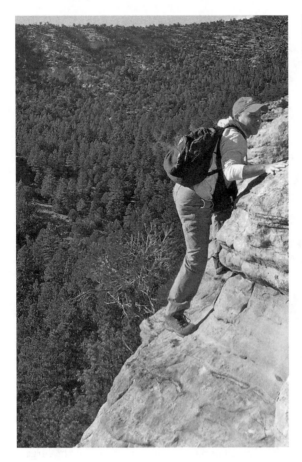

Climbing out of the canyon is easier than it looks.

WCWA is a mere mile long, terminating at a hefty gate to Mount Taylor Ranch. To complicate east–west exploration, canyon walls escalate 700 feet within 0.3 mile of the stream banks.

The hike described here is an improvised route that provides a brief introduction to the WCWA and points out some nearby features worth checking out. There's no need to follow it precisely, so feel free to explore whatever draws your attention. For a deeper exploration, bring a detailed topo map and (ideally) a GPS unit.

From the parking area, begin by crossing the stream. It tends to look like a piddly creek after months of drought, but evidence of flooding suggests it occasionally runs at impressive capacities. Head north along the east bank. Within a quarter-mile you'll cross a shallow drainage cluttered with rocks. Follow it a hundred yards or so up to where it trenches into the cliffside. The strenuous part of this route begins here. The next quarter-mile gains 600 feet in elevation. If you're not in the mood for a bit of scrambling, then you're probably better off taking a stroll farther up the drainage. The Cretaceous-age sandstone is riddled with interesting features.

Those heading up to the ridge above it can explore this little side canyon on the way back down. You'll encounter two bands of vertical rock on the way to the top. Each is easier to scale than it first looks—if you take a moment to scout for a sensible way up. The sloping terrain between them is mostly dirt and loose rock. Game paths are faint through here. We ended up following a fresh trail of elk scat.

Once at the top, you'll have a magnificent view across mesalands clear down to the Sawtooth Mountains east of Pie Town. For even better views, head north another quarter-mile or so to the next peak.

> Expect a few obstacles along the way.

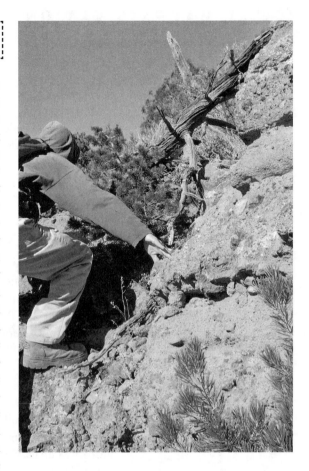

Return the way you came and continue south to a slightly lower peak on the ridge, then start working your way back down into the canyon. About halfway down, angle to your right and aim for the head of the drainage you crossed earlier. It's considerably deeper on this end, so use caution when choosing your way into it. Seeps at the bottom keep the ground muddy in spots, and help sustain a stand of oak. Follow the drainage out and return to the parking area. Before driving off, however, consider extending the hike another half-mile south on the faint remains of an old roadbed alongside the stream. It'll help keep your legs from tightening up during the long drive back to Albuquerque.

NEARBY ACTIVITIES

Bibo is a revived ghost town on the east side of Mount Taylor. Get a burger and suds at the historic **Bibo Bar**, established in 1913. Friendly staff there can best advise on how to enjoy the local sights. (Exploring the area on your own is highly discouraged.) Serving hours are generally from 11 a.m. to 2 a.m. Call (505) 552-9428. To get there, take Exit 114 at Laguna and go west about 1.2 miles to the turnoff for Paguate and Seboyeta. Turn right and drive about 11 miles north to Bibo.

59 EL MALPAIS NATIONAL MONUMENT: SANDSTONE BLUFFS

KEY AT-A-GLANCE INFORMATION

LENGTH: 5.5 miles

DIFFICULTY: Moderate

SCENERY: Overlooks, lava fields, natural arches

EXPOSURE: Morning shade on lower trail

TRAIL TRAFFIC: Popular overlook; low elsewhere

SHARED USE: Low (pets must be leashed)

TRAIL SURFACE: Sand, rock

HIKING TIME: 3 hours

DRIVING DISTANCE: 81 miles

ACCESS: Year-round, dawn–dusk

LAND STATUS: National Park Service

MAPS: USGS Los Pilares

FACILITIES: Restroom at trailhead. No water. Part of the overlook is wheelchair-accessible. Water and wheelchair-accessible restrooms and visitor center at ranger station, 2 miles from the trailhead.

LAST-CHANCE FOOD/GAS: Convenience store–gas station at Exit 89

SPECIAL COMMENTS: El Malpais (BLM) Visitor Center, en route to the trailhead, is a recommended stop. Open 8:30 a.m.–4:30 p.m. daily except Thanksgiving, Christmas, and New Year's Day. (505) 280-2918; nps.gov/elma or nm.blm.gov.

GPS TRAILHEAD COORDINATES

Latitude   34° 56' 42"

Longitude   W107° 50' 18"

IN BRIEF

Most visitors at Sandstone Bluffs seem content with the 30-mile view from the overlook. True, the sea of lava and distant mountain peaks are lovely, but the most impressive sights are along an informal path directly below.

DESCRIPTION

El Malpais (mall-pie-EES) refers to both the national monument and the national conservation area, administered by the National Park Service and the Bureau of Land Management, respectively. Between the two, El Malpais comprises 377,000 acres of public badlands.

Generally speaking, the terms *malpais* and *badlands* are used to describe any land that's inhospitable to humans. In New Mexico, there's usually a lava flow involved that makes them extra bad. Indeed, the lava flow of El Malpais National Monument is a most brutal terrain. And like most dangerous things in nature, its allure is irresistible.

The land wasn't always so bad. The shale and sandstone bluffs of the Colorado Plateau tectonic block quietly formed at the bottom of oceans and lakes for 500 million years. Sedimentary layers are obvious today in white-, tan-, and rust-colored bands running the length of the escarpment like bathtub rings.

Seventy million years ago, the plateau started rising above its neighbors. A north–

Directions _____➤

From I-40 West, take Exit 89 and turn left on NM 117. Go south 10 miles to the signed entrance for Sandstone Bluffs. Turn right and follow the gravel road 1.7 miles southwest to its end.

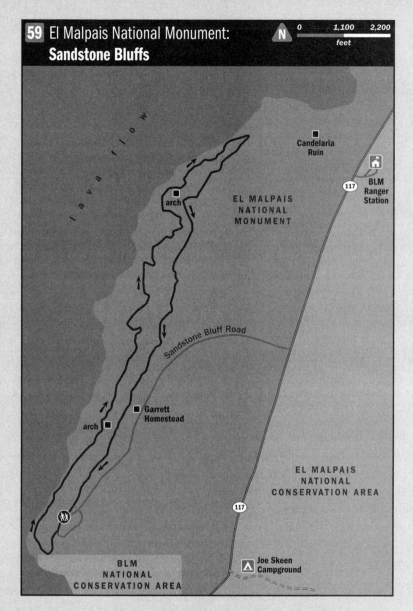

59 El Malpais National Monument: **Sandstone Bluffs**

N

0   1,100   2,200
feet

lava flow

Candelaria Ruin

117

BLM Ranger Station

arch

EL MALPAIS NATIONAL MONUMENT

Sandstone Bluff Road

arch   Garrett Homestead

EL MALPAIS NATIONAL CONSERVATION AREA

117

BLM NATIONAL CONSERVATION AREA

Joe Skeen Campground

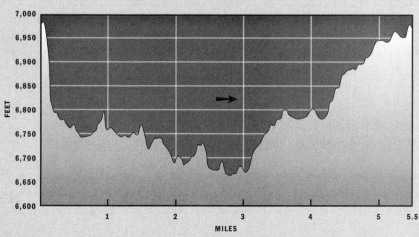

FEET

7,000
6,950
6,900
6,850
6,800
6,750
6,700
6,650
6,600

1   2   3   4   5.5

MILES

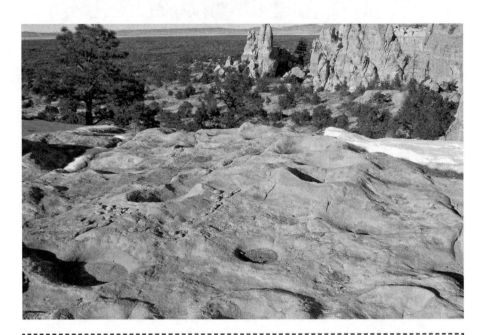

Holes in the sandstone indicate where Moqui marbles (spherical concretions) have been removed.

south rift slowly opened the Rio Grande Valley between 30 and 10 million years ago. But the heaviest volcanic action started in the last 5 million years, with magma swelling into the deep fault in the crust that created Mount Taylor and the Valles Caldera 1–3 million years ago. It still smolders today from Raton to Springerville, Arizona; through the Jemez; and of course, El Malpais: the freshest volcanic field in the southwestern United States. Small cones erupted here at least five separate times between 120,000 and 1000 BC, until the valley filled with a river of lava 40 miles long and 5 miles wide. Stories of the nearby Acoma Pueblo suggest the latest outburst might even have been as recent as AD 1200.

Much of the lava cooled to form edges as sharp as steak knives. Jagged ridges and deep sinkholes further inhibit exploratory options. These vast, enigmatic black fields add credence to legends of lost bounty, including Acoma treasure hidden from Spanish invaders and gold looted in a train robbery, in addition to tales of a private jet said to have crashed and vanished out there with a hefty cash cargo. If nothing else, it's a land of strange phenomena. A phantom homestead occasionally shimmers into view. It's also the only place I've seen snow falling while temperatures hovered steadily at 58°F. In short, El Malpais is wonderfully weird.

Start the hike on the overlook to the immediate west of the parking area. Take a moment to enjoy the views and scout out the terrain below. At first glance you might guess that nothing short of a rappelling line is required to reach the path 200 feet below. Go to the south end for a safe passage down. You might have to poke around the maze of rocks to find it, but you'll know it when you see it—a steep but manageable slope populated with tall pines. There's no discernible path in this short, scrubby section, but a few cairns offer helpful suggestions for picking your way down.

The first mile below is easy navigating. Once on flat ground, hook right to the west face of the base and process northeast. You can follow the faint remains of a doubletrack, or a deer path closer to the wall, but you won't stray off-course because the span between the wall and the lava is 600 feet at most.

It is easy to wander off the path with your neck craned in search of the next magnificent rock feature. Be mindful of what's on the ground to keep from stepping on a cactus, or worse: knobby black crust on the ground is cryptobiotic soil, a living community of cyanobacteria (blue-green algae), soil lichens, mosses, green algae, microfungi, and bacteria. It protects loose soil from erosion, and it's essential for holding the ground in place long enough for other plants to take root. Much of it is older than the tallest ponderosas. Rest assured that any cryptobiotic soil crushed under your boot might grow back in a few centuries.

After a mile of heading northeast, or 1.5 miles into the hike, you'll arrive at a double amphitheater opening to the south. Beyond that, the wall has crumbled down to a half-dozen freestanding rocks and outcrops scattered throughout an area of rumpled terrain about the size of a driving range. The transition to the upper trail is easy in this gap. Stray 100 yards or so to the east and you'll cross it without knowing, so mind your bearings.

Continue northeast with the rocks on your right and you'll stay on course. The bluffs resume after the break, though on this side they're not as uniform. Alcoves, towers, ridges, and buttes multiply your exploratory options. Maintain a straight line and you'll find its end in another half-mile or so, but exploring every nook could easily double that and is well worth the time. In one partially obscured alcove, the largest of three arches reaches across a break in a massive sandstone wall. Just ahead and sharing the same wall, an extraordinary gallery of petroglyphs depicting thunderbirds, scorpions, and other creatures appears alongside the path. A useful waypoint for finding both the arch and the petroglyphs: N 34° 58' 09"; W 107° 49' 41".

Eventually you'll run low on water and/or daylight—remember, the gates close at dusk—and you'll need to start looking for a way back up. If you made it as far north as the ranger station, the transition to the upper trail is easy, but you've got about 2.3 miles and a 300-foot elevation gain ahead of you. Follow deer paths southwest. Again, mind the gap in the wall. It's all too easy to inadvertently drift down to the lower trail only to later face a steep scramble or significant backtracking. Stay above the rim and you'll have no problem returning to the parking area.

NEARBY ACTIVITIES

Garrett Homestead is a partially reconstructed residential structure from the mid-1930s. It stands roadside en route to the overlook.

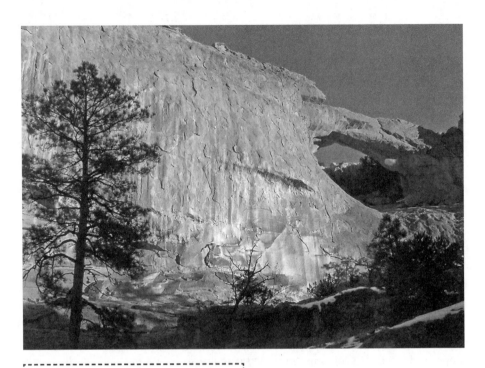

The biggest of three arches at Sandstone Bluffs

Other nearby points of interest are listed below. (Driving distances are in approximate miles south of the Sandstone Bluffs Road/NM 117 junction.)

Zuni–Acoma Trail (6): This ancient trade route traverses four major lava flows in 7.5 miles, one-way. It's a tough hike, but cairns make it easy to follow.

La Ventana (8): With a height of 80 feet and a span of 165 feet, this natural arch is the second-longest in New Mexico. (The state record goes to the inaccessible Snake Bridge in San Juan County.) A paved, wheelchair-accessible trail and picnic area are near the base of the arch.

Narrows Picnic Area (11): Facilities include wheelchair-accessible tables and restrooms. No water. The Narrows Rim Trail begins at the south end of the picnic area. This well-marked 6-mile out-and-back culminates with a view over La Ventana.

Lava Falls (26): A cairned 1-mile loop explores El Malpais's youngest lava flow. Facilities include a restroom and picnic area. No water.

MOUNT TAYLOR: GOOSEBERRY SPRING 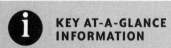 **60**

IN BRIEF

Often snowcapped into mid-spring, Mount Taylor is the massive volcano on Albuquerque's sunset horizon. A classic hike on a designated trail winds through woods and meadows to culminate on the rim of the caldera.

DESCRIPTION

Our final destination stands just 53 miles west of where we began, though at an elevation some 6,300 feet higher. The Navajo know this volcanic peak as *Tsoodzil*, "turquoise mountain." According to their tradition, it's the mountain of the south, one of four sacred peaks that mark the boundaries of *Dinetah*, the Navajo homeland.

Thong trees further indicate a history of local Indian activity. Also called trail trees, water trees, and buffalo trees, they began as flexible saplings that were notched and bent at right angles. The "thong" refers to a Y-shaped stick or leather strap that prevented the tree from growing out of the contorted position. The trees' distinct stairstep trunks pointed the

----

Directions ──────────────────────▶

From I-40 West, take Exit 85 and veer right toward Grants. About 2.5 miles from the exit, turn right on NM 547 and follow it about 13.4 miles up Mount Taylor. (NM 547 is also signed First Street, Roosevelt Avenue, and Lobo Canyon Road.) Do *not* turn at the Lobo Canyon Campground, which is about 4.5 miles too soon. And if you run out of paved road while still on NM 547, you've gone about 100 yards too far. Turn right on FR 193, a maintained dirt road, and follow it 5 miles. The trailhead is on the left. Park in a small lot on the right. (The signed junction of FR 193 and FR 501 is about 200 yards too far.)

KEY AT-A-GLANCE INFORMATION

LENGTH: 6-mile out-and-back

DIFFICULTY: Moderate–strenuous

SCENERY: Ponderosa and aspen, thong trees, meadows, volcanic crater, 100-mile views

EXPOSURE: Some forest shade

TRAIL TRAFFIC: Moderate

SHARED USE: Low (equestrians, mountain bikers; livestock; closed to all motor vehicles except snowmobiles)

TRAIL SURFACE: Gravel, dirt, loose rock

HIKING TIME: 4 hours

DRIVING DISTANCE: 95 miles

ACCESS: Year-round, subject to road closures due to snow or fire

LAND STATUS: Cibola National Forest–Mount Taylor Ranger District

MAPS: Brochure map available from visitor center; USGS Lobo Springs, Mount Taylor

FACILITIES: None

LAST-CHANCE FOOD/GAS: All services available in Grants

SPECIAL COMMENTS: Pack your binoculars for the views and your snowshoes for winter hikes. See longer note at the end of the Description for more details.

GPS TRAILHEAD COORDINATES

Latitude	35° 13' 12"
Longitude	107° 38' 13"

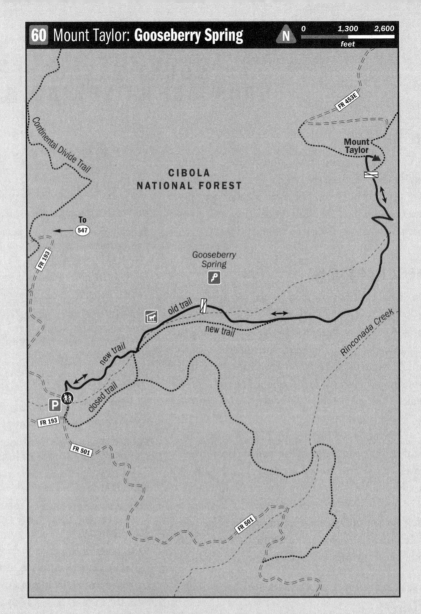

N

0   1,300   2,600
feet

CIBOLA
NATIONAL FOREST

Continental Divide Trail

FR 453E

Mount
Taylor

To
547

FR 193

Gooseberry
Spring

old trail

new trail

new trail

Rinconada Creek

closed trail

P

FR 193

FR 501

FR 501

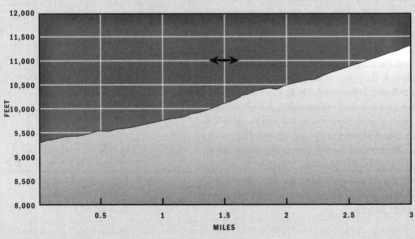

12,000
11,500
11,000
10,500
10,000
9,500
9,000
8,500
8,000

FEET

0.5   1   1.5   2   2.5   3

MILES

way to nearby resources, such as water, food, or medicinal herbs. Subtler modifications coded the details. In short, thong trees are like pages from an old guidebook. Many still stand out among regiments of pencil-straight aspens on Mount Taylor, particularly on north-facing slopes.

The mountains show up on early Spanish maps as *Sierra de la Zebolleta,* or "range of the little onion." Later settlers renamed them in honor of San Mateo. In 1849 an army lieutenant dubbed the central peak for President Zachary Taylor, who soon repaid the favor to New Mexicans by preventing Texas from expanding its state boundaries into the New Mexico Territory. The Anglo name stuck for the mountain, but the range is still referred to as both the Cebolleta Mountains and the San Mateo Mountains.

The area has an extensive history of logging, grazing, and mining, as evidenced by an endless web of roads. (For a driving guide, consult the 2011 Travel Management Decision for the Mount Taylor Ranger District, along with its supplementary map of open roads.)

The hike begins on the north side of FR 193, in a patch of quintessential American woodland. Bluebirds, squirrels, and chipmunks frolic. Aspens bear the paired initials and heart-shaped scars of adolescent affections. To the south, runoff from Gooseberry Spring sometimes streams from the draw and tunnels under the road. You'll see this stream (or its dry bed) again often throughout the hike ahead. And if you miss a right turn on your way down from the peak, you'll end up following it back to the road.

Start on Trail 77, heading north on a pale gravel trail that climbs quickly into denser woods. Gravel soon gives way to a carpet of pine needles. The first 0.5 mile of this new trail holds its form as it winds around rock formations near the edge of the draw, which by this point has assumed the proportions of a canyon. The trail then descends into an eroded meadow where multiple trails converge. The *new* version of Trail 77 crosses the streambed and turns south. After a short climb up to a closed forest road, it hooks northeast and continues its gentle climb. Blue arrows guide you through this junction, and from there the trail is easy to follow. Most hikers prefer this nicely shaded option.

However, if you're curious about the *old* route and you don't mind contending with cattle, turn left after crossing the streambed and follow the ruts northeast. About 0.4 mile upstream, an old corral stands in ruins on the left bank. About 1 mile into the hike, the canyon meadow widens as you approach a drop gate. Go through it and leave it as you found it. Cross back over the streambed and continue northeast into a stand of aspen. Multiple paths branch off to connect with the new version of Trail 77. Take your pick to climb up the north-facing slope of the canyon.

The old and new trails merge near the edge of the meadow on the other side of the aspen woods, where it becomes less a path than a rut. As you follow the tracks uphill, your destination peak comes into view on the left. At this point, you're about halfway there. The rest of the hike is high and exposed so keep an eye out for storm clouds.

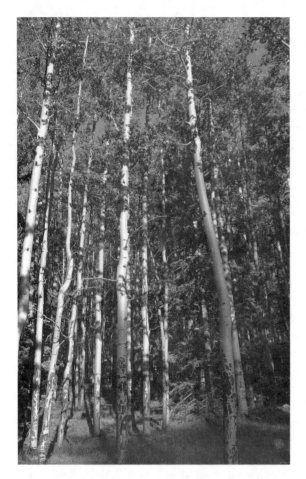

At 1.8 miles, the trail slumps over a saddle on the ridge and curves left. Enjoy a brief stretch of flat terrain while it lasts. Far below to your right, Rinconada Creek begins its winding 14-mile course to the Rio San Jose. The trail eases back over the ridge and crosses the uppermost cut of the arroyo. Note the Z-shaped switchbacks ramping up the southern slope of the peak. Once you get through those, you'll arrive at the gateway in an old fence. From there it's less than 0.25 mile to the peak.

Upon the sacred summit of Tsoodzil, the head of Pogo the Possum is mounted on a steel pole, along with a sign reading MT. TAYLOR ELEV. 11,301 and a box containing a logbook and a thermometer. Take a moment to read past entries and enjoy the view. On a clear day, you can see into both Arizona and Colorado. Closer in to the northeast, a road splits from FR 453 to drop over the rim and slither down to the floor of the caldera. Trekkers should take advantage of the bird's-eye view to scout out potential routes below.

You can extend your hike another mile on a steep, narrow path that winds down to FR 453 near La Mosca Lookout. Water Canyon Trail (76) starts from there and runs 4.5 miles to the east forest boundary, losing 1,500 feet in elevation along the way.

Note: Check with the Mount Taylor Ranger Station or the Northwest New Mexico Visitors Center for road conditions and possible closures. The ranger station is en route at 1800 Lobo Canyon Road and can be reached at (505) 287-8833 or **fs.usda.gov/cibola.** To reach the Northwest New Mexico Visitors Center, turn left from the end of the ramp at Exit 85 and follow the signs about 0.25 mile to the parking lot on the left. You can call the center at (505) 876-2783.

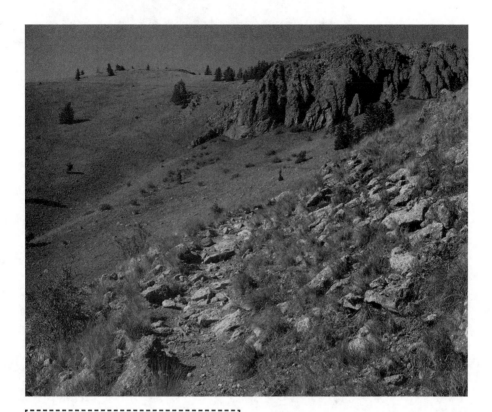

The trail is easy to follow on the upper slopes.

NEARBY ACTIVITIES

Continental Divide Trail: The parking area for Mount Taylor's section of the CDT is on the south side of NM 547 (Lobo Canyon Road) at the forest boundary, about 3 miles past the ranger station. The trail begins with a fork. The right branch visits an overlook above water-sculpted (though usually dry) falls. The left branch is the actual CDT. Casual hikers are content with the first 2 miles or so, which includes a strenuous climb up the west side of Horace Mesa. Views from the top seem endless. By this point the actual divide is about 35 miles west. The Continental Divide National Scenic Trail and the Continental Divide part ways in the northwest corner of El Malpais and don't reunite until they cross well into Colorado.

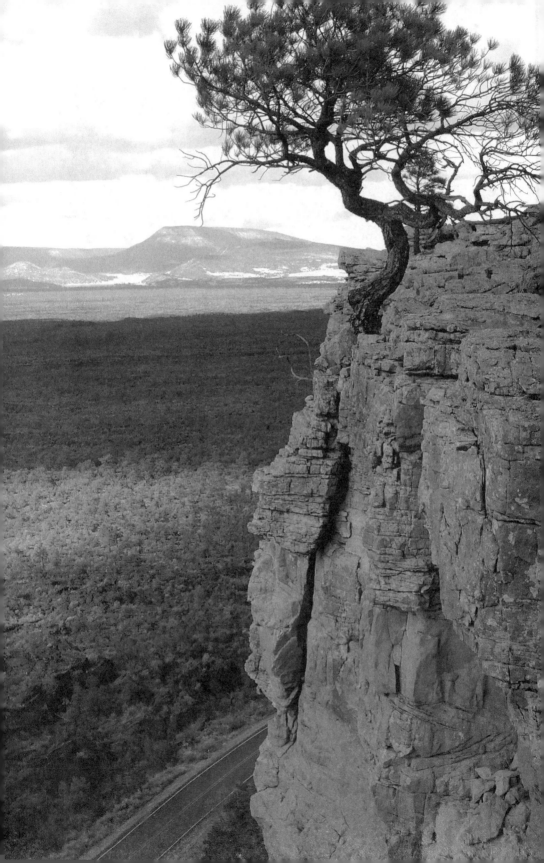

APPENDIXES AND INDEX

APPENDIX A:
PUBLIC LANDS

STATE AND LOCAL AGENCIES

ALBUQUERQUE OPEN SPACE DIVISION
cabq.gov/openspace
3615 Los Picaros SE
Albuquerque, NM 87105
(505) 452-5200

The OSD manages 28,000-plus acres in and around Albuquerque to conserve natural and archaeological resources, provide opportunities for outdoor education and places for high- and low-impact recreation, and define the edges of the urban environment.

BERNALILLO COUNTY OPEN SPACE
bernco.gov/openspace
111 Union Square SE, Suite 200
Albuquerque, NM 87102
(505) 314-0400

With a mission to provide opportunities for education and recreation, BernCo Open Space manages a dozen properties in the East Mountains and in Albuquerque's North and South valleys.

MIDDLE RIO GRANDE CONSERVANCY DISTRICT
mrgcd.com
1930 2nd St. SW
Albuquerque, NM 87102
(505) 247-0234

The MRGCD oversees 1,200 miles of ditches and canals to ensure that the Middle Rio Grande Valley is full of farmlands, wildlife, and recreational opportunities.

NEW MEXICO DEPARTMENT OF GAME AND FISH
wildlife.state.nm.us
3841 Midway Place NE
Albuquerque, NM 87109
(505) 222-4700

The NMGDF manages 56 areas that provide primarily for fishing and hunting, though many include camping, picnicking areas, and trails for hiking and wildlife viewing.

NEW MEXICO STATE LAND OFFICE
nmstatelands.org
310 Old Santa Fe Trail

Santa Fe, NM 87501
(505) 827-5760

The New Mexico State Land Office manages some 9 million surface acres. Hiking, hunting, and horseback riding is allowed by permit on publicly accessible and non-commercial land. Permit applications can be downloaded from the office's website.

NEW MEXICO STATE PARKS

nmparks.com
1220 S. St. Francis Drive
Santa Fe, NM 87505
(505) 476-3355 or (888) NMPARKS

With 35 parks throughout the state, the New Mexico State Parks Division manages more than 118,000 acres, not including water-surface area in 17 reservoirs. Annual day-use passes and camping permits are available to purchase online.

FEDERAL AGENCIES

BUREAU OF LAND MANAGEMENT

nm.blm.gov

The BLM manages 13.4 million surface acres in New Mexico, most of which are open to outdoor recreational activities including backpacking, hiking, biking, whitewater boating, fishing, caving, wildlife viewing, and cultural-site touring.

RIO PUERCO FIELD OFFICE
435 Montano NE
Albuquerque, NM 87107
(505) 761-8700

TAOS FIELD OFFICE
226 Cruz Alta Road
Taos, NM 87571
(575) 758-8851

SOCORRO FIELD OFFICE
901 S. Highway 85
Socorro, NM 87801
(575) 835-0412

NATIONAL PARK SERVICE

nps.gov

NPS boasts more than 1.6 million visitors to the 13 national parks in New Mexico. Also included in the NPS New Mexico inventory: 1,085 National Register of Historic Places listings, 12 National Natural Landmarks, and three World Heritage Sites.

U.S. FISH AND WILDLIFE SERVICE

fws.gov

The USFWS manages seven National Wildlife Refuges that are open for wildlife viewing.

U.S. FOREST SERVICE

www.fs.fed.us

The USFS manages about 9 million acres of New Mexico's most ecologically diverse lands ranging in elevation from 4,000 to more than 13,000 feet.

APPENDIX A:
PUBLIC LANDS (CONTINUED)

CIBOLA NATIONAL FOREST
fs.usda.gov/cibola
2113 Osuna Road NE, Suite A
Albuquerque, NM 87113
(505) 346-3900

Mountainair Ranger District
40 Ranger Station Road
Mountainair, New Mexico 87036
(505) 847-2990

Mount Taylor Ranger District
1800 Lobo Canyon Road
Grants, NM 87020
(505) 287-8833

Sandia Ranger District
11776 Highway 337
Tijeras, NM 87059
(505) 281-3304

SANTA FE NATIONAL FOREST
www.fs.usda.gov/santafe
11 Forest Lane
Santa Fe, NM 87508
(505) 438-5300

Española Ranger District
1710 N. Riverside Drive
Española, NM 87532
(505) 753-7331

Jemez Ranger District
Highway 4
Jemez Springs, NM 87025
(575) 829-3535

Pecos/Las Vegas District
Highway 63
Pecos, NM 87552
(505) 757-6121

OTHER AGENCIES

PUBLIC LANDS INFORMATION CENTER
publiclands.org
301 Dinosaur Trail
Santa Fe, NM 87508
(505) 438-PLIC, (877) 276-9404

Billing itself as "Your One-Stop Source for Recreation Information," the PLIC is a
handy resource for planning outdoor activities in the western states. Their site includes
links to road conditions, weather, fire alerts, and an online store for books and maps.

APPENDIX B:
EVERYTHING ELSE YOU NEED TO KNOW ABOUT NEW MEXICO

GET INVOLVED

ALBUQUERQUE WILDLIFE FEDERATION

abq.nmwildlife.org

Albuquerque Wildlife Federation is an all-volunteer nonprofit organization focused on New Mexico's wildlife and habitat resources. AWF offers monthly meetings featuring guest speakers, and opportunities to participate in restoration projects.

AUDUBON NEW MEXICO

newmexicoaudubon.org
(505) 983-4609

Four chapters of the New Mexico Audubon Council offer programs and field trips throughout the year. Visit the scenic headquarters and hiking trails at the Randall Davey Audubon Center at 1800 Upper Canyon Road in Santa Fe.

NEW MEXICO WILDERNESS ALLIANCE

nmwild.org
(505) 843-8696

The New Mexico Wilderness Alliance is a grassroots environmental organization dedicated to the protection, restoration, and continued enjoyment of New Mexico's wildlands and Wilderness areas. Check their events calendar for hikes and other outings.

SIERRA CLUB

nmsierraclub.org
(505) 243-7767 (Albuquerque Office)

With a mission to "explore, enjoy and protect the planet," the Sierra Club offers numerous opportunities for activism, volunteer programs, and organized hikes throughout New Mexico.

APPENDIX B: (CONTINUED)

GEAR UP

ALBUQUERQUE

REI
rei.com
1550 Mercantile Ave. NE
(505) 247-1191

SPORT SYSTEMS
nmsportsystems.com
6915 Montgomery NE
(505) 837-9400

STONE AGE CLIMBING
climbstoneage.com
4201 Yale Ave. NE
(505) 341-2016

SANTA FE

ALPINE SPORTS
alpinesports-santafe.com
127 Sandoval St.
(505) 983-5155

SANGRE DE CRISTO MOUNTAINWORKS
sdcmountainworks.com
328 S. Guadalupe St.
(505) 984-8221

TRAVEL BUG
mapsofnewmexico.com
839 Paseo de Peralta
(866) 992-0418

VISITOR INFORMATION

ALBUQUERQUE CONVENTION & VISITORS BUREAU
itsatrip.org
(800) 284-2282

NEW MEXICO TOURISM DEPARTMENT
newmexico.org
(800) 733-6396

SANTA FE CONVENTION AND VISITORS BUREAU
santafe.org
(800) 777-2489

For information on just about everything else in Albuquerque, dial 311 from any local phone or visit **cabq.gov/a-z.**

INDEX

Check out this great title from
── Menasha Ridge Press! ──

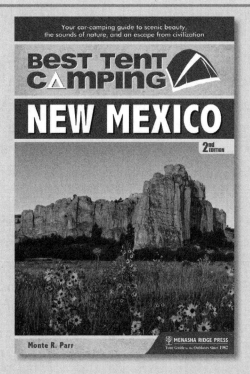

Best Tent Camping: New Mexico

by Monte R. Parr
ISBN: 978-0-89732-502-8
$15.95

6x9, paperback
maps and index

Best Tent Camping: New Mexico is a must-read for campers and adventurers desiring an excursion into the Southwest. New Mexico offers a charm and beauty that is rare. From open Southwestern landscapes with blue mountains visible on the distant horizon to the meadows and streams and pines of Sugarite Canyon State Park in northern New Mexico, and on to White Sands, it is a truly an enchanting journey. This state is full of history, offering ruins and forts from the Spanish-American War, Native American pueblos, archaeology, and cliff dwellings.

Best Tent Camping: New Mexico is an indispensable guide, and the best campgrounds in and around these remarkable areas are described in great detail.

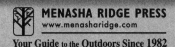

MENASHA RIDGE PRESS
www.menasharidge.com

Your Guide to the Outdoors Since 1982

DEAR CUSTOMERS AND FRIENDS,

SUPPORTING YOUR INTEREST IN OUTDOOR ADVENTURE, travel, and an active lifestyle is central to our operations, from the authors we choose to the locations we detail to the way we design our books. Menasha Ridge Press was incorporated in 1982 by a group of veteran outdoorsmen and professional outfitters. For many years now, we've specialized in creating books that benefit the outdoors enthusiast.

Almost immediately, Menasha Ridge Press earned a reputation for revolutionizing outdoors- and travel-guidebook publishing. For such activities as canoeing, kayaking, hiking, backpacking, and mountain biking, we established new standards of quality that transformed the whole genre, resulting in outdoor-recreation guides of great sophistication and solid content. Menasha Ridge continues to be outdoor publishing's greatest innovator.

The folks at Menasha Ridge Press are as at home on a white-water river or mountain trail as they are editing a manuscript. The books we build for you are the best they can be, because we're responding to your needs. Plus, we use and depend on them ourselves.

We look forward to seeing you on the river or the trail. If you'd like to contact us directly, join in at www.trekalong.com or visit us at www.menasharidge.com. We thank you for your interest in our books and the natural world around us all.

SAFE TRAVELS,

Bob Sehlinger

BOB SEHLINGER